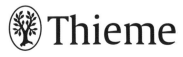

Patient Blood Management

Hans Gombotz, MD
Professor
Former Chairman of the Department of Anesthesiology
and Intensive Care Medicine
General Hospital Linz
Linz, Austria

Kai Zacharowski, MD, PhD, FRCA
Professor and Chairman
Department of Anesthesiology
Intensive Care Medicine and Pain Therapy
University Hospital Frankfurt
Frankfurt am Main, Germany

Donat Rudolf Spahn, MD, FRCA
Professor and Chairman
Institute of Anesthesiology
Section Head Medical
Anesthesiology—Intensive Care Medicine—OR Management
University of Zurich and University Hospital Zurich
Zurich, Switzerland

44 illustrations

Thieme
Stuttgart · New York · Delhi · Rio de Janeiro

Library of Congress Cataloging-in-Publication Data is available from the publisher.

Twenty one subchapters have been previously published in the German language in the following publication: *Patient Blood Management* published and copyrighted 2013 by Georg Thieme Verlag, Stuttgart.

Translator: Sarah Venkata, London, UK
Illustrator: Angelika Brauner, Hohenpeißenberg, Germany

© 2016 Georg Thieme Verlag KG

Thieme Publishers Stuttgart
Rüdigerstrasse 14, 70469 Stuttgart, Germany
+49 [0]711 8931 421, customerservice@thieme.de

Thieme Publishers New York
333 Seventh Avenue, New York, NY 10001, USA
+1-800-782-3488, customerservice@thieme.com

Thieme Publishers Delhi
A-12, Second Floor, Sector-2, Noida-201301
Uttar Pradesh, India
+91 120 45 566 00, customerservice@thieme.in

Thieme Publishers Rio, Thieme Publicações Ltda.
Edifício Rodolpho de Paoli, 25º andar
Av. Nilo Peçanha, 50 – Sala 2508
Rio de Janeiro 20020-906 Brasil
+55 21 3172 2297 / +55 21 3172 1896

Cover design: Thieme Publishing Group
Graphic on back cover: Martina Berge, Bad König, Germany.
© v. Yakobchuk – Fotolia.com (left column) and
Dynamic Graphics (middle column)
Typesetting by Druckhaus Götz GmbH, Ludwigsburg, Germany

Printed in Germany by AZ Druck und Datentechnik, Kempten

ISBN 978-3-13-200441-2   5 4 3 2 1

Also available as an e-book:
eISBN 978-3-13-200451-1

Important note: Medicine is an ever-changing science undergoing continual development. Research and clinical experience are continually expanding our knowledge, in particular our knowledge of proper treatment and drug therapy. Insofar as this book mentions any dosage or application, readers may rest assured that the authors, editors, and publishers have made every effort to ensure that such references are in accordance with **the state of knowledge at the time of production of the book.**

Nevertheless, this does not involve, imply, or express any guarantee or responsibility on the part of the publishers in respect to any dosage instructions and forms of applications stated in the book. **Every user is requested to examine carefully** the manufacturers' leaflets accompanying each drug and to check, if necessary in consultation with a physician or specialist, whether the dosage schedules mentioned therein or the contraindications stated by the manufacturers differ from the statements made in the present book. Such examination is particularly important with drugs that are either rarely used or have been newly released on the market. Every dosage schedule or every form of application used is entirely at the user's own risk and responsibility. The authors and publishers request every user to report to the publishers any discrepancies or inaccuracies noticed. If errors in this work are found after publication, errata will be posted at www.thieme.com on the product description page.

Some of the product names, patents, and registered designs referred to in this book are in fact registered trademarks or proprietary names even though specific reference to this fact is not always made in the text. Therefore, the appearance of a name without designation as proprietary is not to be construed as a representation by the publisher that it is in the public domain.

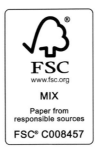

Contents

Foreword

Patient Blood Management (PBM) is a compelling concept to preempt anemia, correct bleeding disorders, and minimize blood loss. This evidence-based, multidisciplinary approach does not only lead to reductions in the use of blood and blood products, and therefore to considerable cost savings, but—more importantly—it also improves patient outcomes and patient safety. Beginning with a state-wide initiative by the Department of Health in Western Australia and several hospital-based programs in the United States and Europe, PBM has evolved into a widely accepted holistic treatment concept that is a must-have for all modern health care systems.

The applicability of PBM is not limited to the perioperative setting; PBM is equally relevant to all medical fields where anemia and bleeding are prevalent and where blood and blood products are commonly administered.

After the very successful publication of this textbook in German, the editors—together with a team of internationally recognized PBM experts—have now produced an updated, expanded edition in the English language.

I am convinced that this edition will be successful in increasing awareness among clinicians and in sharing the topic with others who are interested in patient care. I hope that this new edition will help to drive the implementation of PBM until it becomes the new normal.

Denton A. Cooley, MD
Pioneering cardiovascular surgeon
Founder and Surgeon in Chief of the Texas Heart Institute

Preface

This book provides a detailed account of the modern concept of Patient Blood Management (PBM). The well-received chapters of the original German edition have been revised and expanded for the current English edition, with the additional content including a whole new section on PBM in surgical settings. In reflection of the multidisciplinary and international nature of PBM, authors from many countries with different areas of expertise were invited to contribute. We thereby succeeded in creating interfaces between the various specialist areas and meeting their demands in a better way. The well-balanced selection of authors also guaranteed an overarching and experience-based portrait of the subject matter. Each chapter is evidence-based and represents the opinions of its author(s), which were respected by the editors. Accordingly, editing was mainly restricted to formal aspects. Therefore, discrepancies may exist with regard to certain contentious questions that have not yet been corroborated through investigations, and some issues may remain unresolved.

PBM is a clinical, multidisciplinary, patient-oriented concept that focuses primarily on the treatment or avoidance of anemia, the reduction of blood loss, and the enhancement of a patient's tolerance to anemia to improve patient safety and outcome. Only after these therapeutic options have been exhausted is the transfusion of allogeneic blood products considered. By contrast, the Optimal Blood Use project (www.optimalblooduse.eu) initiated by the European Union aims at administering the right blood product to the right patient at the right time. PBM reaches farther because it has a preventive and corrective impact on the risk factors that normally result in transfusion.

Application of the principles of PBM is indicated not only in the perioperative phase but also in all areas of medicine where treatment involves the use of blood and blood products. The primary goals of PBM are the promotion of patient safety and the improvement of patient outcomes. The concept of PBM was developed by collaboration between international experts and has been implemented in Western Australia and in several American and European centers. As early as 2010, the WHO endorsed PBM as the most important principle underlying patient safety, and the concept is featured on the website of the American Association of Blood Banks (AABB). The European Union launched its own PBM project in 2013, also with a particular focus on patient safety.

The central focus of this book—based on the recognition that there are three modifiable risk factors (blood loss, anemia, and transfusion)—is the presentation and discussion of the three pillars of PBM: avoidance, diagnosis, and treatment of preoperative anemia; reduction of peri-interventional blood loss; and augmentation of the tolerance to anemia in everyday clinical practice. Other important aspects of PBM addressed in this book include the requirements for modern transfusion medicine and surgery in the light of changing demographic trends, the procedures used for ordering blood products, the role of the preanesthesia clinic, the potential impact on the course of disease, the importance of benchmarking, and the potential financial savings and possible consequences for the public health sector.

Since the majority of investigations of PBM to date have focused on the transfusion of red blood cells, one can easily get the mistaken impression that PBM is aimed exclusively at the treatment of anemia and the transfusion of red blood cell concentrates. However, in addition to minimizing diagnostic and interventional blood loss, PBM is also targeted toward the avoidance and treatment of coagulation disorders and, as such, toward the patient-oriented administration of coagulation products and platelet concentrates.

PBM is currently undergoing rapid development and this is set to continue in the foreseeable future. Several unresolved issues—including the extent to which the treatment of anemia improves the course of disease, and the pros and cons of treatment with iron preparations and erythropoiesis-stimulating agents—are still to be clarified in prospective studies.

This book is intended as a reference for those clinicians whose patients, in addition to experiencing the consequences of their underlying disease, are often at risk for anemia, coagulation disorders, and/or major blood loss. With PBM, causal treatment is aimed at eliminating these risks, thus minimizing the side effects of autologous and allogeneic blood transfusion. Hence, PBM is one of the few concepts in modern medicine that improves patient outcomes while also saving costs.

We extend our special thanks to the authors and to the staff at Thieme Publishers, in particular Angelika-M. Findgott, Martina Habeck, Joanne Stead, and Deborah A. Cecere, who made our book on this vitally important topic possible.

Prof. Hans Gombotz, MD
Prof. Kai Zacharowski, MD, PhD, FRCA
Prof. Donat Rudolf Spahn, MD, FRCA

Contributors

Ben Clevenger, MD
Department of Anaesthesia
Division of Surgery and Interventional Science
Royal Free Hospital
London, UK

Jochen Walter Erhard, MD
Professor
Evangelische Klinik Niederrhein gGmbH
Duisburg, Germany

Shannon L. Farmer
School of Surgery
Faculty of Medicine, Dentistry, and Health Sciences
University of Western Australia
Centre for Population Health Research at Curtin
University
Glenn Forest, Western Australia, Australia

Michael Fridrik, MD
Lecturer
Center for Hematology and Medical Oncology
Internal Medicine III
General Hospital Linz
Linz, Austria

Barbara Friesenecker, MD
University Professor
Medical University of Innsbruck
University Clinic for General and Surgical Intensive
Care Medicine
Innsbruck, Austria

Gerhard Fritsch, MD
Salzburg County Hospital
University Hospital for Anesthesiology, Periopera-
tive Medicine and General Intensive Care Medicine
Salzburg, Austria

Christof Geisen, MD
Institute for Transfusion Medicine and Immune
Hematology
Johann Wolfgang Goethe University Hospital
German Red Cross Blood Donation Service
Baden-Württemberg and Hessen
Frankfurt am Main, Germany

Richard S. Goldweit, MD, FACC
Assistant Clinical Professor
Englewood Hospital and Medical Center
Mount Sinai School of Medicine
Englewood, New Jersey, USA

Hans Gombotz, MD
Professor
Former Chairman of the Department of
Anesthesiology and Intensive Care
Medicine
General Hospital Linz
Linz, Austria

Jeffrey Mark Hamdorf, MBBS, PhD, FRACS
Professor
School of Surgery
University of Western Australia
Crawley, Western Australia, Australia

Michael Hiesmayr, MD
University Professor
University Hospital for Anesthesiology, General
Intensive Care Medicine, and Pain Management
Medical University of Vienna
Vienna, Austria

Axel Hofmann, Dr. rer. medic., ME
Institute for Anesthesiology
University of Zurich
Zurich, Switzerland

James Paton Isbister, MBBS, FRACP, FRCPA
Clinical Professor of Medicine
Sydney Medical School
St. Leonards, New South Wales, Australia

Mazyar Javidroozi, MD, PhD
Director of Clinical Research
Department of Anesthesiology
Englewood Hospital and Medical Center
Englewood, New Jersey, USA

Lutz Kaufner, MD
Department of Anesthesiology –
Operative Intensive Care Medicine
Charité – University Medicine Berlin
Campus Virchow Klinikum
Berlin, Germany

Alwyn Kotze, MD
Consultant Anaesthetist and Fellow NIHR CLAHRC
for Leeds, York, and Bradford
Leeds Teaching Hospitals
Leeds, UK

Thomas Kuehlein, MD
Department of General Medicine and Clinical
Research
Heidelberg University Hospital
Heidelberg, Germany

Gerhard Lanzer, MD
University Professor
Medical University of Graz
University Hospital for Blood Group Serology and
Transfusion Medicine
LKH Graz – University Hospital
Graz, Austria

Jeong Jae Lee, MD, PhD
Professor
Department of Obstetrics and Gynecology
Soonchunhyang University Hospital
Yongsan-GU, Seoul, Korea

Rudolf Mair, MD
Department of Anesthesiology and Operative
Intensive Care Medicine
General Hospital Linz;
Faculty of Medicine at the Kepler University of Linz
Linz, Austria

Jens Meier, MD
Professor and Director
Clinic of Anesthesiology and
Intensive Care Medicine
Faculty of Medicine at the Kepler University of Linz
Linz, Austria

Dirk Meininger, MD
Professor
Hospital for Anesthesiology, Operative Intensive
Care Medicine, Trauma, and Pain Management
Main-Kinzig-Clinics
Gelnhausen, Germany

Patrick Meybohm, MD
Adjunct Professor
Clinic of Anesthesiology
Intensive Care Medicine and Pain Therapy
Johann Wolfgang Goethe University Hospital
Frankfurt am Main, Germany

Hannes Mueller, MD
Department of Surgery I
General Hospital Linz
Linz, Austria

Peter Rehak †
Former University Professor
Medical University of Graz
University Hospital for Surgery
Medical Technology and Data Processing Unit
Graz, Austria

Toby Richards
Senior Lecturer in Surgery
Division of Surgery
University College London
London, UK

Arno Schiferer, MD
Clinical Department for Cardiac, Thorax, and
Vascular Surgery,
Anesthesiology and Intensive Care Medicine
Medical University Vienna
Vienna, Austria

Erhard Seifried, MD
Institute for Transfusion Medicine and Immune
Hematology
German Red Cross Blood Donation Service
Baden-Württemberg and Hessen
University Hospital Frankfurt am Main
Frankfurt am Main, Germany

Aryeh Shander, MD, FCCM, FCCP
Chief, Department of Anesthesiology, Critical Care
Medicine
Hyperbaric Medicine and Pain Management
Englewood Hospital and Medical Center
Englewood, New Jersey, USA

Donat Rudolf Spahn, MD, FRCA
Professor and Chairman
Institute of Anesthesiology
Section Head Medical
Anesthesiology – Intensive Care Medicine –
OR Management
University of Zurich and University Hospital Zurich
Zurich, Switzerland

Bruce D. Spiess, MD
Department of Anesthesiology
Virginia Commonwealth University Medical
Center
Richmond, Virginia, USA

Jost Steinhaeuser, MD
University of Heidelberg
Department of General Medicine and Clinical
Research
Heidelberg, Germany

**Simon Charles Bruce Towler, MD, FCICM,
FANPZCA, FAMA**
Medical Co-Director and Intensive Care Specialist
Adjunct Professor at Edith Cowan and Curtin
Universities
Fiona Stanley Hospital
Murdoch, Western Australia, Australia

Christian von Heymann, MD, DEAA
Professor
Department of Anesthesiology – Operative
Intensive Care Medicine
Charité – University Medicine Berlin
Campus Virchow Klinikum
Berlin, Germany

Philippe Van der Linden, MD
Professor
Department of Anesthesiology
CHU Brugmann Hospital
Brussels, Belgium

Christian Friedrich Weber, MD
Clinic of Anesthesiology
Intensive Care Medicine and Pain Therapy
Johann Wolfgang Goethe University Hospital
Frankfurt am Main, Germany

Alexander Weigl, MD
General Hospital Linz
Pharmacy
Linz, Austria

Kai Zacharowski, MD, PhD, FRCA
Professor and Chairman
Department of Anesthesiology
Intensive Care Medicine and Pain Therapy
University Hospital Frankfurt
Frankfurt am Main, Germany

Abbreviations

AABC	Australasian Association for Blood Conservation	INR	International normalized ratio
ACSQHC	Australian Commission on Safety and Quality in Health Care	LDH	Lactate dehydrogenase
		MCH	Mean corpuscular hemoglobin
ANH	Acute normovolemic hemodilution	MCHC	Mean corpuscular hemoglobin concentration
ARDS	Acute respiratory distress syndrome	MCV	Mean corpuscular volume
ASA	American Society of Anesthesiologists	MiECT	Minimally invasive extracorporeal circulation technology
BSE	Bovine spongiform encephalopathy	MIS	Minimally invasive surgery
CABG	Coronary artery bypass graft	MTP	Massive transfusion protocol
CHD	Coronary heart disease	NAT	Nucleic acid testing
CHMP	Committee for Medicinal Products for Human Use	NBA	National Blood Authority
		NOAC	New oral anticoagulant
CI	Confidence interval	NSAID	Nonsteroidal anti-inflammatory drug
CJD	Creutzfeldt-Jakob disease	ONTraC	Ontario Transfusion Coordinators
CPB	Cardiopulmonary bypass	OR	Odds ratio
CRG	Clinical Reference Group	PAD	Preoperative autologous blood donation
CRP	C-reactive protein		
CTR	Crossmatch-to-transfusion ratio	PBM	Patient Blood Management
DAPT	Dual antiplatelet therapy	PCC	Prothrombin complex concentrate
DCS	Damage control surgery	PCR	Polymerase chain reaction
DO_2	Oxygen delivery to the tissues	PEG	Polyethylene glycol
DRG	Diagnosis-related group	PO_2	Partial pressure of oxygen
ECG	Electrocardiography	PT	Prothrombin Time
EPO	Erythropoietin	RBC	Red blood cell
ESA	Erythropoietin-stimulating agent	RCT	Randomized controlled trial
FDA	Food and Drug Administration	rHuEPO	Recombinant human erythropoietin
FFP	Fresh frozen plasma	ROTEM	Rotational thrombelastometry
GP	General practitioner	RPI	Reticulocyte production index
HAA	Haematology Society of Australia and New Zealand, Australian and New Zealand Society of Blood Transfusion, and Australasian Society of Thrombosis and Haemostasis	rVIIa	Recombinant activated factor VII
		SABM	Society for the Advancement of Blood Management
		SHOT	Serious Hazards of Transfusion
		SIRS	Systemic inflammatory response syndrome
Hb	Hemoglobin	sTfR	Soluble transferrin receptor
HBOC	Hemoglobin-based oxygen carrier	TACO	Transfusion-associated circulatory overload
HBV	Hepatitis B virus		
Hct	Hematocrit	TAVR	Transcatheter aortic valve replacement
HCV	Hepatitis C virus	TRALI	Transfusion-related acute lung injury
HES	Hydroxyethyl starch	TRIM	Transfusion-related immunomodulation
HITS	Hospital information technology system		
HLA	Human leukocyte antigens	TTI	Total Transfusion Index
HPA	Human platelet antigen	VKA	Vitamin K antagonists
HR	Hazard ratio	VO_2	Oxygen consumption
ICCTO	International Consensus Conference on Transfusion and Outcome		
ICD	International Classification of Diseases		
ICU	Intensive care unit		

Conflicts of Interest

Shannon L. Farmer

The contributor has reported the following conflicts of interest: Shannon Farmer has received consulting/lecture honoraria or travel support from: Western Australia, Queensland, New South Wales, and South Australia Departments of Health; Australian Red Cross Blood Service; Australian National Blood Authority; Australian Jurisdictional Blood Committee; Medical Society for Blood Management; Society for the Advancement of Blood Management; Fremantle General Practice Network, Western Australia; Thieme Publishers, Stuttgart, Germany; Elsevier Science, USA; Haematology Society of Australia and New Zealand/Australian and New Zealand Society of Blood Transfusion; Novo Nordisk; Vifor Pharma; Johnson & Johnson Ethicon Biosurgery. He is Associate Investigator, Chief Investigator, and Principal Investigator of three government-sponsored research trials and a member of the Expert Panel for the European Commission Patient Blood Management Project.

Michael Fridrik

The contributor has reported the following conflict of interest: Advisory Board: Vifor Pharma.

James Paton Isbister

"I have declared no conflicts of interest. As you know there is always confusion over what is a conflict of interest. I neither presume that being Chair of the Australian Federal Government National Blood Authority Patient Blood Management can be regarded as a 'conflict' nor being on the Advisory Committee of the Australian Red Cross Blood Service nor Chair of a Human Research Ethics Committee. Specifically, in recent years I have not been paid honoraria for lectures or advisory roles to any company."

Axel Hofmann

The contributor has reported the following conflicts of interest: In the past 5 years, Dr. Hofmann has received fees, honoraria, or travel support for consultancy or lecturing from the following companies and organizations: Australian Red Cross Blood Service, Brisbane, Australia; Austrian Institute of Technology, Vienna, Austria; B. Braun Melsungen, Melsungen, Germany; BioMed-zet Life Science, Linz, Austria; CSL Behring, Lisbon, Portugal; CSL Behring, Marburg, Deutschland; Fresenius Kabi, Bad Homburg, Germany; General Hospital Linz, Linz, Austria; Hospira, Leamington Spa, United Kingdom; Janssen-Cilag EMEA, Beerse, Belgium; Johnson & Johnson Ethicon Biosurgery, Somerville, NJ, USA; Johnson & Johnson Medical, North Ryde, Australia; Klinikum Sindelfingen-Böblingen, Sindelfingen, Germany; Landeskliniken-Holding, St. Pölten, Austria; Medical Society for Blood Management, Laxenburg, Austria; National Blood Authority, Canberra, Australia; Physicians World, Mannheim, Germany; Society for the Advancement of Blood Management, Richmond, VA, USA; TEM, Munich, Germany; Institute for Patient Blood Management & Bloodless Medicine and Surgery, Englewood, NJ, USA; United States Department of Health and Human Services, Washington, DC, USA; Vifor Pharma, Glattbrugg, Switzerland; Vifor Pharma Österreich, Vienna, Austria; Vifor Pharma Deutschland, Munich, Germany; Vision Plus, Monza, Italy; Western Australia Department of Health, Perth, Australia.

Mazyar Javidroozi

The contributor has reported the following conflicts of interest: Mazyar Javidroozi has been a consultant and contractor for the Society for the Advancement of Blood Management and Gauss Surgical.

Alwyn Kotze

The contributor has reported the following conflicts of interest: Alwyn Kotze has received funding related to PBM activity from the Health Foundation, an independent UK charity that aims to improve the quality of healthcare. He has also received funding for research and quality improvement unrelated to PBM from the Yorkshire and Humber Academic Health Sciences Network and the Leeds Clinical Commissioning Groups. In addition, he received expenses related to travel, accommodation, and conference attendance for one scientific conference in 2010, from Vifor Pharma.

Patrick Meybohm

The contributor has reported the following conflicts of interest: Support from Vifor Pharma, B. Braun Melsungen, CSL Behring, and Fresenius Kabi for the implementation of Frankfurt's Patient Blood Management Program in four German university hospitals.

Hannes Mueller

The contributor has reported the following conflict of interest: Support from Nycomed Pharma for a case and photo documentation of the clinical use of TachoSil, in March 2012. Nycomed Pharma is the predecessor of Takeda Pharmaceutical Company, the current distributor of TachoSil.

Donat Rudolph Spahn

The contributor has reported the following conflicts of interest: Dr. Spahn's academic department has received grants from the Swiss National Science Foundation, Bern, Switzerland; the Ministry of Health (Gesundheitsdirektion) of the Canton of Zurich, Switzerland for Highly Specialized Medicine; the Swiss Society of Anesthesiology and Reanimation (SGAR), Bern, Switzerland; the Swiss Foundation for Anesthesia Research, Zurich, Switzerland; Bundesprogramm Chancengleichheit, Bern, Switzerland; CSL Behring, Bern, Switzerland; and Vifor, Villars-sur-Glâne, Switzerland. Dr. Spahn was Chairman of the ABC Faculty and is Co-chairman of the ABC-Trauma Faculty, which are both managed by Physicians World Europe, Mannheim, Germany, and sponsored by unrestricted educational grants from Novo Nordisk Health Care, Zurich, Switzerland; CSL Behring, Marburg, Germany; and LFB Biomedicaments, Courtabœuf Cedex, France.

In the past 5 years, Dr. Spahn has received honoraria or travel support for consultancy or lecturing from the following companies: Abbott, Baar, Switzerland; Amgen, Munich, Germany; AstraZeneca, Zug, Switzerland; Bayer (Schweiz), Zürich, Switzerland; Baxter, Volketswil, Switzerland, and Roma, Italy; B. Braun Melsungen, Melsungen, Germany; Boehringer Ingelheim (Schweiz), Basel, Switzerland; Bristol-Myers-Squibb, Rueil-Malmaison Cedex, France, and Baar, Switzerland; CSL Behring, Hattersheim am Main, Germany, and Bern, Switzerland; Curacyte, Munich, Germany; Ethicon Biosurgery, Sommerville, NJ, USA; Fresenius, Bad Homburg, Germany; Galenica, Bern, Switzerland (including Vifor, Villars-sur-Glâne, Switzerland); GlaxoSmithKline, Hamburg, Germany; Janssen-Cilag, Baar, Switzerland; Janssen-Cilag EMEA, Beerse, Belgium; Merck Sharp & Dohme, Luzern, Switzerland; Novo Nordisk, Bagsværd, Denmark; Octapharma, Lachen, Switzerland; Organon, Pfäffikon/SZ, Switzerland; Oxygen Biotherapeutics, Costa Mesa, CA, USA; Photonics Healthcare, Munich, Germany; ratiopharm Arzneimittel Vertriebs-GmbH, Vienna, Austria; Roche Diagnostics International, Reinach, Switzerland; Roche Pharma (Schweiz), Reinach, Switzerland; Schering-Plough International, Kenilworth, NJ, USA; Tem International, Munich, Germany; Verum Diagnostica, Munich, Germany; Vifor Pharma Deutschland, Munich, Germany; Vifor Pharma Österreich, Vienna, Austria; Vifor (International), St. Gallen, Switzerland.

Disclaimer: "None of the above listed companies and/or entities have been directly or indirectly involved in discussing and/or developing this manuscript or parts thereof. Moreover, none of the above listed companies and/or entities have financially contributed to this endeavor in whatever form, neither directly nor indirectly. Therefore it is beyond my capacity to tell whether any of the above listed companies and/or entities do or do not have a direct financial interest in the subject matter or materials discussed in this manuscript."

Christian Friedrich Weber

The contributor has reported the following conflicts of interest: Christian Weber has received speaker's honoraria from CSL Behring, Roche, TEM International, and Verum Diagnostica.

Kai Zacharowski

The contributor has reported the following conflicts of interest: In the past 3 years, Professor Zacharowski has received honoraria or travel support for consultancy or lecturing from the following companies: Abbott, Aesculap Akademie, AQAI, Astellas Pharma, AstraZeneca, Aventis Pharma, B. Braun Melsungen, Baxter Deutschland, Biosyn, Biotest, Bristol-Myers Squibb, CSL Behring, Dr. F. Köhler Chemie, Dräger Medical, Essex Pharma, Fresenius Kabi, Fresenius Medical Care, Gambro Hospal, Gilead, GlaxoSmithKline, Grünenthal, Hamilton Medical, HCCM Consulting, Heinen + Löwenstein, Janssen-Cilag, med update, Medivance EU BV, MSD Sharp & Dohme, Novartis Pharma, Novo Nordisk Pharma, P. J. Dahlhausen, Pfizer Pharma, Pulsion Medical Systems, Siemens Healthcare, Teflex Medical, Teva, TopMed Medizintechnik, Verathon Medical, and Vifor Pharma.

Professor Zacharowski's academic department has received unrestricted educational grants from B. Braun Melsungen, Fresenius Kabi, CSL Behring, and Vifor Pharma.

October 2015

Chapter 1

Introduction

1.1 PBM: A Concept to Improve Patient Safety and Outcome

H. Gombotz, A. Hofmann

1.1.1 The Triad of Anemia, Blood Loss, and Transfusion: Three Independent Risk Factors for an Adverse Outcome

▶ **Anemia.** Anemia, characterized by a subnormal concentration of circulating red blood cells (RBCs), is prevalent in many different surgical populations and in critically ill patients. In patients undergoing elective surgery, the frequency of preoperative anemia ranges from 5% to 75%, with a higher incidence in older patients (Kulier and Gombotz 2001, Myers et al 2004, Gombotz et al 2007, Kulier et al 2007, Musallam et al 2011, Baron et al 2014). Anemia is a strong and independent predictor of adverse outcomes such as average hospital length of stay and the composite outcome of morbidity and mortality (Carson et al 1996, Nemergut et al 2007, Musallam et al 2011). One of the main contributing factors to this clinically significant condition is an absolute iron deficiency (Guralnik et al 2004). Various other factors including functional iron deficiency, chemotherapy, radiation, certain medications, menorrhagia, and congenital disorders can also cause anemia.

▶ **Perioperative blood loss.** Perioperative blood loss is an independent predictor for the same adverse outcomes as those seen with anemia (Carson et al 1988, Rao et al 2005, Walsh et al 2013). Blood loss can be attributable to surgery, diagnostic or therapeutic interventions, trauma, obstetric complications, long-term anticoagulant therapy, and other reasons (Gombotz and Knotzer 2013). In nonanemic patients, acute blood loss or severe hemorrhage can lead to immediate, serious sequelae (Karkouti et al 2008b, Karkouti et al 2009, Walsh et al 2013, Hogervorst et al 2014). In patients with preexisting anemia, the tolerance to blood loss may be even lower.

▶ **Transfusion.** For decades, transfusion has been considered to be the optimal treatment for anemia and/or blood loss. However, although the administration of RBCs can be lifesaving in hemodynamically unstable patients, there is little evidence of clinical benefit in hemodynamically stable patients, the group that receives the vast majority of all RBC transfusions (Bernard et al 2009, Refaai and Blumberg 2013a). Although transfusions result in corrected laboratory values, they do not treat the actual cause of anemia, nor do they stop any bleeding.

Moreover, stored blood that is transfused has limited oxygen off-loading capacity (Napolitano et al 2009). Animal models have shown that the morphological changes of RBCs during storage lead to impaired tissue perfusion followed by diminished oxygenation and inadequate removal of carbon dioxide (Tsai et al 2010, Yalcin et al 2014). These rheological changes might explain the observation of a dose–response relationship between ischemic events and RBC transfusions (Murphy et al 2007, Koch et al 2008, Lacroix et al 2015).

In addition, there is a link between transfusion and cancer recurrence. The causality is still under debate, but the findings of several clinical studies are suggestive of a causal relationship (Amato and Pescatori 2006, Al-Refaie et al 2012, Riedl et al 2013, Boehm et al 2014, Luan et al 2014, Wang et al 2014).

The relationship between transfusion-related immunomodulation (TRIM) and postoperative infection has also been the subject of scientific controversy for decades. However, in this case, the causal link has now been confirmed (Refaai and Blumberg 2013b). Retrospective and prospective observational studies in various patient populations have shown a dose–response relationship between transfusion and nosocomial infections (Lacroix et al 2007, Bernard et al 2009, Carson et al 2013, Curley et al 2014). Moreover, a meta-analysis of randomized controlled trials (RCTs) comparing the use of liberal versus restrictive transfusion thresholds showed an increase in hospital-acquired infections with liberal transfusions (Rohde et al 2014).

In preparation of the 1st International Consensus Conference on Transfusion and Outcome (ICCTO), the ICCTO research group applied the Bradford Hill criteria for establishing causation to assess the link between transfusion and adverse outcomes, using the evidence available at the time (Isbister et al 2011). The Bradford Hill criteria include strength, consistency, specificity, temporality, biological gradient or dose–response relationship (i.e., increased exposure results in increased risk), and biological plausibility of the findings. Sir Austin Bradford Hill and Sir Richard Doll used this methodology to establish the causal link between tobacco smoking and lung cancer (Darby et al 2006). When applying the Bradford Hill criteria to transfusion and adverse outcomes, the ICCTO research group found strong evidence for a causal link. Meta-analyses of RCTs and systematic literature reviews have corroborated this finding, showing that the use of liberal—as opposed to restrictive—transfusion thresholds leads to significantly higher morbidity and mortality (Carson et al 2012b) (see Chapter 1.3).

Although perceived as beneficial by many clinicians, transfusion is in fact an independent, dose-dependent, and additive risk factor for morbidity, increased hospital length of stay, and mortality in most clinical settings (Spiess 2004a, Murphy et al 2007, Bernard et al 2009, Ferraris et al 2012, Howard-Quijano et al 2013, Carson 2014, Isil et al 2015). Patients at the limits of their cardiovascular reserve, such as those undergoing cardiac surgery, may constitute an exception—they have been shown to benefit from the higher hemoglobin levels achieved with a liberal transfusion threshold (Murphy et al 2015). Overall, however, anemia, blood loss, and transfusion constitute a triad of independent risk factors for adverse outcomes (Ranucci et al 2013, Farmer et al 2013b) (**Fig. 1.1**).

> **Note**
>
> Anemia, blood loss, and transfusion constitute a triad of independent predictors of an adverse outcome.

This triad constitutes a vicious circle: blood loss and bleeding induce anemia or exacerbate preexisting anemia; anemia triggers transfusion; and transfusion—as shown in several studies—increases the risk of rebleeding, potentially leading to further blood loss (Blair et al 1986, Henriksson and Svensson 1991, Hearnshaw et al 2010, Jairath et al 2010, Restellini et al 2013, Villanueva et al 2013b). The intention of breaking this cycle by modifying the potential risk factors has led to the concept of PBM.

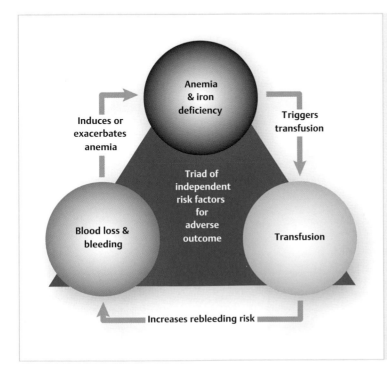

Fig. 1.1 Triad of independent risk factors for an adverse patient outcome. Reprinted from Farmer et al 2013 b with permission from Elsevier.

1.1.2 PBM: Improving Outcomes by Preempting the Impact of the Triad

Rationale behind PBM

The rationale behind PBM is that improved patient safety and optimal clinical outcomes can be achieved when optimization and preservation of the patient's own blood take priority over the transfusion of donor blood.

> **Note**
>
> To achieve an optimal clinical outcome, optimization and preservation of the patient's own blood takes priority over the transfusion of donor blood.

This can be achieved by preempting the detrimental mechanisms within the triad: each of the three risk factors is modifiable and should be addressed as early as possible in the course of treatment. The clinical measures addressing these risks are grouped into the so-called *three pillars of PBM*:
1. Optimization of the patient's endogenous RBC mass.
2. Proactive and timely bleeding management (minimization of diagnostic, interventional, and surgical blood loss).
3. Optimization of the patient's tolerance to anemia by maximizing oxygen delivery while reducing the metabolic rate, and harnessing the patient's ability to tolerate anemia by strictly adhering to physiological transfusion thresholds.

> **Note**
>
> PBM is based on three pillars. Together, they address and minimize each risk factor for an adverse patient outcome in the triad:
> 1. Optimization of the endogenous RBC mass through the targeted stimulation of erythropoiesis and the treatment of modifiable underlying disorders.
> 2. Minimization of diagnostic, interventional, and surgical blood loss to preserve the patient's RBC mass.
> 3. Optimization of the patient-specific tolerance to anemia through strict adherence to physiological transfusion thresholds.

In most clinical scenarios, implementation of the first two pillars is sufficient to address all three risks in the triad. Through optimizing a patient's RBC mass and reducing blood loss, the hemoglobin value of most patients is kept above the threshold where transfusion might be considered. However, addition of the third pillar can further reduce the transfusion rate (Meier and Gombotz 2013).

1.1.3 PBM in the Surgical and Nonsurgical Setting

The concept of PBM was initially developed in the surgical setting. By applying the three-pillar approach to the pre-, intra-, and postoperative phases, the model further evolved to the multidisciplinary, multimodal nine-field matrix shown in **Fig. 1.2**. Each of the fields includes a set of clinical measures that can be combined, and tailored to specific patient needs and procedures and to the expertise of a given organization.

Most PBM scenarios can be managed by a team of PBM-trained anesthesiologists, surgeons, and—in some cases—intensive care specialists. A smaller number of scenarios also require support from hematologists, gastroenterologists, radiologists, or other specialists.

> **Note**
>
> Each field of the multidisciplinary, multimodal nine-field matrix of PBM includes a set of clinical measures that can be combined and tailored to specific patient needs and procedures.

The principles of PBM can also be applied to procedures that have traditionally been associated with major blood loss and hemorrhage, and to medical settings where transfusion has been intrinsic to treatment. Furthermore, PBM is not confined to the transfusion of RBCs. Its principles can be expanded to preempt the transfusion of platelets, fresh frozen plasma (FFP), and other blood products that also carry risk.

> **Note**
>
> PBM was first developed in elective surgery but the principles can be applied in a modified form to obstetric, pediatric, and emergency surgery, trauma management, and other medical settings.

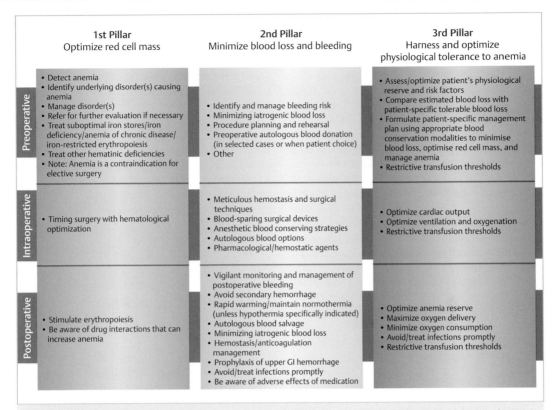

	1st Pillar Optimize red cell mass	2nd Pillar Minimize blood loss and bleeding	3rd Pillar Harness and optimize physiological tolerance to anemia
Preoperative	• Detect anemia • Identify underlying disorder(s) causing anemia • Manage disorder(s) • Refer for further evaluation if necessary • Treat suboptimal iron stores/iron deficiency/anemia of chronic disease/iron-restricted erythropoiesis • Treat other hematinic deficiencies • Note: Anemia is a contraindication for elective surgery	• Identify and manage bleeding risk • Minimizing iatrogenic blood loss • Procedure planning and rehearsal • Preoperative autologous blood donation (in selected cases or when patient choice) • Other	• Assess/optimize patient's physiological reserve and risk factors • Compare estimated blood loss with patient-specific tolerable blood loss • Formulate patient-specific management plan using appropriate blood conservation modalities to minimise blood loss, optimise red cell mass, and manage anemia • Restrictive transfusion thresholds
Intraoperative	• Timing surgery with hematological optimization	• Meticulous hemostasis and surgical techniques • Blood-sparing surgical devices • Anesthetic blood conserving strategies • Autologous blood options • Pharmacological/hemostatic agents	• Optimize cardiac output • Optimize ventilation and oxygenation • Restrictive transfusion thresholds
Postoperative	• Stimulate erythropoiesis • Be aware of drug interactions that can increase anemia	• Vigilant monitoring and management of postoperative bleeding • Avoid secondary hemorrhage • Rapid warming/maintain normothermia (unless hypothermia specifically indicated) • Autologous blood salvage • Minimizing iatrogenic blood loss • Hemostasis/anticoagulation management • Prophylaxis of upper GI hemorrhage • Avoid/treat infections promptly • Be aware of adverse effects of medication	• Optimize anemia reserve • Maximize oxygen delivery • Minimize oxygen consumption • Avoid/treat infections promptly • Restrictive transfusion thresholds

Fig. 1.2 The multidisciplinary, multimodal nine-field matrix of PBM. RBC, red blood cell. Reproduced from Hofmann et al 2007 with permission from the Department of Health, Western Australia.

1.1.4 Brief History of PBM

The renowned heart surgeon and founder of the Texas Heart Institute, Denton Cooley, was one of the first people to develop an individualized multimodal approach to blood conservation to perform complex heart surgery without the use of RBC transfusion. The positive patient outcomes associated with this approach led to the development of comprehensive hospital-wide "blood conservation programs." One of the early programs was established at Kaleeya Hospital in Fremantle, Western Australia, in 1990. The success of this program ultimately led to the implementation of a state-wide PBM program in Western Australia (Farmer et al 2013b).

In 1994, the anesthesiologist Aryeh Shander and the clinical nurse Sherri Ozawa established a pilot program at Englewood Hospital and Medical Center in Englewood, NJ. They have reported extensively on the improved patient outcomes resulting from their programmatic approach to PBM, and their approach has become a model for numerous programs and initiatives around the world (Shander et al 2010).

The term *Patient Blood Management* was coined by the Australian hematologist James Isbister during a board meeting of the Medical Society for Blood Management in Prague (Farmer and Leahy 2014). He and his colleagues advocated the use of this terminology to ensure a focus on management of the patient's own blood as opposed to the management of donor blood. In 2007, the term first appeared in the literature (Isbister 2007). In 2008, Isbister—together with colleagues from Europe—published the article "Patient blood management: the pragmatic solution for the problems with blood transfusions" (Spahn et al 2008); this was the first publication with PBM in the title. Since then, the number of PBM-related publications has been growing constantly, the articles spanning many different disciplines (Spahn et al 2008, Thomson et al 2009, Spahn 2010, Emmert et al 2011, Gombotz 2011, Ranucci et al 2011a, Gombotz 2012, Goodnough and Shander 2012, Kotze et al 2012, Meier et al 2012, Shander et al 2012a, Shander et al 2012b, Spahn et al 2012, Bruhn 2013, Farmer et al 2013b, Gombotz and Knotzer 2013, Goodnough et al 2013, Gross et al 2013, Liumbruno et al 2013, Mukhtar et al 2013, Shander et al 2013, Shaz et al 2013, Spahn et al 2013b, Cohn et al 2014, Leahy et al 2014).

The pre-, intra-, and postoperative phases of blood conservation were first described by Martyn and colleagues (2002), and the three-pillar concept of blood conservation was first mentioned in a peer-reviewed paper by Gombotz and colleagues in 2007, followed by a number of publications where this concept was referred to as the *three pillars of PBM* (Hofmann et al 2011). In 2008, Farmer and Hofmann combined the three phases of surgery and the three pillars of PBM to create the multidisciplinary, multimodal nine-field matrix of PBM for a PBM Program run by the Department of Health in Western Australia (Hofmann et al 2011, Hofmann et al 2012, Farmer et al 2013b). They also developed the concept of the triad of risk factors based on a review of the literature in which they identified three clinical risk factors that can be modified by PBM (Farmer et al 2013b).

The Department of Health in Western Australia was the world's first health authority to implement PBM across the public health system of an entire state or country. Other Australian health authorities followed with similar projects, and currently PBM is being implemented nationwide with the support of leading clinicians, hospital managers, and health authorities (Spahn et al 2008, Hofmann et al 2012, Spahn et al 2012, Farmer et al 2013b).

Managed by the National Blood Authority and endorsed by the Australian National Health and Patient Research Council, five of six modules of the national Patient Blood Management Guidelines for Australia have now been developed and published online (www.blood.gov.au/pbm-guidelines). In these guidelines, the PBM Program in Western Australia is acknowledged as a pilot program that addresses many of the challenges of program implementation.

In 2010, the World Health Assembly of the WHO adopted the concept of PBM with Resolution WHA63.12: "…PBM means that before surgery every reasonable measure should be taken to optimize the patient's own blood volume, to minimize the patient's blood loss and to harness and optimize the patient-specific physiological tolerance to anemia following the WHO's guide for optimal clinical use (three pillars of PBM)" (WHO 2010b).

In 2014, the European Commission announced a pilot program for the implementation of PBM in five European teaching hospitals (www.europe-pbm.eu). A number of institutions in North America, Europe, and the Asian-Pacific Region are currently establishing PBM as the standard of care. An increasing number of transfusion medicine specialists and leading professional organizations—e.g., the American Association of Blood Banks (www.aabb.org/pbm)—are supporting the concept.

1.1.5 Definition of PBM

Several descriptions and definitions of PBM have been published:
- "PBM is the timely application of evidence-based medical and surgical concepts aimed at achieving better patient outcome by relying on a patient's own blood rather than on donor blood" (Hofmann et al 2011).
- "Evidence-based PBM is aimed at achieving better patient outcome by relying on a patient's own blood rather than on donor blood" (Hofmann et al 2012).
- "PBM…employs a patient-specific perioperative/peri-event, multidisciplinary, multimodal team approach to managing the patient's own blood and haemopoietic system. PBM views a patient's own blood as a valuable and unique natural resource that should be conserved and managed appropriately" (DHWA 2011).
- "PBM improves patient outcome by improving the patient's medical and surgical management in ways that boost and conserve the patient's own blood" (http://blood.gov.au/patient-blood-management-pbm).
- "Patient blood management aims to improve clinical outcome by avoiding unnecessary exposure to blood components. It includes the three pillars… These principles apply in the management of any hematologic disorder. Patient blood management optimizes the use of donor blood and reduces transfusion-associated risk" (NBA 2011).

- "Professional definition: PBM is the timely application of evidence-based medical and surgical concepts designed to maintain hemoglobin concentration, optimize hemostasis and minimize blood loss in an effort to improve patient outcome" (www.sabm.org).
- "Public description: PBM is the scientific use of safe and effective medical and surgical techniques designed to prevent anemia and decrease bleeding in an effort to improve patient outcome" (www.sabm.org).

The various descriptions and definitions of PBM convey the idea that PBM

- Is evidence-based.
- Is a multimodal concept.
- Is an individualized, patient-specific therapeutic approach.
- Is multidisciplinary.
- Is applicable in surgical and nonsurgical settings.
- Improves patient outcomes.
- Improves patient safety/reduces transfusion-associated risks.
- Is based on three pillars.
- Involves the management of the patient's *own blood* as opposed to management of the patient with *somebody else's (donor) blood.*

In an attempt to integrate all of these aspects, the following universal definition is proposed: PBM is an evidence-based, integrated, multidisciplinary, multimodal approach to individually manage and preserve a patient's own blood in surgical and nonsurgical settings by correcting anemia, reducing blood loss, and harnessing and optimizing the physiological tolerance to anemia, thus minimizing or avoiding transfusion and improving patient safety and outcomes.

1.1.6 The Potential Impact of PBM

In 2011, the total number of blood units collected worldwide was approximately 92 million (WHO 2011a); the number of whole blood units and RBCs transfused was probably 10% lower (approximately 83 million). On the backdrop of this massive consumption, PBM has huge potential given the high prevalence of untreated preoperative anemia and the unmet need for bleeding management protocols—apart from protocols relating to massive bleeding (Spahn et al 2007)—and their system-wide implementation, together with a be-havior-based transfusion practice that is still too liberal. Year after year, the implementation of PBM could improve the outcomes of millions of patients and help to avoid millions of allogeneic transfusions with all the associated adverse effects.

The cost of RBC transfusions to U.S. health care providers is estimated at $14 billion per annum; however, the true costs might be much higher because of transfusion-related adverse outcomes (Shander et al 2010, Hofmann et al 2013, Vamvakas 2013). A retrospective cohort study using data from the 2004 Nationwide Inpatient Sample database found that, after adjustment for confounders, the average hospital costs per patient were $17,194 higher for those who had received a transfusion than for those who had not. In terms of 2014 dollars, this would be more than $57 billion for a study population of 2.33 million inpatients who received a transfusion. A retrospective cohort study conducted in Western Australia showed that, after adjustment for potential confounders, the total hospital-associated cost of RBC transfusion reached $72 million; the study included 89,996 multiday acute-care inpatients, 4,805 of whom had received a transfusion (Trentino et al 2015).

These amounts are of macroeconomic relevance and a significant share of these costs could be reallocated, resulting in better cost-effectiveness ratios when applying PBM (Shander et al 2010).

The Austrian Benchmark Study (Gombotz et al 2007) was the first study to indicate the enormous value of PBM in elective surgery. This study showed that 97.6%, 97.4%, and 96.9% of all RBC transfusions in patients undergoing total hip arthroplasty, knee arthroplasty, or coronary artery bypass (CABG) surgery, respectively, can be predicted by the following three parameters, which can all be modified through PBM (Gombotz et al 2007):

- Preoperative hemoglobin value.
- Blood loss.
- Transfusion trigger.

These results, and the fact that most transfusions are given to hemodynamically stable patients, indicate that with PBM fully implemented, RBC transfusion will become obsolete in many clinical scenarios or it will only have a minor role. PBM programs in different parts of the world have already demonstrated significant reductions in the number of transfusions with comparable or improved patient outcomes (Moskowitz et al 2010, Kotze et al 2012, Frank et al 2014b).

A number of other factors are also in favor of PBM. One is the constant threat posed by emerging and re-emerging blood pathogens, even though the problems with HIV, hepatitis B virus (HBV), and hepatitis C virus (HCV) seem to have been eliminated, albeit at an enormous cost (Goodnough et al 1999a, Goodnough et al 1999b). Besides, a shortage of allogeneic blood in high-income countries has been predicted because of a decline in blood donations, against a background of an aging population (Greinacher et al 2011). The failure to comply with existing guidelines and the broad variability in blood consumption are a drain on health budgets, in addition to presenting an increased health risk (Sanguis Study Group 1994, Gombotz et al 2007, Bennett-Guerrero et al 2010, Gombotz et al 2014). Process cost analysis has revealed that treatment with blood products is one of the most expensive forms of modern-day therapy (Shander et al 2007, Abraham and Sun 2012, Gombotz 2012).

>
>
> **Note**
>
> The high prevalence of untreated preoperative anemia and the unmet need for bleeding management protocols and their implementation, together with a transfusion practice that is too liberal, indicate that PBM represents a huge opportunity to improve patient outcomes and avoid millions of transfusions every year. The PBM approach is further supported by the inherent risks posed by new and re-emerging bloodborne pathogens, by blood supply pressures, and by the escalating costs associated with transfusion.

1.1.7 Clinical Practice: First Steps toward Reducing the Patient-specific Transfusion Risk

When implementing a PBM program, the identification and management of patients with a high transfusion probability can quickly yield initial results. Three principal steps can effectively achieve this aim:

- Identification of the procedures with the highest transfusion rates/indices (see Chapter 1.6). For hospitals with a patient-level database on transfusions and blood ordering processes, it should be relatively easy to capture this kind of information.
- Calculation of the mean blood loss experienced during these procedures from the hospital's retrospective patient-level database with a representative number of cases (see Chapter 2.3). **Note:** the calculated perioperative blood loss takes account of the amount of blood in swabs, hematomas, etc., and is therefore more accurate than blood loss estimates.
- Calculation of the individual patient's preoperative blood volume, based on the preoperative hemoglobin level, body weight, height, and gender. After deducting the hospital's empirically collected, procedure-specific mean blood loss from the patient's preoperative blood volume, the postoperative hemoglobin level can be predicted by using the Mercuriali algorithm. If the predicted hemoglobin level is close to, or below, the target hemoglobin level, PBM is clearly indicated. The target hemoglobin level or the transfusion threshold is set in accordance with the respective clinical picture and the transfusion guidelines of the pertinent societies (see Chapter 2.3).

>
>
> **Note**
>
> By empirically devising and calculating the mean perioperative blood loss for selected procedures, and by using patient-specific data such as the preoperative hemoglobin level, body weight, height, and gender, patients can be identified in whom PBM is indicated.

For many institutions that wish to introduce PBM, the routine correction of anemia in patients undergoing a procedure that is associated with high blood loss might be the first step toward a change in practice. With some structural adjustments, this step can be implemented almost immediately. The adaptation of treatment modalities to systematically reduce blood loss and bleeding might require more time, particularly if this involves surgical training. However, in a fully developed PBM program, anemia should be corrected always and in every patient because it is listed as a disease in the International Classification of Diseases (ICD-10), and blood loss should always be minimized. The ultimate goal is an institution-wide change in the transfusion culture (Oliver et al 2009).

1.1.8 PBM versus Optimal Blood Use—Two Different Approaches

Knowledge of the manifold nature of the problems related to transfusion has led the majority of high-income countries to formulate guidelines, and introduce hemovigilance registries and recommendations, for the optimal use of blood products; an example is the EU Optimal Use of Blood program (www.optimalblooduse.eu) (Hofmann et al 2011). These programs must not be confused with PBM, which involves the proactive and routine identification of patients with anemia and/or those at risk of clinically significant blood loss in order to provide them with a management plan aimed at reducing these risks. As a result, PBM leads to a reduction in the *demand* for allogeneic RBC transfusions. By contrast, the concept of optimal blood use is product-centered. It is geared toward the provision of a pathogen-free blood *supply* and the minimization of blood component wastage, while its clinical scope is limited to the implementation of an optimal transfusion threshold (**Table 1.1**).

>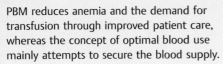
>
> **Note**
>
> PBM reduces anemia and the demand for transfusion through improved patient care, whereas the concept of optimal blood use mainly attempts to secure the blood supply.

Conclusion

To achieve optimal clinical outcomes and improve patient safety, the management and preservation of the patient's *own blood* has to take priority over the management of the patient with *donor blood*. This can be achieved by an evidence-based, multidisciplinary, multimodal, patient-specific treatment concept that is based on three pillars: (1) optimization of the (preoperative) endogenous RBC mass through the stimulation of erythropoiesis; (2) minimization of diagnostic, interventional, and operative blood loss to preserve the patient's RBC mass; and (3) optimization of the patient's physiological tolerance to anemia and strict adherence to physiological transfusion thresholds to further reduce the odds of RBC transfusion. When used in combination, these three pillars help to minimize the impact of the triad of independent risk factors for adverse outcomes (anemia, blood loss, and RBC transfusion).

The principles of PBM were first developed for elective surgery but can be applied in a modified form to obstetric, pediatric, and emergency surgery, trauma management, and medical settings. The consistent implementation of this three-pillar strategy improves the course of disease and patient safety, and leads to a substantial reduction in the use of allogeneic blood components compared with current transfusion practices.

Table 1.1 Comparison of the EU Optimal Blood Use program and the Patient Blood Management (PBM) concept (Gombotz and Knotzer 2013)

	Optimal blood use	PBM
Approach	Centered on the supply of blood products	Centered on patient outcomes
Minimization of the transfusion rate	?	Yes
Optimization of the treatment regimen	No	Yes
Treatment of perioperative anemia	No	Yes
Minimization of blood loss	No	Yes
Anticoagulation management	No	Yes
Increase of anemia tolerance	No	Yes
Remuneration	Yes	No

1.2 Requirements of Modern Transfusion Medicine

C. Geisen, M. M. Mueller, E. Seifried

1.2.1 Hemotherapy—from Blood Donation to Transfusion

The quality of modern hemotherapy does not depend solely on the quality of the blood components administered. Hemotherapy must be understood as a complex process ranging from blood donation through blood testing, indication assessment, blood sampling from the recipient, and compatibility testing to transportation to the storage site and the clinical user. Within this chain, failure of the weakest link poses risks to the patient (**Fig. 1.3**) (Isbister 1994).

Blood Donation

Blood donors make an important voluntary and unremunerated contribution to society. Donor selection is based on medical assessment using a medical history form completed by the donor, medical interview, medical examination (at least blood pressure, pulse, temperature), and laboratory analysis (hemoglobin measurement) (e.g., Standards for Blood Banks and Transfusion Services 2014, Norfolk 2013).

> **Note**
>
> Only donors who meet the minimum requirements set out in national guidelines will be permitted by the physician to donate blood.

Preparation of Blood Components

▸ **Blood components.** Blood transfusion in high-income countries is limited to the transfusion of blood components. RBCs, platelets, and plasma are separated from whole blood by centrifugation or collected directly from the donor through automated apheresis. Apheresis can also be used to obtain granulocytes or hematopoietic stem cells from peripheral blood.

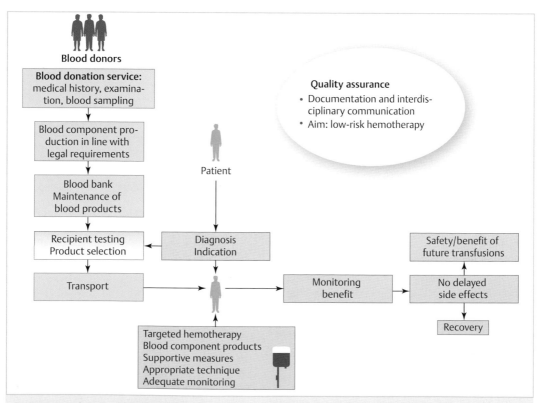

Fig. 1.3 Hemotherapeutic chain—hemotherapy as a process. Data source: Geisen et al 2012.

► **Further processing.** Standard blood products can be processed further, depending on the indication. This includes irradiating blood preparations to prevent transfusion-associated graft-versus-host disease, washing cellular preparations to prevent incompatibility reactions (caused by residual plasma from the donor) in sensitized individuals, and producing separated or concentrated blood components, e.g., for use in neonatology.

Note

The use of the different blood components should be based on an individualized risk–benefit analysis, corroborated by evidence from clinical trials. Specific recommendations are given in guidelines such as the United Kingdom's Handbook of Transfusion Medicine (Norfolk 2013) and the Cross-Sectional Guidelines for Therapy with Blood Components and Plasma Derivatives of the German Medical Association (BAEK 2011a).

Red Blood Cell Concentrates

► **Indication.** The administration of RBC concentrates continues to be a causal therapy—with the fastest onset of efficacy—for life-threatening anemic hypoxia. The indication for transfusion must be based on strict criteria adapted to the individual patient.

Note

The clinical symptoms of anemic hypoxia determine the actual indication of RBC transfusion (physiological transfusion triggers).

However, the symptoms of anemic hypoxia are nonspecific and may be difficult to identify under clinical conditions. There are no absolute or generally valid critical transfusion thresholds that can be defined for the hemoglobin level or the hematocrit. Any decision-making regarding transfusion must take into consideration not only the laboratory values, but also the duration, severity, dynamics, and cause of anemia as well as the patient's previous history, age, and clinical status. More detailed information on the indications for, and administration of, RBC concentrates is provided in the 2011 edition of Cross-Sectional Guidelines for Therapy with Blood Components and Plasma De-

rivatives of the German Medical Association (BAEK 2011a).

► **Storage.** RBC concentrates are stored at +4°C ±2°C for 28–49 days depending on the production process and in accordance with the manufacturer's instructions. In recent years, there has been an extensive discussion about the extent to which the complex morphological and biochemical changes occurring during storage can affect the clinical efficacy and side effects of transfused RBC concentrates (Roback 2011). Despite a plethora of published studies, it has not yet been possible to provide definitive answers, for two reasons: first, the studies carried out were retrospective or prospective observational studies, and second, not all influencing factors were taken into account (van de Watering 2011a, van de Watering 2011b). The first RCT in this area, which addressed mortality as the primary outcome, failed to show an improved clinical outcome in premature infants transfused with fresh RBCs compared with standard blood products (Fergusson et al 2012). In a 2015 study, the transfusion of fresh RBCs, as compared with standard-issue RBCs, did not decrease the 90-day mortality among critically ill adults (Lacroix et al 2015). Several other large RCTs assessing the effect of RBC storage time on mortality or multiple organ dysfunction are currently in progress and may help to shed more light on the influence of storage time (Flegel et al 2014).

Note

The question as to whether there is a causal link between the shelf life of RBC concentrates and the occurrence of adverse reactions can ultimately only be resolved by prospective randomized clinical trials.

Platelet Concentrates

Platelet concentrates contain more than 2×10^{11} platelets. Their volume is between 200 mL and 350 mL. The platelets are resuspended in either plasma or an additive solution. They are stored at +22°C ±2°C under continuous agitation.

► **Product types.** Platelet concentrates are isolated either from whole blood donations through pooling of four buffy coats from donors with the same ABO and Rhesus D group, or through platelet apheresis from a single donor (Schrezenmeier and Seifried 2010).

> **Note**
>
> In nonrefractory recipients, pooled platelet concentrates and apheresis platelet concentrates are comparable in terms of safety, tolerability, and efficacy (**Table 1.2**) (Schrezenmeier and Seifried 2010, BAEK 2011a).

For supply reasons, both product types should be available. That way, products from donors compatible for human leukocyte antigen (HLA) and/or human platelet antigen (HPA) can be promptly administered to immunized recipients, while keeping available a supply of platelet concentrates with special characteristics.

▶ **Indication.** Thresholds for the therapeutic administration of platelet concentrates and for their prophylactic administration before procedures and interventions are provided in the 2011 edition

of the Cross-Sectional Guidelines of the German Medical Association (BAEK 2011a).

Therapeutic Plasma

Various types of therapeutic plasma are available for clinical use. The efficacy of the various product types—FFP, methylene-blue-/light-treated plasma, lyophilized human plasma, and pooled solvent/detergent-treated plasma—is broadly similar. Plasma is transfused in an ABO-compatible fashion (BAEK 2011a).

▶ **Indication.** Plasma is used for the replacement of deficient coagulation factors (provided the missing factors are not available as factor concentrates) and for plasma exchange therapy. The specific indications have been narrowed in recent years (Shepard and Bukowski 1987, Bell et al 1991, Rock et al 1991) and are available in the 2011 edition of the Cross-Sectional Guidelines of the German Medical Association (BAEK 2011a) (see also Chapter 1.5).

Table 1.2 Comparison of the main characteristics of pooled platelet concentrates isolated from the buffy coat of whole blood donations and apheresis platelet concentrates

Characteristic		Buffy-coat pooled platelet concentrates (leukocyte-depleted)	Apheresis platelet concentrates
Quality criteria	Platelet count	++	++(+) [a]
	Residual leukocytes	Low	Low
	Residual plasma	Low	High
Adverse reactions	Transfusion reactions	No difference	
	Allosensitization/refractoriness	No difference	
	Bacterial contamination	No difference	
Efficacy	Platelet increment		
	• Random transfusion	No difference [b]	
	• Allosensitized patients (HLA/HPA antibodies)	(+)	+++
	Hemorrhage	No difference	
	Time to next transfusion	No difference	
Donor	Donor complications	No	Possible

Abbreviations: HLA, human leukocyte antigen; HPA, human platelet antigen.
[a] On using platelet apheresis, higher platelet counts can be obtained. Most blood donation services collect double or triple apheresis platelet products if the platelet count is adequate; hence, the platelet count per therapeutic unit is comparable.
[b] The platelet increment is highly dependent on the clinical status of the recipient.

1.2.2 Quality Assurance in Clinical Hemotherapy

Blood Donation Centers

Institutions that collect blood and blood components, produce blood products, and/or store and supply them, are legally required to have an effective quality assurance system in place that meets stringent safety and utility requirements.

Health Care Centers

In many countries, inpatient and outpatient centers that administer blood products are also required to set up a quality assurance system. Quality assurance comprises the entire spectrum of staffing, organizational, technical, and normative measures designed to maximize the quality of patient care and to improve it in line with the state of the art in medical science. In hemotherapy, quality indicators for the analysis and use of blood products must be defined. In addition, the qualifications and duties of the responsible persons must be defined. The quality assurance measures and operating procedures must be summarized in a quality management manual.

1.2.3 Safety of Blood Products—Adverse Reactions

▶ **Classification.** Based on their pathophysiological mechanisms, any adverse reactions associated with the use of blood products can generally be classified as immune-mediated or nonimmune-mediated transfusion reactions or as transfusion-related infections (**Table 1.3**). Another classification system is based on the time course; it distinguishes between acute side effects, e.g., immediate-type hemolytic reactions, and delayed side effects, e.g., delayed-type hemolytic reactions (**Table 1.3**). The International Haemovigilance Network provides useful definitions of adverse reactions on its website (www.ihn-org.com).

▶ **Mandatory notification.** Serious transfusion reactions must be reported to the manufacturer of the blood product and to the respective competent authority. Examples of reports in which the reported data are evaluated include the United Kingdom's Serious Hazards of Transfusion (SHOT) report (Bolton-Maggs et al 2013) and the annual hemovigilance report by the Paul Ehrlich Institute in Germany (Funk et al 2012a).

▶ **Incidence.** Next to acute (allergic) transfusion reactions, transfusion-related acute lung injury

Table 1.3 Classification of adverse reactions to blood products according to their pathologic mechanism and time of onset after the transfusion

Mechanism	Acute onset	Delayed onset
Immune-mediated adverse reaction	• Acute hemolytic transfusion reaction • Immunogenic TRALI • Febrile nonhemolytic transfusion reaction • Allergic transfusion reaction	• Delayed hemolytic transfusion reaction • ta-GvHD • PTP • Transfusion-associated immunomodulation
Nonimmune-mediated adverse reaction	• Nonimmunogenic TRALI • TACO • Hyperkalemia • Citrate toxicity • Hypothermia	• Transfusion hemosiderosis
Infection	• TTBI	• TTVI • Transfusion-transmitted parasitic infection • Transfusion-related vCJD

Abbreviations: PTP, posttransfusion purpura; ta-GvHD, transfusion-associated graft-versus-host disease; TACO, transfusion-associated circulatory overload; TRALI, transfusion-related acute lung injury; TTBI; transfusion-transmitted bacterial infection; TTVI, transfusion-transmitted viral infection; vCJD, variant Creutzfeldt–Jakob disease.

(TRALI) and hemolytic transfusion reaction are the most commonly reported serious transfusion-associated adverse reactions.

> **Note**
>
> In Germany, the risk of immunogenic TRALI has been significantly reduced since 2009 through the exclusive use of therapeutic plasma from male donors or from women with no history of pregnancy (Funk et al 2012a, Funk et al 2012b, PEI 2011).

Approximately 70% of hemolytic transfusion reactions that result in death are attributable to AB0-incompatible transfusions. Under-reporting is likely. The main reasons for mismatched transfusions are failure to identify the intended recipient, misidentification at the time of collecting the blood specimen for pretransfusion laboratory analysis, and errors when administering the transfusion, such as product mix-ups (Lippi and Plebani 2011, Stainsby et al 2005, Bolton-Maggs et al 2013, Wallis 2006).

> **Note**
>
> The majority of serious transfusion reactions are caused by errors. Therefore, it is imperative to establish and verify identity at each step of the transfusion chain!

Infections

Different pathogens (viruses, bacteria, or parasites) can be transmitted via blood products.

Transfusion-transmitted Viral Infections

▸ **Serology tests.** Typical transfusion-transmitted viral infections include HBV, HCV, and HIV-1 infections. It was already known in the 1970s that blood product recipients can develop posttransfusion hepatitis (Barker and Gerety 1976). Since the middle of the 1970s, all blood products are screened using the HBV surface antigen (HBsAg) test for the direct detection of HBV. However, the diagnostic window is approximately 38–40 days.

▸ **Nucleic acid tests.** To complement serology screening tests (antibody/antigen tests), highly sensitive tests for the direct detection of viral genomes were introduced into the screening program in the late 1990s. Nucleic acid testing (NAT) is based on nucleic acid amplification techniques (e.g., real-time polymerase chain reaction [PCR] or transcription-mediated amplification) (Busch and Dodd 2000, Roth et al 2000). Germany was one of the first countries to implement this technology for blood donor screening, with significant improvements in the safety of blood products (Roth et al 1999). By 2009, more than 300 million NAT tests for HCV and HIV-1 and approximately 100 million NAT tests for HBV had been performed worldwide (Roth et al 2012). The tests resulted in the identification of 1,728, 680, and 244 blood donors who were infected with HBV, HCV, and HIV-1, respectively, and who would not have been identified with any other method.

Anti-HBc testing was introduced as an additional screening parameter in various countries (e.g., introduction in Germany in 2006) to detect occult HBV infections. Blood donors with an occult HBV infection are potentially infectious because the HBV concentration might be below the detection limit of existing screening methods (Schmidt et al 2006).

▸ **Success of nucleic acid testing.** Since blood donor screening for HCV by mini-pool NAT became mandatory in Germany in 1999, only one transfusion-related transmission of HCV has been observed. Likewise, the number of transmitted HIV-1 infections has markedly declined. However, in 2007 and 2010 there were isolated cases of false-negative PCR results. The amplification efficiency of the PCR technique had been reduced because of virus genome mutations in the primer/probe regions, leading to HIV-1 remaining undetected in donor plasma (Schmidt et al 2009). In two of five cases, this gave rise to the transmission of HIV-1 to a recipient (Chudy et al 2012). This diagnostic gap will be closed by using an HIV-1 NAT system with two target regions (dual-target approach).

▸ **Cost-effectiveness of the "dual-safety" strategy.** Apart from the evident successes achieved with the introduction of mini-pool NAT to blood donor screening, evaluation of health economic data has also highlighted the cost-effectiveness of the modern dual-safety strategy based on infection serology and NAT. This is reflected in increases in quality-adjusted life years gained thanks to the avoidance of transfusion-related HBV, HCV, and HIV transmission (**Fig. 1.4**) (Jackson et al 2003, Nübling et al 2009).

>
>
> **Note**
>
> The residual risk of transfusion-transmitted viral infection is currently estimated at 1:10.8 million for HCV, 1:4.3 million for HIV-1, and 1:360,000 for HBV, based on blood products from the German Red Cross (Hourfar et al 2008).

Transfusion-transmitted Bacterial Infections

Compared with transfusion-transmitted viral infections, bacterial contamination presents a resid-

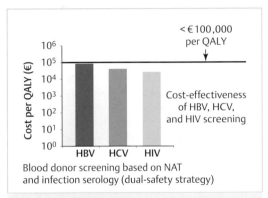

Blood donor screening based on NAT and infection serology (dual-safety strategy)

Fig. 1.4 Cost of blood donor screening per QALY gained, based on NAT and infection serology. HBV, hepatitis B virus; HCV, hepatitis C virus; HIV, human immunodeficiency virus; NAT, nucleic acid testing; QALY, quality-adjusted life years.

ual infection risk that is higher by a factor of 10–100 (**Fig. 1.5**) (Blajchman and Goldman 2001, Hourfar et al 2008, Schrezenmeier et al 2007). That said, unless lethal septicemia occurs, bacteria do not cause chronic illness like the earlier mentioned viruses and the clinical relevance is therefore not easily comparable. Platelet concentrates are at particular risk of bacterial contamination because they are stored at room temperature, thus providing good growing conditions for numerous bacterial strains.

▶ **Initial specimen diversion technique and shelf life restriction.** The initial specimen diversion technique was introduced worldwide at the beginning of this century to reduce the risk of bacterial transmission (de Korte et al 2002, de Korte et al 2006). This means that subsequent to venipuncture, the first 30 to 40 mL of blood are diverted into a separate bag. Bacteria introduced by the needle puncture will thus be removed again with the initial blood flow. This technique has helped to reduce the residual bacterial infection risk by around 50%.

Studies carried out worldwide found that the prevalence of bacterial contamination of platelet concentrates is 1 in 2,000. The incidence of serious septic reactions to platelet concentrate transfusions is reported to be between 1 in 50,000 and 1 in 150,000. For Germany, the Paul Ehrlich Institute reported a total of 12 deaths because of bacterial transmission via blood components between 1997 and 2009 (with a total of approximately 50 million transfused blood products). Although platelet concentrates constitute less than 8% of all transfused units, they were implicated in six cases, with most of these platelet concentrates

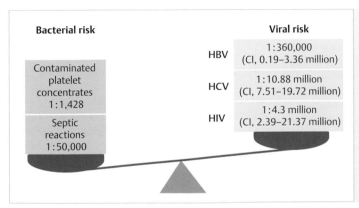

Fig. 1.5 Residual infection risk in transfusion medicine in Germany. HBV, hepatitis B virus; HCV, hepatitis C virus; HIV, human immunodeficiency virus. Data from Geisen et al 2012.

having been transfused at the end of their shelf life. Consequently, the maximum shelf life for platelet concentrates in Germany was reduced from 5 days to 4 days.

► **Detection and inactivation procedures.** Worldwide, culture methods (de Korte 2011) (e.g., BacT/Alert or Bactek) or rapid test methods including PCR-based detection methods (Dreier et al 2009, Sireis et al 2011) are the main methods currently used to screen for bacterial contamination. As an alternative, pathogen inactivation methods—e.g., Mirasol (AuBuchon et al 2005), Intercept (Osselaer et al 2009), and Theraflex (Seltsam and Müller 2011)—are being developed. Methods based on a photochemical or photodynamic functional principle lead to the irreversible destruction of DNA, thus preventing pathogen growth. A drawback that persists to the present day is that different pathogen inactivation procedures are needed for different blood products.

> **Note**
>
> The risk of transfusion-transmitted bacterial infections was significantly reduced through introduction of the initial specimen diversion technique, the reduction of the maximum shelf life for platelet concentrates from 5 days to 4 days, and the introduction of detection techniques for bacterial contamination.

Transfusion-associated "Proteinopathies"

Transfusion-associated Variant Creutzfeldt–Jakob Disease

Creutzfeldt–Jakob disease (CJD), a disease that has been known for several decades but is very rare, belongs to the group of diseases associated with irreversible damage to the central nervous system and involves the deposition of pathological prion proteins. To date, there is no spontaneous cure or treatment. CJD remains an important health problem because of the emergence of a new variant of this disease in the United Kingdom in 1996. Variant CJD (vCJD) has been linked to foodborne transmission to humans of an infectious agent contracted through the consumption of meat products derived from cattle infected with bovine spongiform encephalopathy (BSE), also known as classi-

cal BSE, which was first reported in the United Kingdom in 1986.

► **Epidemiology.** vCJD is very rare. By February 2015, 229 people had contracted vCJD worldwide, 177 of whom in the United Kingdom, 27 in France, 5 in Spain, 4 each in Ireland and the United States, 3 in the Netherlands, 2 each in Italy, Portugal, and Canada, and 1 each in Japan, Taiwan, and Saudi Arabia (NCJDRSU 2015). The number of vCJD cases in the United Kingdom peaked in 2000 with 28 deaths. There has since been a sharp decline in the disease rate, with a drop to fewer than five new infections per year worldwide. So far, no cases of vCJD have occurred in Germany, Austria, or Switzerland, but the emergence of new cases in other countries cannot be ruled out.

► **Bloodborne transmission.** Animal experiments have demonstrated that bloodborne transmission of prions is in principle possible. Four human cases (including one "subclinical case") where prions are thought to have been transmitted in non-leukocyte-reduced RBC concentrates have been reported in the United Kingdom. This must be viewed as proof of the potential human-to-human transmissibility of the vCJD agent through blood. The patients had received blood products from donors in whom vCJD was diagnosed 17, 18, 20, and 41 months after the implicated donation. It should be noted, however, that these patients themselves were exposed to the same risk factors for vCJD as their donors so that the connection to blood transfusion is not definitive.

► **Measures.** It can be assumed that new vCJD infections from the food chain have been effectively suppressed since 1996. One of the measures contemplated to block any ongoing hypothetical transmission chain and the persistence of vCJD via blood products was the exclusion of transfusion recipients from blood donation. This measure was introduced in some countries (the United Kingdom, the Netherlands, Switzerland, and France, although in the last case this measure had already been imposed in 1998 in the wake of cases of viral transmission). However, a model calculation based on pessimistic assumptions showed that the general exclusion of transfusion recipients would not essentially impact epidemiological trends, and any potential effect in terms of preventing isolated cases would, at most, be minimal.

Since exclusion of a significant number of blood donors would have a negative effect on the blood supply, the exclusion of transfusion recipients from blood donation was not implemented in Germany.

Some countries have opted to indefinitely defer individuals from donation who spent time in the United Kingdom (or in Europe) during the critical time window. In the United Kingdom, patients born after the emergence of vCJD receive non-European plasma products.

Any secondary transmission could be suppressed as far as possible if a screening test were available. No such test is available at present, nor will it be in the foreseeable future. Therefore, top priority should be given to the development of such test methods.

Alzheimer's Disease—a "Novel Transfusion-associated Proteinopathy"?

At the beginning of 2012, media reports caused a sensation with headlines suggesting that researchers studying Alzheimer's disease had found evidence that this type of dementia can be transmitted through RBC transfusion. American neuroscientists were reported to have transmitted Alzheimer's disease through blood from a mouse with a model of this condition to another healthy mouse (Morales et al 2012).

Even though the experiments in transgenic, predisposed mice did produce evidence of an accelerated induction of cerebral amyloid deposition that was potentially transfusion-mediated, it remains unclear whether this led to the development of the disease in the animal models. There is convincing evidence that Alzheimer's disease belongs to a group of "protein misfolding diseases" subsumed under the newly coined collective term *proteinopathies* (de Calignon et al 2012, Soto 2012). In these diseases, misfolded proteins (in Alzheimer's disease this is amyloid β) with an altered structure serve as a "template" for the misfolding of normally folded proteins; the misfolded proteins then form aggregates that are thought to damage brain tissue. Based on this hypothesis, misfolded amyloid β serves as a "seed" (Jucker and Walker 2011). Hence, certain parallels to prion diseases (CJD, vCJD) can be drawn (**Table 1.4**), but these have not yet been studied in detail, let alone proven. In a recent evaluation of the potential infectivity of proteins associated with Alzheimer's or Parkinson's disease (i.e., amyloid β, tau, and α-synuclein) in 796 recipients of cadaveric human growth hormone, a population with a markedly elevated risk of vCJD, no cases of Alzheimer's or Parkinson's disease were identified (Irwin et al 2013).

Table 1.4 Comparison of vCJD and Alzheimer's disease

Parameter	vCJD	Alzheimer's disease
Human-to-human transmission	Yes	No evidence
Causative agent	Prions	Amyloid β (amyloid plaques); induction of the pathology unknown
Dose of exposure	Clear relationship with incubation period and probably with illness	Unknown
Bloodborne transmission	Yes	Preliminary experiment data
Latency before disease onset	17–41 months	Unknown
Blood donor selection criteria	Yes, but evidence base uncertain	No evidence
Screening test	Under development	Not available
Elimination	Difficult to inactivate, but can be reduced in plasma products	Unknown

Abbreviation: vCJD, variant Creutzfeldt–Jakob disease.

> **Note**
>
> There is no evidence of human-to-human transmissibility of Alzheimer's disease. The available evidence of experimental bloodborne transmission must be viewed as provisional, but should be urgently reviewed in light of the experience with vCJD. Experimental and epidemiological data are needed to that effect. To date, there is no epidemiological evidence of a link between transfusions and Alzheimer's disease but, equally, no specific studies have been carried out to address this question.

1.2.4 Outlook

Demographic Trends

The European population is aging rapidly (WHO Regional Office for Europe 2012). The group aged 65 years or older constituted 15% of the total population by the end of 2010 and is projected to comprise more than 25% by 2050, so it is the fastest-growing segment of the population. A similar demographic change is expected for the United States; the population aged 65 and older increased from 8.1% of the total population in 1950 to 12.8% in 2009 and is projected to reach 20.2% in 2050 (Shrestha and Heisler 2011).

> **Note**
>
> According to the projected demographic changes, the drop in the proportion of younger potential donors will coincide with a growing need for blood products because of more invasive treatments for the expanding group of older people (**Fig. 1.6**) (Seifried et al 2011).

Modern Treatment Methods

Modern methods of treatment will help to restrict the consumption of blood and blood products. Various perioperative measures are already in use, such as blood salvage from the surgical site, use of controlled hypotension, and optimized perioperative anticoagulation management. Thanks to technological advances, it is now increasingly possible to avail of minimally invasive surgery for procedures involving a risk of bleeding. Targeted therapeutic antibodies, tyrosine kinase inhibitors, and novel targeted cancer drugs will, in some cases,

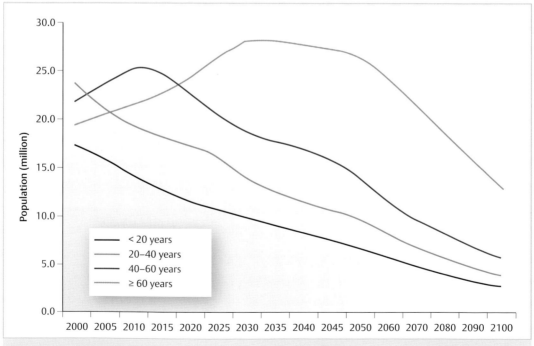

Fig. 1.6 Demographic trends in Germany, 2000–2100. Data from Birg 2003.

replace myelosuppressive chemotherapy regimens, thus reducing the need for blood. At present, hemoglobin- or perfluorocarbon-based oxygen carriers are rarely used because of side effects and intolerance reactions, but the development of erythropoietin and thrombopoietin analogues has meant that blood products can be avoided for certain indications.

In parallel with the development of recombinant proteins, which have already replaced some plasma-derived therapeutic proteins, a similar trend can be expected for cellular blood components. Even the exvivo production of RBCs seems increasingly more realistic thanks to advances in stem cell research. However, at present the development of universally deployable RBC concentrates from stem cells appears difficult, if not impossible, given the large number of clinically relevant blood groups, the broad genetic diversity of blood group alleles, and the resulting diversity of potential alloantibodies in transfused patients. RBC production from stem cells is currently performed on a laboratory scale. There are still many problems to be resolved in this respect, including: industrial-scale production in compliance with Good Manufacturing Practice; prevention of pathogen transmission from immortalized stem cell cultures; avoidance of malignant transformation; quality control of manufactured products (e.g., absence of nucleated RBCs); and approval and monitoring criteria. To produce RBC concentrates from stem cells of Good Manufacturing Practice quality using the current production processes, several hundred liters of high-grade culture medium—and commensurate financial resources—would be needed (Seifried et al 2011).

> **Note**
>
> Novel therapeutics and conventional blood products must be evaluated in comparative clinical trials so that evidence-based treatment recommendations can be further developed.

Conclusion

Life expectancy in high-income countries has continued to increase for various reasons, including high-performance medicine. Hemotherapy is one of the key elements of modern treatment concepts. Without the transfusion of RBC and platelet concentrates and of therapeutic plasma, it would not be possible to carry out high-dose chemotherapy for hematologic and solid tumors, hematopoietic stem cell transplantation, organ transplantation, major surgical procedures, or modern trauma management. Accordingly, the annual requirement for blood products has continued to rise during the last decades in many countries. The demands made on modern transfusion medicine include the assurance that hemotherapy is as safe as possible and that the clinical indications for the use of blood products are based on evidence. However, the safety of hemotherapy is not determined by blood products alone but also, to a large extent, by the quality of the transfusion process. Hemovigilance data from the United Kingdom (SHOT) and Germany (Paul Ehrlich Institute) show that there is still room for improvement, in particular as regards the indications for and the use of blood products (Funk et al 2012b, Bolton-Maggs et al 2013). Thanks to the development of modern screening methods, stringent donor selection criteria, and pathogen inactivation methods, blood products today have reached a safety level never witnessed before in the history of medicine.

1.3 Transfusion and Patient Outcomes

S. Farmer, A. Hofmann, J. Isbister

1.3.1 Introduction

Any review of the literature on transfusion and patient outcomes is sobering. In nonbleeding patients, evidence for the benefit from transfusion is scant—even in critically ill patients. Of concern is the large and growing body of literature showing that transfusion is independently associated with adverse patient outcomes in a dose-dependent manner (**Table 1.5**) (Hofmann et al 2011, Isbister et al 2011).

Table 1.5 Studies reporting a dose-dependent increase in adverse outcomes associated with red blood cell transfusion

Author/Year	Setting/population	Sample size	Dose-dependent adverse outcomes
Chaiwat et al 2009	Trauma	14,070	ARDS
Salim et al 2008	Traumatic brain injury	1,150	Mortality, ARDS, ARF, acute respiratory failure, bacteremia or fungemia, MOF, pulmonary embolism, pneumonia, sepsis
Bochicchio et al 2008	Trauma	1,172	Infection, ICU & hospital LOS, mechanical ventilation, mortality
Weinberg et al 2008	Trauma	1,624	Morbidity, mortality
Charles et al 2007	Trauma	8,215	Mortality
Malone et al 2003	Trauma	15,534	Mortality
Claridge et al 2002	Trauma	1,593	Infection
Moore et al 1997	Trauma	513	MOF
Parsons et al 2013	ICU	124	Decreased muscle strength
Zilberberg et al 2007	ICU	4,892	ARDS
Gong et al 2005	ICU	688	ARDS, mortality
Shorr et al 2005	ICU	4,892	Bloodstream infections
Corwin et al 2004	ICU	4,892	Mortality, ARDS, ICU & hospital LOS
Taylor et al 2006	ICU	2,085	Nosocomial infections, ICU & hospital LOS, mortality
Kneyber et al 2007	Pediatric ICU	295	Mortality
Shaw et al 2014	Cardiac surgery	3,516	Mortality
Horvath et al 2013	Cardiac surgery	5,158	Infection
Mikkola et al 2012	Cardiac surgery	2,226	Stroke
Stone et al 2012	Cardiac surgery	1,491	Mortality
van Straten et al 2010	Cardiac surgery	10,425	Mortality
Hajjar et al 2010	Cardiac surgery	512	Morbidity, mortality
Karkouti et al 2009	Cardiac surgery	3,460	Acute kidney injury
Scott et al 2008	Cardiac surgery	1,746	Postoperative LOS
Murphy et al 2007	Cardiac surgery	8,500	Infection, ischemic events
Kulier et al 2007	Cardiac surgery	5,065	Cardiac and noncardiac adverse events
Banbury et al 2006	Cardiac surgery	15,592	Septicemia, bacteremia, superficial & deep sternal wound infection
Koch et al 2006b	Cardiac surgery	11,963	In-hospital mortality, renal failure, postoperative ventilatory support, postoperative infections, cardiac & neurologic morbidity, overall postoperative morbidity
Koch et al 2006c	Cardiac surgery	10,289	Long-term (10-year) survival
Koch et al 2006a	Cardiac surgery	7,321	Functional recovery
Rogers et al 2006	Cardiac surgery	9,218	Infections
Chelemer et al 2002	Cardiac surgery	533	Bacterial infections

Continued ▶

Table 1.5 Continued

Author/Year	Setting/population	Sample size	Dose-dependent adverse outcomes
Leal-Noval et al 2003	Cardiac surgery	738	Infections, pneumonia
Ferraris et al 2012	Noncardiac surgery	941,496	Morbidity, mortality, resource use
Ferraris et al 2011b	Thoracic surgery	8,728	Morbidity, mortality
Al-Refaie et al 2012	Cancer surgery	38,926	Mortality, complications, hospital LOS
Linder et al 2013	Nephrectomy	2,318	Mortality
Bernard et al 2009	General surgery	125,177	Morbidity, mortality
Beattie et al 2009	Noncardiac surgery	7,759	Mortality
Bursi et al 2009	Vascular surgery	359	Mortality, MI, composite MI/mortality
Dunne et al 2002	Noncardiac surgery	6,301	Pneumonia, hospital LOS, mortality
Gauvin et al 2008	Pediatrics	1,100	Mortality
Jagoditsch et al 2006	Rectal surgery	597	Mortality
Xenos et al 2012	Colorectal surgery	21,943	VTE
Chang et al 2000	Colorectal surgery	1,349	Infections
Vignali et al 1996	Colorectal surgery	267	Infections
Ho et al 2007	Spinal surgery	1,046	Delayed infections
Carson et al 1999	Hip fracture surgery	9,598	Infections, pneumonia
Palmieri et al 2006	Burns	666	Infections, mortality

Abbreviations: ARDS, acute respiratory distress syndrome; ARF, acute renal failure; ICU, intensive care unit; LOS, length of stay; MI, myocardial infarction; MOF, multisystem organ failure; VTE, venous thromboembolism.

1.3.2 The Literature on Transfusion Outcomes

Most studies evaluating the clinical efficacy of transfusion have failed to demonstrate a benefit.

▶ **Oxygen transport.** Napolitano et al (2009) reviewed 20 studies that evaluated the clinical effect of RBC transfusion on oxygen delivery (DO_2) and oxygen consumption (VO_2). Although transfusion universally increased the hemoglobin level and it increased the DO_2 in most studies (15 of 20), it increased the VO_2 in only 3 of the 20 studies.

> **Note**
>
> RBC transfusion increases the hemoglobin level and the DO_2; an increase in the VO_2 can rarely be demonstrated.

▶ **Surgery, trauma, internal medicine, and critical care.** Based on a systematic review and analysis of the literature on transfusion and outcomes published over the preceding 13 years, the 2009 International Consensus Conference on Transfusion and Outcome used the RAND/UCLA Appropriateness Method to determine the appropriateness (defined as "likely to improve the patient's health outcome") of allogeneic RBC transfusion in 450 clinical scenarios in which transfusion is typically considered (Shander et al 2011a). The patient populations included surgery, trauma, internal medicine, and critical care. To avoid the confounding of critical bleeding, the analysis was confined to patients who were nonactively bleeding and relatively stable. Based on the available literature, the 15-member international multidisciplinary expert panel concluded that transfusion was likely to improve the patient's health outcome in only 11.8% of the 450 scenarios. In 59.3% of the scenarios, transfusion was found to be inappropriate, that is, not likely to improve patient health outcomes, or that is was even likely to harm the patient. In 28.9 % of scenarios, the findings were inconclusive, with more research required to make definitive conclusions.

▶ **Massive bleeding.** Intuitively, transfusion is seen to be of benefit in the critically bleeding patient. However, even in this setting, it is difficult to get a clear picture of the benefits and harms of transfusion. In a review of systematic reviews evaluating the outcomes of transfusion in trauma, Curry and colleagues (2011) concluded that RBC transfusion "offers life-saving potential" in exsanguinating patients. However, they stated that their systematic review of the literature provided little evidence of benefit for transfusion in that setting. A great deal of the literature has shown that, while transfusion may be part of the solution in the initial hemorrhagic setting, it may also become part of the problem and may itself contribute to a negative outcome later on. Studies in trauma patients have shown transfusion to be independently associated with increased infection (Hill et al 2003, Dunne et al 2006), multiple organ failure (Ciesla et al 2005, Moore et al 1997), acute respiratory distress syndrome (ARDS) (Silverboard et al 2005, Croce et al 2005, Chaiwat et al 2009), systemic inflammatory response syndrome (SIRS) (Dunne et al 2004, Beale et al 2006), and mortality (Malone et al 2003, Bochicchio et al 2008). This is clearly a difficult patient population in which to separate out all factors that may contribute to a poor outcome. However, the consistency of the literature demonstrating a contributory negative effect of transfusion warrants serious questions about its efficacy; further research is needed to address this issue.

▶ **Children with anemia and/or malaria.** Some evidence for benefit in extreme situations comes from two nonrandomized observational studies from Kenya, Africa, in children with severe anemia and/or malaria. The first study by Lackritz et al (1992) compared transfused versus nontransfused patients in a cohort of 2,433 children admitted to a rural district hospital. When 678 children under the age of 3 years and with severe anemia (hemoglobin < 5 g/dL) were analyzed, a subgroup was identified in whom transfusion was associated with reduced mortality. This subgroup was made up of: (1) Patients with a hemoglobin level < 3.9 g/dL

transfused on day 0 or day 1 of admission. There was no difference thereafter in transfused versus nontransfused patients irrespective of the hemoglobin level at admission. (2) Patients with a hemoglobin level < 4.7 g/dL along with respiratory distress. There was no difference in children without respiratory distress irrespective of the hemoglobin level at admission. Overall, transfusion given to children with a hemoglobin level ≥ 3.9 g/dL was associated with an increased risk of death. However, the results of this study are difficult to translate to other clinical settings because whole blood was used, and blood used in this setting was mostly from family member donations and thus relatively fresh. Also, most children presenting with acute malaria are hypovolemic and no information was given on fluid management in nontransfused children.

The second study by English et al (2002) involved a cohort of 9,968 children. The analysis included 1,516 children with severe anemia (hemoglobin < 5.9 g/dL), comparing transfused children with nontransfused children. Overall, there was no difference in mortality between the two groups (8 % in each group; n = 984 transfused and n = 532 nontransfused). An association between transfusion and lower mortality was identified in a subgroup of 75 patients who had malaria or anemia, prostration, respiratory distress, and a hemoglobin level < 4.0 g/dL (mortality: 89 % [8 of 9] in the nontransfused group versus 23 % [15 of 65] in the transfused group). Again, whole, relatively fresh blood was used from family donors and no information was given on other fluid management measures.

With the exception of two RCTs in children in Africa with severe malarial anemia, RCTs in transfusion medicine have not evaluated the safety and efficacy of transfusion compared with no transfusion (placebo) or with some other modality. In the two African RCTs, Holzer et al (1993) randomized 116 children aged between 2 months and 6 years with severe malarial anemia (hemoglobin between 4 g/dL and 5.7 g/dL) to receive either malaria treatment and a whole-blood transfusion (donated by relatives), or malaria treatment alone. Bojang et al (1997) randomized 114 children aged between 6 months and 9 years with severe malarial anemia (hemoglobin between 4 g/dL and 5 g/dL), and without clinical signs of respiratory distress, to receive either a whole-blood transfusion or oral iron. Meremikwu and Smith (2000) combined the data from these two trials in a Cochrane Collaboration review and meta-analysis. The combined data showed there was no significant difference in mortality between the transfused and the non-transfused children (relative risk, 0.41; 95% confidence interval [CI], 0.06–2.70; p = 0.4). There were, however, significantly more severe adverse events in the transfused group compared with the non-transfused group (relative risk, 8.60; 95% CI, 1.11–66.43; p = 0.04).

▶ **Restrictive versus liberal transfusion threshold.** Apart from these two trials, RCTs in transfusion medicine have been confined to comparing one transfusion strategy with another (i.e., a restrictive versus a liberal transfusion threshold with thresholds mostly based on a single hemoglobin value). These studies have almost universally found no evidence for benefit from a liberal transfusion threshold, including in elderly patients with preexisting, or risk factors for, cardiovascular disease. Many studies favor a restrictive strategy, resulting in reduced transfusion and, in some cases, improved patient outcomes.

A systematic review and meta-analysis of 19 RCTs published between 1990 and February 2011 with a total of 6,264 patients compared restrictive (hemoglobin 7.0–10.0 g/dL) versus liberal (hemoglobin 9.0–13.0 g/dL) transfusion thresholds. It found no benefit from a liberal transfusion policy in any outcome measure, including functional recovery (Carson et al 2012a). Patient populations included cardiac, vascular, orthopaedic, acute blood loss and/or trauma, critical care, and leukemia patients undergoing chemotherapy (one trial). Restrictive transfusion reduced the risk of receiving an RBC transfusion by 39% (risk ratio, 0.61; 95% CI, 0.52–0.72). The in-hospital mortality was 23% lower (risk ratio, 0.77; 95% CI, 0.62–0.95) and infections were 19% lower (risk ratio, 0.81; 95% CI, 0.66–1.00) with restrictive transfusion. The increased mortality and infection rates in liberal transfusion led the investigators to conclude that this "raises the possibility of harm associated with liberal transfusion."

An RCT (n = 921) comparing a restrictive transfusion strategy (hemoglobin < 70 g/dL) versus a liberal strategy (hemoglobin < 90 g/dL) in acute upper gastrointestinal bleeding resulted in significant reductions in transfusion and improvement in patient outcomes in the restrictive group compared with the liberal group (Villanueva et al

2013a). The restrictive group had significantly improved survival at 6 weeks (hazard ratio [HR] for death, 0.55; 95% CI, 0.33–0.92; p = 0.02), reduced rates of rebleeding (HR, 0.62; 95% CI, 0.43–0.91; p = 0.01) and adverse events (HR, 0.73; 95% CI, 0.56–0.95; p = 0.02), and a reduced hospital length of stay (restrictive 9.6 ± 8.7 days versus liberal 11.5 ± 12.8 days; p = 0.01).

Salpeter et al (2014) conducted an updated systematic review and meta-analysis of RCTs published between 1996 and April 2013 comparing restrictive versus liberal thresholds. The investigators conducted a primary meta-analysis to evaluate the clinical outcomes of more restrictive (hemoglobin < 7 g/dL) transfusion thresholds and a secondary meta-analysis to evaluate the outcomes of less restrictive thresholds (7.5–10.0 g/dL), as well as a systematic review of observational studies to evaluate even more restrictive thresholds. Three trials met the inclusion criteria for the primary analysis with a total of 2,364 patients, which included adult critical care, pediatric critical care, and acute upper gastrointestinal bleeding. The more restrictive threshold significantly reduced the percentage of patients transfused (40% less) and the volume transfused per patient (2 units less). Restrictive thresholds resulted in significantly reduced incidences of acute coronary syndrome (risk ratio, 0.44; CI, 0.22–0.89), pulmonary edema (risk ratio, 0.48; CI, 0.33–0.72), rebleeding (risk ratio, 0.64; CI, 0.45–0.90), and bacterial infection (risk ratio, 0.86; CI, 0.73–1.00), and significantly reduced rates of in-hospital mortality (risk ratio, 0.74; CI, 0.60–0.92), 30-day mortality (risk ratio, 0.77; CI, 0.61–0.96), and total mortality (risk ratio, 0.80; CI, 0.65–0.98). The number needed to treat to save one life was 33.

The secondary meta-analysis of less restrictive thresholds included 19 trials with a total of 4,572 patients. In this analysis, there was no significant difference in outcomes between the groups. When the trials from the primary and secondary analysis were pooled (n = 6,936 patients), a restrictive transfusion threshold significantly reduced the rates of pulmonary edema (risk ratio, 0.68; CI, 0.51–0.90), bacterial infections (risk ratio, 0.84; CI, 0.73–0.95), rebleeding (risk ratio, 0.64; CI, 0.47–0.88), in-hospital mortality (risk ratio, 0.73; CI, 0.59–0.89), and 30-day mortality (risk ratio, 0.83; CI, 0.69–0.99).

The investigators' systematic review of observational studies showed that in surgical patients, the critically ill, and those with acute bleeds, hemoglobin levels of 5–6 g/dL are well tolerated when combined with supportive care. The observational literature produced no evidence of cardiac ischemia or inadequate oxygenation until hemoglobin levels decreased below 3–4 g/dL. The authors' conclusion from their review was "there is no randomized trial evidence that RBC transfusions improve oxygen delivery or clinical outcomes in any setting."

Rohde and coauthors (2014) published a systematic review and meta-analysis evaluating the effect of transfusion thresholds on hospital-acquired infection. Of 20 trials meeting the eligibility criteria, 17 trials with a total of 7,456 patients were included in the meta-analysis. The included trials were published between 1998 and 2014. The restrictive hemoglobin thresholds for transfusion ranged from 6.4 g/dL to 9.7 g/dL and the liberal thresholds from 9.0 g/dL to 13.0 g/dL. Overall, there was no significant difference in the risk of hospital-associated infection between the two transfusion strategies. However, serious infections were significantly reduced in the restrictive strategy compared with the liberal strategy. The risk ratio for serious infection was 0.84 (95 % CI, 0.73–0.96; I^2 = 0 %, τ^2 < 0.0001). The number needed to treat with restrictive strategies to prevent serious infection was 48 (95 % CI, 36–71). In a subset analysis of seven trials using exclusively leukocyte-reduced blood, the risk of serious infection remained significantly smaller with restrictive transfusion thresholds.

A 2015 systematic review and meta-analysis of RCTs comparing restrictive versus liberal thresholds, which included 31 trials and a total of 9,813 patients, found no benefit from liberal transfusion thresholds in terms of the mortality and overall morbidity (Holst et al 2015). However, this analysis also showed an increase in infectious complications with a liberal transfusion strategy.

The most recent RCT at the time of publication of the systematic review compared a postoperative restrictive transfusion threshold (hemoglobin < 7.5 g/dL) with a liberal transfusion threshold (hemoglobin < 9.0 g/dL) in 2,003 patients undergoing cardiac surgery (Murphy et al 2015b). No benefit for a liberal transfusion threshold was found in terms of the primary outcome (serious infection or an ischemic event within 3 months of randomization). The authors' suggestion of a possible benefit for liberal transfusion in terms of 90-day mortality in this trial needs to be viewed with caution because this was not a primary endpoint and it was not presaged by any of the periprocedural complications (Spertus 2015).

However, RCTs do not directly assess the effects of transfusion on patient outcome in the short or long term. There are at least two factors that limit, and possibly confound, their ability to do so. First, these trials are essentially comparing less transfusion with more transfusion, rather than comparing transfusion with no transfusion or placebo. In all trials included in meta-analyses, a considerable percentage of patients in the restrictive transfusion threshold group are still transfused and so are exposed to the same potential adverse outcome of transfusion. In some trials, the transfusion rate does not differ much between the groups. For example, in a cardiac surgery trial the transfusion rate was 60 % in the restrictive group and 64 % in the liberal group (Bracey et al 1999). Of interest, Hajjar et al (2010) and colleagues in their RCT comparing restrictive (maintaining hematocrit ≥ 24 %) versus liberal (maintaining hematocrit ≥ 30 %) transfusion thresholds after cardiac surgery found no significant difference in outcomes between the two groups. However, their analysis showed that patients who received an RBC transfusion postoperatively had higher rates of complications and a dose-dependent increase in 30-day mortality, regardless of whether the restrictive or the liberal strategy was used.

A second factor limiting the ability of RCTs to directly assess transfusion outcomes is that patients are often randomized during a specific period of their hospital stay, e.g., during their stay in the intensive care unit (ICU) or during the postoperative period, whereas outcomes are related to the patient's entire episode of care, e.g., the inhospital period, outcome after 30 or 60 days (Bracey et al 1999, Hébert et al 1999b, Lacroix et al 2007, Carson et al 2011). Accordingly, units transfused to patients prior to randomization or after the investigated subsection of their stay, and unaccounted for in the analysis, introduce a significant potential confounder and limit the ability of trials to directly assess the overall effect of transfusions on outcome during the entire episode of care. In the TRICC trial by Hébert et al (1999a), 1,045 units were transfused prior to randomization to 418 patients who were then assigned to a restrictive strategy, and 966 units were transfused to the 420 patients eventually assigned to the liberal group. In the FOCUS trial by Carson et al (2011), 531 units were transfused to 1,009 patients before they were assigned to a restrictive strategy, with 452 units transfused to 1,007 patients who were eventually assigned to the liberal group.

A study by Horvath et al (2013) illustrates the possible magnitude of this potential confounding effect. Their prospective multicenter study assessing the relationship between transfusion and infection in cardiac surgery identified that 48% of patients received an RBC transfusion. Of these, 27% received transfusions only in the operating room, 38% received transfusions only postoperatively, and 35% received transfusions both intra- and postoperatively. One RCT appears to address this potential confounder by randomizing patients immediately after admission and excluding any patients transfused 90 days prior to admission (Villanueva et al 2013a).

What can be concluded from the meta-analyses of RCTs to date is that liberal transfusion strategies appear to offer no benefit but may be associated with an increase in certain adverse patient outcomes.

The only studies that have attempted to directly assess transfusion outcomes are large retrospective and prospective observational studies comparing transfused patients with nontransfused patients after controlling for potential confounding variables. With very few exceptions, the vast majority of these studies have shown transfusion to be independently associated with increased mortality (Hopewell et al 2013) and a long list of morbid events and adverse outcomes (Hofmann et al 2011, Isbister et al 2011).

> **Note**
>
> With very few exceptions, the vast majority of studies have shown transfusion to be independently associated in a dose-depended manner with increased mortality and a long list of morbid events and adverse outcomes.

▶ **Risk–benefit ratio.** Scores of these studies have now been published and—after adjusting for numerous risk factors known to be associated with poor patient outcomes—transfusion remains independently associated with increased mortality, ICU admission, ICU and hospital length of stay, and morbidity including increased incidences of infec-

tion, septicemia, ischemic events (including stroke, myocardial infarction, and renal impairment/failure), thromboembolism, atrial fibrillation, vasospasm, low-output heart failure, cardiac arrest, prolonged ventilation, multiple organ failure, SIRS, ARDS, and reoperation for bleeding. These adverse outcomes have been reported in a wide range of patient populations including cardiac and noncardiac surgery, acute coronary syndrome, critically ill, burns, pediatrics, and trauma (Thomson et al 2009). In many studies, this risk-adjusted association is seen to be dose-dependent with increased exposure associated with increased risk (see **Table 1.5**).

In a systematic review and meta-analysis of cohort studies assessing the independent effect of transfusion on patient outcomes, Marik and Corwin (2008) classified risks versus benefits as follows: (1) the risk of transfusion outweighs the benefit, (2) a neutral effect of transfusion, and (3) the benefit of transfusion outweighs the risk. The outcome measures were mortality, infection, multiorgan dysfunction syndrome, and ARDS. The studies covered a broad spectrum of high-risk patients including trauma, surgical (general, cardiac, orthopaedic, neurosurgery), cardiac, and general ICU. Forty-five studies including 272,596 patients (median 687 patients per trial) were analyzed. In 42 of 45 studies, the risks of RBC transfusion outweighed its benefits, two studies were neutral, and in one study benefit outweighed risk. In 17 of 18 studies, transfusion was an independent predictor of death (pooled odds ratio [OR] in 12 studies, 1.7; 95% CI, 1.4–1.9). In 22 of 22 studies, transfusion was an independent risk factor for nosocomial infection (pooled OR in 9 studies, 1.8; 95% CI, 1.5–2.2). Transfusion was also associated with an increased risk of multiorgan dysfunction syndrome (three studies) and ARDS (pooled OR in 6 studies, 2.5; 95% CI, 1.6–3.3).

A systematic review and meta-analysis to assess the outcomes of transfusion in anemic patients with myocardial infarction identified 10 studies (9 observational studies and 1 RCT) with a total of 203,665 patients (Chatterjee et al 2013). RBC transfusion was independently associated with an increased all-cause mortality (risk ratio, 2.91; 95% CI, 2.46–3.44; $p < 0.001$) and a significantly higher risk of subsequent myocardial infarction (risk ratio, 2.04; 95% CI, 1.06–3.93; $p = 0.03$). The risk for increased mortality was independent of the baseline hemoglobin level, the nadir hemoglobin, and the change in hemoglobin during hospital stay. The weighted absolute risk increase for mortality was 12% and the number needed to harm was 8 (95% CI, 6–17). In a subgroup analysis, the risks of RBC transfusion were mitigated in patients with myocardial infarction with ST-segment elevation (risk ratio, 2.89; 95% CI, 0.54–15.58; $p = 0.22$) and in patients with hemoglobin levels < 10.0 g/dL (risk ratio, 1.72; 95% CI, 0.39–7.63; $p = 0.47$).

▶ **Patient outcome in large observational studies.** In one of the largest studies to date, involving a cohort of 8,004,571 patients discharged from 1,004 hospitals in 2004, Morton and colleagues (2010) conducted a retrospective analysis to assess in-hospital outcomes associated with RBC transfusion. Based on the sampling design, an estimated 38.66 million discharges in the United States in 2004 were associated with 2.33 million (5.8%) transfusions. In the 10 most common primary procedures involving a transfusion, after adjustment for age, gender, comorbidities, admission type, and diagnosis-related group, transfusion was independently associated with a 1.7-times increased odds of death ($p < 0.0001$), a 1.9-times increased odds of infection ($p < 0.0001$), and a hospital length of stay increased by 2.5 days.

A number of recent studies have shown that transfusion even of a single unit may have a negative impact on patient outcomes. Bernard and colleagues (2009) analyzed 125,223 patients from the American College of Surgeons National Surgical Quality Improvement Program database to assess the impact of transfusing 1 or 2 units of leukocyte-reduced RBCs on outcomes in patients undergoing major surgery. After adjusting for transfusion propensity and important risk factors (> 30 risk variables), the transfusion of 1 unit of RBCs was significantly associated with an increased risk of mortality (OR, 1.32; $p < 0.05$), composite morbidity (OR, 1.23; < 0.05), pneumonia (OR, 1.24; $p < 0.05$), and sepsis/septic shock (OR, 1.29; $p < 0.05$). The risk of surgical-site infection was not significantly increased with a single unit (OR, 1.02). The transfusion of 2 units increased the risks associated with these factors (OR, 1.38, 1.40, 1.25, and 1.53, respectively; $p \leq 0.05$), as well as significantly increasing the risk of surgical-site infection (OR, 1.25; $p < 0.05$).

Ferraris and colleagues (2012) used the ACS NSQIP database to evaluate the effect of a single unit on patient outcomes in noncardiac surgery. Of

48,291 patients who received intraoperative RBC transfusions, 15,186 (31.4%) received a single unit of RBCs during their operation. When matched with nontransfused patients using logistic regression (55 variables) and propensity score analysis, patients receiving 1 unit of RBCs intraoperatively had significantly increased risks of mortality (5.2 vs. 6.1%; $p = 0.005$), wound problems (9.7% vs. 11.4%; $p < 0.001$), systemic sepsis (8.2% vs. 10.6%; $p < 0.001$), pulmonary complications (11.7% vs. 15.3%; $p < 0.001$), postoperative renal dysfunction (5.5% vs. 6.8%; $p < 0.001$), composite morbidity (30.1% vs. 34.2%; $p < 0.001$), and prolonged postoperative hospital length of stay (10.3 vs. 11.8 days; $p < 0.001$). A note of caution: the ACS NSQIP database does not capture all units administered and may therefore be subject to the same confounding as noted earlier with some RCTs.

Paone and colleagues (2014) used the Michigan Society of Thoracic and Cardiovascular Surgeons Quality Collaborative data warehouse containing data from all 33 hospitals that perform adult cardiac surgery in the state of Michigan to assess the impact of receiving just 1 or 2 units of RBCs on outcomes. Of the 22,785 consecutive patients included in the cohort, 16,835 patients received 0, 1, or 2 units of RBCs. In a multivariate analysis, the transfusion of 1 or 2 units was independently associated with an increased mortality (OR, 1.90; CI, 1.23–2.91; $p = 0.003$). Propensity score analysis yielded similar results (OR, 1.86; CI, 1.21–2.87; $p = 0.005$). Transfusion of these small quantities of RBCs was also independently associated with increased risks of stroke, renal failure, atrial fibrillation, initial ventilator time, prolonged ventilation, reoperation for bleeding, ICU and postoperative length of stay, and a reduced rate of patients discharged home.

Chaiwat and colleagues (2009), in a prospective multicenter study of trauma patients, found that each additional unit of RBCs transfused conferred a 6% higher risk of ARDS (adjusted OR, 1.06; 95% CI, 1.03–1.10) and a 5% increased risk of in-hospital mortality (adjusted OR, 1.05; 95% CI, 1.0–1.1).

Paone and colleagues tested the hypothesis that sicker patients being transfused would explain the increased mortality associated with RBC transfusion in 31,818 patients undergoing isolated CABG surgery, using the Society of Thoracic Surgeons' risk adjuster *predicted risk of mortality*. Overall, the transfusion of 1 or more units of RBCs increased the risk of operative mortality sixfold

(OR, 6.19; p < 0.0001). Although the association between transfusion and mortality lessened with adjustment for the predicted risk of mortality, it remained highly significant at an almost threefold increase (OR, 2.99; p < 0.0001). Adjustment with propensity score analysis and multiple logistic regression yielded similar results (OR, 2.88; p < 0.0001, and 3.05; p < 0.001, respectively).

▶ **Transfusion in cancer patients.** Multiple mechanisms have been proposed to explain the adverse outcomes associated with transfusion, including the biophysical and biochemical changes that take place during storage, and TRIM (Tinmouth et al 2006, Reynolds et al 2007, Tsai et al 2010, Donadee et al 2011, Gladwin et al 2012, Refaai and Blumberg 2013b, Yalcin et al 2014). The causal link between TRIM and postoperative infection is considered to be established, whereas the causal link between TRIM and cancer recurrence is uncertain but likely (Refaai and Blumberg 2013b). There are mixed results in studies assessing the latter; however, the majority show RBC transfusion to be associated with a decreased survival in cancer patients, with many demonstrating an increased risk of disease recurrence (Amato and Pescatori 2006, Yao et al 2008, Churchhouse et al 2012, Al-Refaie et al 2012, Halabi et al 2013, Liu et al 2013, Linder et al 2014, Wang et al 2014).

A retrospective cohort study (n = 504,208) investigated the associations between transfusion and venous thromboembolism, arterial thromboembolism, and mortality in hospitalized patients with cancer from 60 U.S. medical centers (Khorana et al 2008). In a multivariate analysis, transfusions were independently associated with an increased risk of in-hospital mortality (RBCs: OR, 1.34; 95% CI, 1.29–1.38; platelets: OR, 2.40; 95% CI, 2.27–2.52). RBC transfusion and platelet transfusion were also independently associated with an increased risk of venous thromboembolism (RBCs: OR, 1.60; 95% CI, 1.53–1.67; platelets: OR, 1.20; 95% CI, 1.11–1.29), and arterial thromboembolism (RBCs: OR, 1.53; 95% CI, 1.46–1.61; platelets: OR, 1.55; 95% CI, 1.40–1.71).

Acheson and colleagues (2012) published a systematic review and meta-analysis of prospective and retrospective observational studies examining transfusion outcomes in patients undergoing colorectal cancer surgery. The analysis included a total of 20,795 patients observed for more than 59 months, representing a total of 108,838 patient years. The investigators reported that allogeneic RBC transfusion was associated with increased all-cause mortality (OR, 1.72; 95% CI, 1.55–1.91; p < 0.001), cancer-related mortality (OR, 1.71; 95% CI, 1.43–2.05; p < 0.001), combined recurrence, metastasis, and death (OR, 1.66; 95% CI, 1.41–1.97; p < 0.001), postoperative infection (OR, 3.27; 95% CI, 2.05–5.20; p < 0.001), surgical re-intervention (OR, 4.08; 95% CI, 2.18–7.62; p < 0.001), and a longer hospital length of stay (mean value, 17.8 ± 4.8 vs. 13.9 ± 4.7 days; p = 0.005).

Castillo and colleagues (2010) investigated the association between transfusion and non-Hodgkin lymphoma, the development of which is known to be associated with immune dysregulation. The investigators conducted a literature review and meta-analysis of observational studies that included a total of 5,904 cases and 10,107 controls. This study demonstrated a 20% increased risk of developing non-Hodgkin lymphoma associated with a history of RBC transfusion (relative risk, 1.2; 95% CI, 1.07–1.35; p < 0.01).

▶ **Impact of observational studies.** Of course, retrospective and prospective observational studies need to be interpreted with caution as there may be unknown confounders not identified even by the most elegant statistical analysis. Additionally, some of these studies suffer the same potential confounding as stated earlier for RCTs, namely, measuring only transfusions given within a specific time during the patient's hospital stay (Dixon et al 2013) or using databases that do not capture all transfusions administered during the hospital stay (Ferraris et al 2012). These limitations can result in a significant number of patients who received transfusions being classified as "nontransfused" in the analysis, thus possibly underestimating the overall adverse outcome of transfusion.

Despite these limitations, in recent times large observational studies have been acknowledged as an important tool in identifying safety issues (Vlahakes 2006). While the evidence from RCTs may be sufficient to establish the efficacy of a new drug, these trials are rarely large enough to identify harmful side effects. It has been suggested that large observational studies (phase 4 clinical testing) that compare the occurrence of adverse events in patients who received a specific treatment versus those who did not could serve as an alternative to evidence from RCTs to identify safety issues.

It is worth noting that Sir Austin Bradford Hill, a pioneer of the RCT design, and epidemiologist Sir Richard Doll established the causal link between tobacco use and lung cancer without an RCT. Bradford Hill proposed nine criteria for the establishment of causality from an association when it is not possible to perform a randomized trial. These became known as the *Bradford Hill criteria*. They include strength, consistency, specificity, and temporality of association, biological gradient (a dose–response relationship with increasing exposure resulting in increasing risk), and biological plausibility. Isbister and colleagues (2011) applied the Bradford Hill criteria to the literature on transfusion and outcomes and concluded that all criteria were met in relation to transfusion and adverse outcomes.

Note

All Bradford Hill criteria for establishing a causal link were met when applying the criteria to the literature on transfusion and adverse outcomes.

Conclusion

A review of the literature on transfusion outcomes reveals a paucity of evidence for benefit and a large and growing body of literature demonstrating transfusion to be a strong independent, dose-dependent risk factor for adverse patient outcomes.

Intuitively, however, RBC transfusion has a life-saving role in extreme situations including severe anemia and hemorrhagic shock. Hard clinical evidence to support this is lacking, probably because of the difficulty in performing clinical trials in the complex setting of this patient group. Although potentially lifesaving in critically bleeding patients and part of the answer in hemorrhagic shock, transfusion may also become part of the problem, as indicated by the current literature; large cohort studies show that transfusion in this patient population to be associated with adverse outcomes in a dose-dependent manner. Further research is required to look at the early and ongoing management of critically bleeding patients including: strategies to arrest bleeding, management of coagulopathy, establishment of the optimal physiological, biochemical, and metabolic parameters, optimization of resuscitation, management of the microcirculation, and maximization of hematopoiesis.

In nonactively bleeding patients (the greatest percentage of patients in whom transfusions are given), the vast majority of the literature demonstrates transfusion to be associated with increased morbidity, hospital and ICU length of stay, and mortality.

An exhaustive review of the literature on the effect of transfusion on patient outcomes conducted to develop modules 1 and 2 of the PBM guidelines issued by the National Blood Authority in Australia similarly identified transfusion's strong association with adverse patient outcomes. Accordingly, the guideline developers advocated a "precautionary approach to RBC transfusion" and recommended that health care services implement multidisciplinary, multimodal PBM programs (NBA 2012).

The PBM concept proposed in this book adopts just such an approach. It preempts and significantly reduces the need for transfusion by addressing modifiable risk factors—factors that contribute to the greatest majority of transfusions in daily clinical practice (Hofmann et al 2011, Farmer et al 2013b).

Salpeter and colleagues (2014), in their review of restrictive versus liberal transfusion thresholds, raised this sobering question: "With millions of blood transfusions given yearly over the past century, it would be hard to calculate how many deaths may have been caused by transfusion." All those responsible for patient care would do well to note the reminders in two editorials. Corwin (1999) wrote: "It is clear that the transfusion of RBCs may not only *not* help, but may in fact do harm to the critically ill patient." In a more recent editorial, Corwin and Carson (2007) stated that "red-cell transfusion should no longer be regarded as 'may help, will not hurt' but, rather, should be approached as 'first, do no harm.'"

1.4 Outcomes after Platelet Transfusion

B. D. Spiess

1.4.1 Introduction

▶ **Platelet physiology.** Platelets (thrombocytes) are small (1–3 µm) cells that have functions in both coagulation/thrombosis and inflammation (Spiess 2000, Rinder 2006). Platelet physiology is complex and highly dependent on the microvascular environment. Platelets are only found in mammals and it is believed this is an evolutionary adaptation to the risk of hemorrhage at childbirth —a mammalian risk.

In their "resting state," platelets circulate as spherical cells that roll and tumble within the flow of the bloodstream. They are marginated by their size toward the walls of vessels, the larger blood cells being forced to the center of the bloodstream, and they continuously interact with the glycocalyx of the vascular endothelium (Spiess 2000, Rinder 2006). (The glycocalyx is a complex carbohydrate and protein barrier secreted by the endothelial cells that forms a highly interactive surface between blood and the endothelial cell membrane. Its health appears to have a great deal to do with vascular biology, normal function, and chronic disease states such as atherosclerosis.)

It is far beyond the scope of this chapter to review all the complex interactions associated with the flow, tumbling, and rolling of platelets and their adherence to the endothelial surface. In the following, a small, incomplete summary of platelet biology is presented so that the reader can put the effects of platelet storage lesions in context.

▶ **Endothelial cells.** Platelets stimulate healthy endothelial cells by interacting with cell-membrane-linked proteo-glycosaminoglycans on the endothelial-cell surface. These transmembrane proteins enable endothelial cells to sense shear stress. In areas of high shear or turbulence, it is this interaction between platelets and the glycocalyx that leads to endothelial cells responding to stress (Spiess 2000, Rinder 2006).

Endothelial cells maintain the blood environment in a liquid state (Spiess 2000, Rinder 2006, Reitsma et al 2007, Collins et al 2013). This is a very active process. The glycocalyx has a surface charge and a very large surface area, giving endothelial cells a "nonwettable" surface. The proteoglycosaminoglycans, which are actively secreted and maintained by the endothelial cells, form a matrix for the attachment of constantly building and eroding carbohydrate chains of varying composition. The length of the carbohydrate chains varies as the shear stresses denude the endothelial-cell surface (Spiess 2000, Reitsma et al 2007, Collins et al 2013), and the side chains of the carbohydrate matrix will undergo higher or lower levels of acidification by sulfhydryl groups depending on factors as yet unknown. It is these sulfhydryl groups that give the glycocalyx its strong negative charge, which repels the surface of platelets.

Further, a certain pentasaccharide sequence binds circulating antithrombin creating activated heparin–antithrombin complexes, which in turn bind serine proteases as anticoagulants. The surface of platelets has various glycoprotein binding sites for serine proteases; ultimately it is at the GPIIb/IIIa binding site where they interconnect with fibrinogen/fibrin. A platelet plug is formed by platelets interacting, conjugating, and connecting their surface membranes. Finally, through the biochemical reactions of the platelet membrane receptors, the intrinsic and extrinsic cascade of serine proteases, and the eventual covalent cross-linking of fibrin with factor XIII, an insoluble clot is created.

▶ **Platelet activation.** The change from a resting platelet to the formation of a platelet plug and, eventually, a fully developed clot is a complex process (Spiess 2000, Rinder 2006). Platelets have the ability to respond to various levels of stimulation in a graded response. The more stimulation, the more receptors on their surfaces are activated and the stronger the response. This graded response is energy-dependent and highly regulated (Spiess 2000, Rinder 2006). As a result, platelets have the ability to undergo a partial shape change and to release certain chemoattractants for other platelets, monocytes, and leukocytes without being completely activated.

One of the very first things that happen when there has been endothelial cell injury is for the endothelial cells to lose their anticoagulant activity and to become inflammatory and prothrombotic instead. The production of nitric oxide by endothelial cells is reduced or ceases altogether as the endothelial cell becomes prothrombotic (Spiess 2000, Rinder 2006, Reitsma et al 2007, Collins et al 2013). The glycocalyx is shed, tissue factor is released, and intercellular adhesion molecule 1 (ICAM-1) is expressed. ICAM-1 causes platelets to roll, stick, and begin to interact with von Willebrand factor (Spiess 2000, Rinder 2006, Reitsma et al 2007, Collins et al 2013).

Platelets contain α granules and dense granules (Spiess 2000, Rinder 2006). The contents of these granules include chemoattractants along with stimulant and prothrombotic factors. When a platelet is stimulated to a certain degree, it can partially release these compounds, but when it is fully/maximally stimulated, it degranulates spewing all the compounds out into the surrounding milieu. The granule membrane moves to the exterior of the cell and fuses with the cell membrane, while the platelet cytoskeleton contracts in a reaction driven by actin and myosin. The platelet spreads in an ameboid fashion, changing from a rounded disk to a splattered sphere that appears flat and highly irregular in shape.

1.4.2 Platelet Blood Banking

▶ **Platelet preparation and storage.** Platelets are harvested by differential centrifugation of citrate-anticoagulated whole blood, leading to platelet-rich plasma and/or a buffy coat product (Murphy and Gardner 1969, Devine and Serrano 2010, Shrivastava 2009). Collection by apheresis involves the use of an automated system that harvests blood from a patient's arm, isolates the platelets by centrifugation, and returns the RBCs and the majority of the plasma to the donor. The magnitude of the G-force used for centrifugation determines the quality of the platelet concentrate. Today, white blood cell reduction is usually performed when platelets are harvested, but platelet concentrates still contain more white blood cells than any other allogeneic blood product. Platelets are suspended in plasma from the donor, and this plasma—because of the way it is spun (allowing for a mixing of the buffy coat with the platelets)—has the highest lipid content of any blood product.

Platelet-rich plasma is supplied either as single-donor apheresis platelets or as pooled platelets (usually from three to five donors). In the United States, there is a significant move toward the use of single-donor apheresis platelets. The percentage used is now almost 80% in the United States, and it is up to 100% in some European countries.

Platelet units are maintained at room temperature on a platelet agitator that rocks the bags, constantly mixing the plasma and platelets. According to the U.S. Food and Drug Administration, platelets may be stored for up to 5 days (Murphy and Gardner 1969, Spiess 2000, Reitsma et al 2007, Vassallo 2009, Shrivastava 2009, Devine and Serrano 2010, Collins et al 2013). The storage time is limited to avoid bacterial contamination of the platelet units. Other countries allow platelet storage for up to 7–9 days. The risk of bacterial contamination, either from skin organisms during harvest or because of latent sepsis in the donor

(an event that is extremely rare), is estimated at 1:2,000 units transfused (Blajchman et al 2005). Efforts to decrease this risk include pH measurement, culture of platelet products, and the use of pathogen inactivation processes. Pathogen inactivation processes involve the use of DNA lysing agents and light activation; the activating compounds will then need to be washed out again. The use of DNA lysis technology in this context has not yet been licensed.

> **Note**
>
> The risk of bacterial contamination of platelet concentrates is estimated at 1:2,000 units transfused.

▶ **Platelet quality.** There is no ideal test for the viability or reaction to aging of platelets in storage bags. The processes involved in the harvesting and storage of platelets seem to cause platelet activation (Murphy and Gardner 1969). Expression analysis of surface ligands such as CD 62P, CD 63, and thromboxane B2 showed that there is a progressive release of these compounds over time (Murphy and Gardner 1969, Rinder et al 1991, Divers et al 1995, Spiess 2000, Vassallo 2009, Shrivastava 2009, Devine and Serrano 2010). The release of agents stored in α granules—including β-thromboglobulin and platelet factor 4—also increases from day 3. As platelets age, they lose parts of their cell membrane and bud off platelet particles. These are highly inflammatory and prothrombotic. CD 40 L is another ligand that is dislodged from the surface of platelet membranes; it is a chemokine with proinflammatory properties (Murphy and Gardner 1969, Shrivastava 2009, Devine and Serrano 2010). Messenger RNA and mitochondrial DNA are released as well (Seghatchian and Krailadsiri 2001). These nucleotide fragments are also thought to be highly inflammatory.

Evaluation of the shape/morphology of platelets is widely used to assess the extent of platelet activation (Murphy and Gardner 1969, Shrivastava 2009, Devine and Serrano 2010). As platelets age, they lose their discoid shape forming spicules and becoming flatter. A simple method to evaluate platelet viability is to test whether they swirl in the bag (Murphy and Gardner 1969, Shrivastava 2009, Devine and Serrano 2010).

Note

Platelets that do not swirl in the bag have been activated and have lost their ability to function, and are of very poor quality.

In radiolabelled studies, transfused allogeneic platelets stay in the circulation for a much shorter time than do normal native platelets (Murphy and Gardner 1969, Rothwell 1998, Shrivastava 2009, Devine and Serrano 2010, Van der Meer et al 2010). At 4–5 days of storage, at least 20% of the platelets in a blood bank bag are already dead upon infusion (Murphy and Gardner 1969, Shrivastava 2009, Devine and Serrano 2010). Over the subsequent 2 days of storage, another 20% will die. The normal in vivo platelet life span in healthy individuals is only 9–10 days, so storage outside the body for 5–7 days already takes up a considerable part of their normal life span. Infused platelets have a short life span and a tendency toward apoptosis.

▶ **Crossmatching.** Of note, platelets have the same blood type antigens on their surface as do RBCs. Few surgical groups use typed platelets, but there is evidence that the use of crossmatched platelets is associated with fewer hemodynamic changes, and crossmatching clearly improves platelet survival, especially in immunosuppressed patients (Vassallo et al 2014).

Note

The use of crossmatched platelets is associated with fewer hemodynamic changes, and crossmatching clearly improves platelet survival.

1.4.3 Risk–Benefit Profile of Platelet Transfusions

The use of any pharmaceutical or transfusion therapy should improve the patient outcome more often than not. If a patient is bleeding because of a low platelet count or profoundly depressed platelet function, platelet transfusion may be effective and even lifesaving. However, in most circumstances, platelet transfusions are given either as a prophylactic measure or as "shotgun" therapy with no specific clinical indication. In bleeding patients with thrombocytopenia or platelet dysfunction, platelet transfusion may reduce the bleeding be-

cause of its procoagulant effect. If, however, the transfusion is given inappropriately or in anticipation of bleeding, it is likely that the risks of transfusion outweigh the benefits (i.e., the reduced risk of bleeding).

In cardiac surgery, the use of platelet transfusion varies considerably depending on the institution where the surgery is performed (Stover et al 1998, Snyder-Ramos et al 2008). Therefore, the driving force behind the use of platelet transfusions for heart surgery is local culture. Clinical practice is highly variable because viscoelastic testing—although demonstrated to be effective—and the use of algorithm-driven transfusion decision trees have not been widely adopted in the fields of anesthesia and surgery. The reader is referred elsewhere to find out more about the effectiveness of these techniques (Welsby et al 2006, Johansson et al 2008, Weber et al 2012).

In some clinical scenarios, the use of prophylactic platelet transfusions is effective, as will be discussed in the following.

▶ **Hematology/oncology.** Hematology/oncology has adopted a level of 10,000 platelets/mL as the recommended cutoff below which most clinicians will infuse platelet units. The standard use of a cutoff of 50,000 platelets/mL for invasive procedures is not backed by evidence. Some procedures such as neurosurgery procedures desire even higher platelet counts, but again there is no solid evidence on which to base these recommended clinical triggers. A recent Cochrane Database review notes there is no evidence base to support any of these numbers (Estcourt et al 2012). In an RCT of patients with a hematologic malignancy, patients who received no prophylactic platelet transfusion had a shorter time to a first bleeding episode and more days with severe bleeds than did those who received prophylactic transfusions (Stanworth et al 2014). One center demonstrated that it is possible to lower the transfusion threshold even further (to 1,000–5,000 platelets/mL), and perhaps there are subsets of transplant patients who should only receive platelet transfusions if they are bleeding (Zeller et al 2014). In a study of adults with leukemia, patients who received fewer platelet transfusions had an improved survival (Blumberg et al 2008). Indeed, in a Cox multivariate analysis, platelet transfusion—in addition to patient age—emerged as an independent variable associated with early death.

It is unclear whether platelet biology and thrombocytopenia are markers of disease severity (they probably are), but those who are more ill tend to receive more platelet transfusions (Blumberg et al 2008); perhaps it is the physician's anxiety that more ill patients will bleed more that drives the use of platelet transfusions. However, in the study in adults by Blumberg, platelet transfusion was an independent predictor of early death, so the clinical practice of early prophylaxis needs to be reviewed and clinicians need to realize that the liberal use of platelet transfusions might well be increasing the patient's risk for transfusion-related side effects (Blumberg et al 2008).

In adults with cancer, the use of platelet transfusions is associated with early and severe deep venous thrombosis. Cancer by itself increases thrombotic risks. The use of RBC transfusions and/or platelet transfusions was strongly associated with deep venous thrombosis (Khorana et al 2008). This makes a great deal of sense because stored platelet concentrates have a high concentration of platelet buds, and those live platelets are partially activated and are therefore "looking" for places to adhere. The take-home message from this body of work is that the platelet count alone should not be used as a trigger for transfusion in cancer patients (Khorana et al 2008).

> **Note**
>
> The routine transfusion of platelets for invasive procedures if the platelet count drops below 50,000 platelets/mL is not backed by evidence. In addition, the platelet count alone should not be used as a trigger for transfusion, at least not in cancer patients.

▶ **Neonatal transfusion.** Neonatal transfusions are fraught with risk. We know that RBC transfusions in neonates are associated with necrotizing enterocolitis (Stanworth 2012, Curley et al 2014a, Gunnink et al 2014). As neonates become progressively more thrombocytopenic, there is a risk (perceived or real) of cerebral bleeding. When this does happen, it is a devastating event. A 660-patient multicenter trial investigating neonatal platelet transfusion is currently under way, with neonates born before 34 weeks of gestation randomized to receive transfusions if their platelet count drops below either 50,000/mL or 25,000/mL (Curley et al 2014a). The neonates will be followed

for 28 days and mortality, sepsis, and major bleeds (particularly head bleeds) will be the major outcomes. Early thrombocytopenia after birth is usually seen in patients with intrauterine growth retardation and immature bone marrow, whereas delayed thrombocytopenia is related to sepsis and/or enterocolitis.

▶ **Liver transplantation.** The number of liver transplantations grew rapidly during the 1990s, and at present approximately 3,000–5,000 transplants are performed each year. End-stage hepatitis is characterized by thrombocytopenia because of portal venous congestion and the splenic sequestration/destruction of platelets. In hepatic transplantation, a low preoperative platelet count is strongly associated with both intraoperative bleeding and overall blood usage. Patients who receive more than 20 units of blood have a particularly high mortality, and blood transfusion overall has a strong association with early mortality (Cywinski et al 2014). That said, the use of platelet transfusions is also associated with early hepatic-artery thrombosis (Arshad et al 2013).

Most centers performing significant numbers of liver transplantations use some kind of viscoelastic testing for the assessment of overall clot strength and platelet function. Different institutions use different algorithms to determine the need for transfusion. However, it makes a great deal of sense in this context to use platelet transfusions only when surgical bleeding is under control, and only to a level at which viscoelastic testing indicates a return to normal function. Excessive platelet transfusion and prophylactic transfusions treating a laboratory value may contribute to the risk of graft thrombosis because implanted livers tend to have dysfunctional endothelial layers.

▶ **Trauma.** Trauma is a different scenario altogether. The coagulopathy after major trauma—in particular battlefield trauma—is unique. Trauma-induced coagulopathy is characterized by a massive release of tissue factor, thrombin activation, and consumption of platelets, fibrinogen, and serine proteases. The massive stimulation of platelets and serine proteases increases fibrinolysis in 30–50% of patients, and the degree of coagulopathy is a predictor of survival. Research from the battlefields in Iraq and Afghanistan has shown that the early transfusion of blood products, an intervention known today as *massive transfusion*, appears to reduce the severity of trauma-induced coagulopathy.

Whether the use of 1 unit of RBCs transfused with 1 unit of FFP and 1 unit of platelets is better or worse than any other ratio is difficult to say. However, a number of both military and civilian studies have shown an improved survival with early transfusion of both platelets and FFP. The best improvement in outcome was with the use of warm fresh whole blood. Indeed, the proposed 1:1:1 massive transfusion protocol can be considered as an effort to recreate whole blood (Simms et al 2014).

The military has a "walking blood bank"—if urgently needed, fresh whole blood is harvested from military personnel at nearby first- or second-echelon evacuation hospitals (Berséus et al 2012). However, the civilian medical world has steadfastly resisted any movement toward the consideration of fresh whole blood as an on-demand emergency commodity. That said, trauma coagulopathy is now being studied with the help of large U.S. Army and National Institute of Health grants, with a focus on the early use of FFP. The use of platelet transfusions (unit number and time of transfusion) has yet to be studied methodically.

▶ **Cardiac surgery.** Transfusion for heart surgery is widely variable across the United States and around the world (Stover et al 1998, Snyder-Ramos et al 2008, McQuilten et al 2014). It has been estimated that 40–60% of all transfusions for heart surgery are unnecessary. The real proportion is probably even larger. These estimates are for RBC transfusions. The use of platelet transfusions has varied from 0–5% of patients at one institution to more than 95% at others (Stover et al 1998, Snyder-Ramos et al 2008, McQuilten et al 2014). The numbers have not changed tremendously over the past 20 years (Stover et al 1998, Snyder-Ramos et al 2008, McQuilten et al 2014). At some centers, however, the tendency to transfuse platelets for heart surgery may well have increased because of the use of P2Y12 platelet inhibitors. There is no doubt that the use of aspirin in conjunction with P2Y12 inhibitors has decreased the restenosis rate of percutaneous stents, and it is a matter of debate how long these drugs should be withheld prior to elective coronary surgery. The pressure for "clinical impression" driving the transfusion of platelets among cardiac teams has increased. Given the high variability in the use of

platelet transfusion in cardiac surgery and the general lack of guidance in this context, one has to ask whether the use will improve or worsen outcome.

In the 1990s, the Multicentered Study of Perioperative Ischemia followed 100 CABG patients at 24 U.S. sites (Stover et al 1998). The frequency of platelet transfusion ranged from 0% to 79% of patients depending on the site of surgery. Surgical site was the leading factor associated with platelet transfusion. This observational study was later repeated on a much larger scale at 60 centers around the world. The finding was the same: there was a high variability in the frequency of platelet transfusions. A substudy using the same database examined the perioperative use of aspirin to reduce graft thrombosis (Mangano 2002). This study included patients who received aspirin and those who did not. Among patients who did not receive aspirin immediately after heart surgery (native platelet function), those who received a platelet transfusion had a risk of death that was four times higher than the risk in those who did not receive a platelet transfusion (Mangano 2002).

In a large database collected for human trials of the drug aprotinin, blood transfusion and coagulation therapy was carefully controlled (Spiess et al 2004). These studies focused on the risk of bleeding in patients undergoing CABG surgery, and some also investigated the risk of thrombosis. In these studies, transfusion protocols were used, although no data are available on how well the protocols were followed. The data were collected in the early to mid-1990s and the findings may therefore not be applicable today. Some of the platelet transfusions were leukocyte-reduced, but it is likely that the vast majority were not leukocyte-reduced. The database yielded 1,720 patients, of whom 14.4% (n = 284) received platelet transfusions (Spiess et al 2004). Those who were transfused were older and more likely to have had a myocardial infarction or congestive heart failure. In a univariate analysis, there was a striking relationship between platelet transfusion and thrombotic stroke. In a multivariate propensity score analysis (which is different from propensity matching) to account for confounding variables, platelet transfusion was significantly associated with postoperative infection, the use of two or more vasopressors, stroke, and death. The OR for death was increased by 476% (OR, 4.76; 95% CI, 1.65–13.73; p = 0.009). The take-home message from this observational study is that platelet transfusion should be targeted to patients with bleeding or demonstrated platelet, fibrinogen, or serine protease deficits (Spiess et al 2004).

The findings from these studies are in contrast to those from studies using more recent data and from centers where the use of leukocyte-reduced platelet transfusions is standard (e.g., in Canada) (Karkouti et al 2006). In their single-center study, Karkouti et al examined 11,459 patients undergoing any type of cardiac surgery over a 10-year period. Nineteen percent (n = 2,174) of these patients received a platelet transfusion after cardiac surgery. There was a highly significant univariate relationship between platelet use and various adverse outcomes. The group also performed a propensity score case–control analysis and found that use of RBC transfusions and use of platelet transfusions were closely linked. The authors felt strongly that the propensity score case–control analysis enabled them to separate the effects of RBC transfusion from the effects of platelet transfusion and that the univariate risk associated with platelet transfusion no longer existed after these adjustments (Karkouti et al 2006).

At the Cleveland Clinic in the United States, similar findings to the Canadian study were noted in 32,298 patients undergoing a wide range of heart procedures: there was no multivariate connection between platelet transfusion and adverse outcomes (McGrath et al 2008). This group found that approximately 12 % of patients received platelet transfusions. Those who received a platelet transfusion were also very likely to receive an RBC transfusion. To control for confounders, the group then used propensity score matching and identified a subset of 2,774 patients in their database who had similar risks but had not received a platelet transfusion. The patients who received platelets had a much higher return rate to the operating room for bleeding than did those who had not received platelets (7 % vs. 2.5 %; p = 0.001). This can be explained by the fact that patients who are bleeding are more likely to receive platelets. With this type of propensity matching, the researchers actually found that patients who received platelets had a lower in-hospital mortality, fewer serious infections, and a lower rate of neurologic events. In a very small propensity-matched cohort with no RBC transfusions and only platelet transfusions, the effect of no platelets versus platelets was not significantly different (McGrath et al 2008).

Another study combined data from two RCTs to look at the effects of FFP, platelet, and RBC transfusion in cardiac surgery (Bilgin et al 2011). Unlike many other studies, this group found that RBC transfusions were less strongly associated with adverse outcomes, compared with transfusions of FFP or platelets. White blood cell-containing RBC transfusions were significantly associated with postoperative infections. Perioperative plasma transfusions were associated with all-cause mortality. Platelet transfusions, if containing white blood cells, were related to both serious infections and mortality (Bilgin et al 2011).

▶ **Other associated risks.** Platelet and plasma transfusions are associated with a higher incidence of TRALI than that seen after RBC transfusion alone in medicine patients. Data from patients admitted to an ICU at the Mayo Clinic in the United States showed that TRALI is very common indeed: it occurs in approximately 1/75–200 patients transfused (Rana et al 2006).

A number of studies have shown that the supernatants from RBC and platelet concentrates can cause pulmonary vascular leakage (Rana et al 2006). Platelet transfusions have particularly high levels of cytokines, interleukin-6, and tumor necrosis factor (TNF-α). In addition, the level of CD40L is very high (Vamvakas and Carven 2002). As discussed earlier (section 1.4.2), CD40L is a platelet surface ligand that serves as a chemoattractant for neutrophils. CD40L is an independent inflammatory mediator that can lead to TRALI (Vamvakas and Carven 2002). Based on platelet biology, it therefore seems that platelet transfusions are particularly inflammatory (Vamvakas and Carven 2002, Sahler et al 2012).

Conclusion

The question whether platelet transfusions are associated with, or cause, worse outcomes has not been settled. Certainly, in situations where patients are not bleeding, the use of platelet transfusions seems particularly risky and unwarranted. The use of transfusion algorithms based on viscoelastic testing or other modalities has proven highly effective in reducing the unwarranted use of blood products. Notwithstanding the data from bone marrow transplant recipients, the prophylactic transfusion of platelets seems to have little benefit. In patients with normal or increased coagulation function, the transfusion of proinflammatory platelets might well tip the balance toward a thrombotic state (particularly in cancer patients). Based on the available evidence, it is hard to prove whether this is always the case, or to which patient groups it applies.

In a study using rotational thromboelastometry in slightly over 100 patients, the use of an algorithm not only reduced the transfusion rate but it also decreased the mortality (Weber et al 2012). In cardiac surgery, the right thing to do is to use the best coagulation data system possible (thromboelastography or rotational thromboelastometry) in conjunction with the platelet count and the fibrinogen level. However, these testing techniques should be vetted with a multidisciplinary PBM strategy and algorithm-driven judicious (rare) use of platelets and plasma. The entire team should buy into the strategy to help to reduce unnecessary platelet transfusions.

Today, at our institution (Virginia Commonwealth University Medical Center) the use of plasma is being replaced by that of four-factor prothrombin complex concentrates. The belief is that by doing so, the risk of inflammation-mediated TRALI reactions will be reduced. It is also believed that if the algorithms are strictly applied and if platelet transfusions in cardiac surgery are reserved for patients who are bleeding, the risks associated with the use of this inflammatory product will be greatly reduced.

Medicine tends to be risk-averse. Yet, we continue to transfuse platelets when there is very little evidence for their effectiveness, and even in cases where they might be helpful (e.g., in severe thrombocytopenia) little work has been done to identify those who are at risk for bleeding (Kander et al 2014, Shander and Gernsheimer 2014). Platelets are grossly overprescribed, probably based upon an ill-founded belief that platelet transfusion will avert bleeding or that it is highly effective. Neither is true, and we are increasingly learning about adverse events associated with unwarranted transfusions.

1.5 Use of Plasma in PBM—Effectiveness and Outcomes

A. Shander, M. Javidroozi

1.5.1 Introduction

PBM calls for the evidence-based and appropriate use of all available treatment modalities with an emphasis on preventive measures in a proactive, concerted, and multidisciplinary effort to improve the patient outcome. Allogeneic blood components should be used if they cannot be safely and effectively replaced or if their use cannot be avoided by using other modalities, and only if clinically indicated and likely to offer benefits that outweigh the risks (Shander et al 2011a, Gross et al 2013, Shander et al 2013). Plasma—commonly referred to as *fresh frozen plasma*, or *FFP*—is no exception, and its use under a PBM strategy should comply with the following principles:

- Clinical use (indication and dosing) should remain within the realm of the established evidence-based guidelines; and
- Safer and/or more effective alternatives (including preventive measures) should always be considered whenever possible.

▶ **Plasma preparations.** FFP is defined as plasma that is separated from donated whole blood or collected directly through apheresis and frozen quickly within a specified time period (often within 8 hours after collection, although the exact specification may differ from country to country). Another related plasma product, *FP24*, is often used in the United States; this is plasma that has been frozen within a longer interval (24 hours) following collection.

Whole blood–derived plasma is produced by centrifugation of a unit of whole blood, and thus the volume is typically around half the volume of the whole blood sample (200–250 mL). The volume can be larger for FFP units collected through apheresis. Given that FFP is collected with minimal processing from blood (no dilution or concentration steps), the concentration of the various coagulation factors is—at least in theory—expected to be the same as that in the plasma of the donor. Nonetheless, the level of some labile and sensitive factors such as factor VIII and, to some degree, factor V gradually diminishes following removal from the body. This issue is more prominent for

FP24 units given the longer time elapsed between collection and freezing. Additionally, the freeze-and-thaw cycle that FFP undergoes prior to transfusion may result in precipitation and removal of some factors, a phenomenon that is exploited in making cryoprecipitate from plasma. Properly maintained in frozen condition, FFP units can be stored for long periods of time. Once thawed, they should be stored refrigerated at 4 °C and used either within 24 hours, or labeled and used beyond the 24-hour window but within 5 days (*5-day plasma* or *thawed plasma*). Lastly, *liquid plasma* is plasma that is collected and never frozen, making it ready for immediate use, e.g., in trauma (Price 2009).

▶ **Dosage.** When indicated, plasma should be given in a dose calculated to achieve a factor concentration of at least 30% of normal plasma, or about 10 to 20 mL/kg (with the upper range usually reserved for actively bleeding patients), to provide an effective supply of coagulation factors. An even higher dose of up to 30 mL/kg has been recommended by some for "toxic" warfarin patients. The recommended dose of plasma translates to 4 to 8 units in an average male adult, as opposed to the conventional practice of transfusing just 1 to 2 units of plasma, which is likely to fail to achieve the intended effect on coagulation while still exposing patients to the risks of allogeneic plasma (ASATF 2015).

>
>
> **Note**
>
> The conventional practice of transfusing 1 to 2 units of FFP fails to achieve the intended effect on coagulation.

▶ **Plasma versus factor concentrates.** Given the relatively "crude" and uncontrolled nature of plasma, it is primarily used for replacement therapy to correct coagulation factor deficiencies for which no specific factor concentrate is available. This means that with the advent and increasing availability of more and more recombinant and concentrated factors, the clinical scenarios in which plasma is indicated and should be used are expected to become increasingly limited. Whenever available, individual factor concentrates offer several advantages over plasma since they can address deficiencies more specifically and effectively, they allow delivery of larger amounts of needed factors in much smaller volumes, and they are devoid of other unneeded and potentially harmful agents that can be present in donor plasma (ranging from the donor's antibodies to pathogenic agents) (Pandey and Vyas 2012).

>
>
> **Note**
>
> Clinical scenarios in which plasma is indicated, and should be used, are expected to become increasingly rare.

▶ **Potential complications.** Plasma shares many of the risks of other allogeneic blood components. TRALI is one of the most common serious complications of transfusion and among the leading causes of transfusion-related mortality (even though it is most likely underreported). While the underlying pathogenesis is not yet fully understood and it is likely to result from an interplay between the transfused blood component and the recipient's body, TRALI is often linked to plasma transfusion (or residual plasma present in other blood components), underscoring the role of factors present in plasma in causing the condition (Kenz and Van der Linden 2014).

Transfusion-associated circulatory overload (TACO) is another transfusion complication that can be of concern specifically in patients receiving plasma, given that multiple units of plasma are often needed to achieve therapeutic levels of factors. In a study of over 600 U.S. hospitals, more than 3% of patients who received plasma experienced fluid overload; these patients had a 29% longer hospital length of stay, and the mean cost of hospital care per admission was more than $14,000 higher (Magee and Zbrozek 2013). Other risks include hemolytic, allergic/anaphylactic and febrile reactions, alloimmunization, and the rare but nonzero risk of transmission of pathogens (Pandey and Vyas 2012). More importantly and as is the case with other allogeneic blood components, a large (and growing) body of evidence links plasma transfusions with unfavorable outcomes such as increased risk of morbidity and mortality and poor functional outcomes in various patient populations (Shander et al 2011b, Shiba et al 2013, Anglin et al 2013). These risks and complications are among the reasons why PBM strategies should seek to improve plasma transfusion practices.

1.5.2 Use(s) and Misuse(s) of Plasma

Overall, the clinical use of plasma has been on the increase in the United States in recent years, giving rise to concerns over its overuse and the appropriateness of plasma transfusions in the clinical arena (Pandey and Vyas 2012, Puetz et al 2012). According to the principles of PBM, the use of plasma must remain limited to evidence-based indications in appropriate scenarios and along with other alternatives, with an emphasis on preventive measures that can safely reduce its need.

▶ **Current practice.** Plasma is used commonly in a number of prophylactic and therapeutic scenarios. In a nationwide study of patients admitted to 29 ICUs over a period of 8 weeks, 12.7% of patients received plasma, with the leading indications including bleeding (48%), prophylaxis with no planned procedure (36%), and prophylaxis prior to a procedure (15%). Quite alarmingly (as will be discussed below), 31% of plasma transfusions were given to patients without a prolonged prothrombin time (PT), and 41% were given to patients with a mildly (< 2.5 times) increased international normalized ratio (INR) without recorded bleeding. Furthermore, plasma transfusion resulted in limited correction of the INR and many aspects of plasma usage were associated with wide variation between centers (Stanworth et al 2011). Another single-center study in a surgical ICU reported an overall 30% rate of plasma transfusion, with nearly half of the orders being considered inappropriate (Lauzier et al 2007).

The prophylactic administration of plasma is usually considered in patients with coagulopathy or factor deficiency (but no active bleeding) who are scheduled for surgery or invasive procedures, in an effort to reduce the risk of bleeding. The therapeutic use of plasma is usually considered in patients with multiple coagulation factor deficiencies (or factor deficiencies for which no specific factor concentrate is available) who are actively bleeding, or when the patient plasma is being exchanged (plasmapheresis or exchange plasma transfusion as part of the treatment for thrombotic thrombocytopenic purpura).

▶ **Bleeding patients with multiple coagulation factor deficiencies.** Plasma is commonly used in actively bleeding patients with multiple coagulation factor deficiencies. Multiple factor deficiency is typically an acquired condition and can result from decreased production (e.g., liver failure, warfarin), increased consumption (e.g., disseminated intravascular coagulation [DIC]), or blood loss and dilution (e.g., profuse bleeding leading to extensive intravenous resuscitation and massive transfusion with packed RBC units, which are largely devoid of plasma).

▶ **Vitamin K antagonist reversal.** For patients receiving vitamin K antagonists (VKA) such as warfarin, coagulopathy on its own is not a sufficient ground for plasma transfusion, and as long as there is no bleeding, an increased INR can be safely and effectively managed with stopping the VKA and administering vitamin K (oral or intravenous administration depending on the setting and the required time line). Plasma can be a reasonable urgent treatment in patients who had received oral VKA therapy and subsequently experienced central nervous system bleeding spontaneously or due to trauma. However, plasma is not indicated in patients with central nervous system bleeding who have not been receiving oral VKA therapy and in the absence of coagulopathy (Shander et al 2014a). Use of plasma in patients who have developed bleeding in the context of VKA therapy should be accompanied by vitamin K administration, as plasma can only provide a temporary relief and the ultimate management relies on aiding the liver to resume production of vitamin-K-dependent factors. Prothrombin complex concentrates—especially formulations that contain all four vitamin-K-dependent factors—are likely to be superior to plasma for urgent warfarin reversal as they have a better safety profile and can supply the deficient factors more effectively and quickly in a smaller infusion volume. The effectiveness of prothrombin complex concentrates versus plasma for the urgent reversal of warfarin in bleeding patients has been studied in a number of populations (e.g., patients with intracranial or gastrointestinal bleeding) and the results generally favor prothrombin complex concentrates (Goodnough and Shander 2011, Cabral et al 2013, Edavettal et al 2014, Karaca et al 2014), but more studies are needed to better establish their safety and efficacy compared with plasma (Goodnough and Shander 2011, Shander et al 2014a).

> **Note** !
>
> Prothrombin complex concentrates are generally more effective than plasma for the urgent reversal of warfarin in bleeding patients.

▶ **Massively bleeding patients.** The use of plasma as a part of predefined fixed-ratio transfusion protocols has gained much interest in recent years especially in the United States. As briefly alluded to earlier, massively bleeding patients who receive large amounts of intravenous fluids and packed RBC units are at risk of dilutional coagulopathy, which could further hinder effective hemostasis resulting in a vicious cycle of more bleeding, more transfusion, and more severe coagulopathy. It has been suggested that these patients may benefit from a balanced transfusion approach including a combination of packed RBCs, platelets, and plasma in a fixed ratio (e.g., 1:1:1), with some studies showing survival benefits, but the optimal ratio remains a matter of debate (Malone et al 2006, Mitra et al 2010). On the other hand, aggressive plasma transfusion in massively transfused patients who do not have coagulopathy does not improve the outcome of the patients (Mitra et al 2012). Although some have suggested that these balanced protocols may allow better hemostasis and a reduced overall use of allogeneic blood components in other settings (Palmieri et al 2013, Pasquier et al 2013), such usage of plasma in routine cases (other than massively transfused patients) amid no evidence of coagulopathy and/or bleeding cannot be recommended based on currently available evidence (Godier et al 2011, Stansbury et al 2009).

▶ **Prophylactic use.** Despite its widespread use, little if any evidence supports the prophylactic use of plasma. Prophylactic use of plasma is often (inappropriately) justified based on the presence of coagulopathy in patients scheduled for an invasive procedure. Coagulopathy is commonly defined by a PT or activated partial thromboplastin time of ≥ 1.5 the normal value, or an INR of ≥ 2. Nonetheless, these thresholds are arbitrary numbers and their real clinical significance is undetermined (Solbeck et al 2012, Veelo et al 2012). Moreover, even if normalizing the INR were a clinically justifiable cause (which it is not), plasma itself can have a raised INR as high as 1.3, and therefore it cannot be reasonably expected to be able to normalize a patient's INR on its own.

In a systematic review of 25 studies, there was no significant increase in the risk of bleeding associated with abnormal (increased) PT and INR tests compared with normal test results among patients undergoing bronchoscopy, central vein cannulation, arteriography, liver biopsy, or transjugular biopsy, leading the authors to conclude that there was insufficient evidence to support the common assumption that abnormal PT and INR results are predictive of clinically significant bleeding (Segal and Dzik 2005).

> **Note**
>
> No significant increase in the risk of bleeding has been found in association with abnormal (increased) PT and INR values in patients undergoing bronchoscopy, central vein cannulation, arteriography, liver biopsy, or transjugular biopsy.

In a multicenter trial, 81 critically ill patients with an INR of 1.5–3 who were planned to have central vein cannulation, percutaneous tracheostomy, chest tube placement, or abscess drainage were randomized to receive no or 12 mL/kg plasma prophylactically. Plasma transfusion resulted in improvement of the INR to < 1.5 in more than half of the transfused patients, but the incidence of bleeding complications was small and did not differ between the study arms. Of note, this trial fell short of recruiting its planned sample size of 400 patients because of enrollment difficulties, which resulted in an inability to demonstrate the noninferiority of no plasma over plasma transfusion. However, a trend toward noninferiority (with patients receiving plasma having a 5% higher rate of bleeding) was shown in a post hoc analysis, and plasma transfusion was associated with an increased incidence of ventilator-associated pneumonia and a prolonged duration of mechanical ventilation (Müller et al 2015).

Although more studies are needed to better describe the bleeding risk in patients with higher levels of coagulopathy and the impact of plasma in preventing the bleeding, currently available evidence does not support the prophylactic use of plasma for patients with a mildly (≤2) elevated INR (ASATF 2015).

► **Unwarranted use.** Plasma should not be used for volume expansion, to prime a cardiac bypass circuit (Miao et al 2014), to increase the concentration of plasma proteins (e.g., albumin, immunoglobulins), or to "accelerate" the recovery and healing process. As indicated earlier, inappropriate plasma transfusion is likely to delay recovery and prolong the hospital length of stay, and there is no evidence that it can benefit patients in any way in this aspect. Similarly, the prophylactic use of plasma as a "hemostatic" agent in the absence of coagulopathy is not warranted because it has not been shown to be able to reduce blood loss, whereas it exposes patients to the risks of allogeneic plasma (Ferraris et al 2011a).

1.5.3 PBM and Sensible Use of Plasma

As discussed earlier, the rising clinical use of plasma has fueled concerns that many of these plasma transfusions are not justified or likely to improve the outcomes of the patients (Puetz 2013). Plasma units are commonly given prophylactically in response to laboratory findings, which correlates poorly with the clinical risk of bleeding, and worse, transfused plasma units often fail to achieve any significant improvements in these laboratory measures (let alone improvements in the clinical condition of the patient). With little if any benefits and real risks, and in the context of more pressure to improve the quality of care at reduced costs, PBM offers several opportunities to improve the clinical use of plasma.

► **Alternative treatment modalities.** A quick look at the indications of plasma discussed here can provide us with a road map for integrating the use of plasma as part of a PBM program. Almost all prophylactic uses of plasma can be replaced by other modalities with adequate planning and foresight. A very common scenario is a mildly coagulopathic patient on warfarin scheduled for an invasive procedure. When there is no urgency and/or active bleeding and with enough time available, adjustment of the VKA dose and administration of vitamin K (oral or intravenous) can restore the coagulation profile to normal levels, eliminating the use of plasma. Preoperative management of coagulopathy in this context shares many features with the management of anemia in PBM. Rather than allowing anemia to go undetected or ignoring

it in the weeks and days leading to elective surgery when there is still time to treat it, PBM calls for the active screening and management of anemia in the preoperative period (Goodnough et al 2011). The same approach can be reasonable for coagulopathic patients scheduled for an elective procedure.

Note

With adequate planning and foresight, almost all prophylactic uses of plasma can be replaced by other modalities.

► **Improving transfusion practice.** In a short-term study in 47 ICUs, it was shown that whereas implementation of national transfusion guidelines can improve the clinical use of packed RBCs to some extent, plasma transfusion practices may not enjoy similar levels of improvement (Westbrook et al 2010). Another study in a large tertiary center reported alarming deviation in the indications and dose of transfused plasma units from the guidelines across departments, and the authors called for increased training of the clinicians and measures to enforce the available guidelines (Pybus et al 2012). On the other hand, another long-term single-center study has shown that an institutional program of active engagement and interdiction of plasma transfusions that involved reviewing all plasma orders, discouraging any orders placed with an INR < 2 without active bleeding, and promoting vitamin K administration in patients taking VKA was able to reduce the use of plasma by 80%, while the rate of unexpected bleedings did not increase and the mortality rate actually dropped (Tavares et al 2011). A reduction of 60% in plasma usage was observed in another study after establishing the prospective monitoring of transfusion practices, which also resulted in significant cost savings (Sarode et al 2010). It is evident that the mere availability of evidence-based guidelines may have limited impact on improving plasma transfusion practices, whereas the active implementation of the guidelines as part of clinical-decision support systems and other similar approaches can have a more far-reaching impact (Goodnough et al 2014b).

Inclusion of transfusion data as part of quality measures is another approach to improve plasma transfusion practice (Shander and Goodnough

2010). Such measures are indispensable in the successful widespread implementation of PBM.

▶ **Strategies to preserve a patient's own plasma.** Although more studies are needed to better define and quantify their impact on plasma transfusions and patient outcomes, many whole blood-sparing PBM strategies are effective in preserving a patient's own plasma, reducing the need for allogeneic plasma. Examples include preoperative autologous donation (PAD) and acute normovolemic hemodilution (ANH). In PAD, the patient undergoes successive phlebotomies in the weeks leading to an elective procedure and the collected autologous blood is stored until the day of surgery to be used if needed. In ANH, the autologous blood is collected on the day of surgery in the operating room and replaced with intravenous fluids to avoid hypovolemia. The autologous blood is stored at the bedside to be used whenever needed during or after the surgery (Goodnough and Shander 2012, Shander et al 2013). Both techniques can preserve autologous whole blood containing plasma, which could in theory substitute the need for plasma to some extent.

Understandably, these techniques are not without controversies. PAD is faced with logistical constraints and runs the risks of blood wastage, storage lesions, and transfusion errors, in addition to increased risks of anemia and transfusion because of the aggressive phlebotomies, among other issues. ANH seems to be beneficial in carefully selected patients, but it also faces the issue of wastage. Although the controlled hemodilution achieved during ANH may be expected in theory to negatively affect coagulation, studies do not support this notion (Guo et al 2013). On the other hand, the impact of transfused autologous whole blood on restoring coagulation and reducing the use of allogeneic blood components (including plasma) is less clear (Shander and Perelman 2006).

The evidence supporting the safety and efficacy of the other available autotransfusion technique—cell salvage—is much stronger (Carless et al 2010b), but it should be remembered that the washed units from cell salvage are largely devoid of plasma. Nonetheless, evidence indicates that the transfusion of autologous cell salvage blood does not adversely affect coagulation, and it is effective in reducing transfusion of allogeneic blood components, including plasma (Niranjan et al 2006). Use of hemostatic agents, use of minimally inva-

sive approaches, avoidance of hypothermia (if not otherwise indicated), and aggressive monitoring and control of operative bleeding are other measures used in PBM that can preserve a patient's plasma as well as other blood components from being wasted and lost (Shander et al 2009, Shander et al 2013).

Conclusion

Emerging evidence supports the notion that PBM modalities are associated with an improved patient outcome, while reducing the reliance on allogeneic blood components (Goodnough et al 2014a, Gross et al 2013). Given its risks, costs, and limited ability to improve the coagulation status and clinical outcome of patients, the use of plasma should only be considered when clearly indicated and in the absence of other alternatives. This is often in sharp contrast to practices commonly seen in the clinic, underscoring the importance of PBM strategies. PBM offers several opportunities for improving the quality of care through more appropriate use of allogeneic blood components including plasma and their alternatives, and through preventive measures that can reduce or eliminate the need for them.

1.6 Key Role of Benchmarking Processes in PBM

A. Hofmann, S. Farmer

1.6.1 Definitions and Explanations

Benchmarking is a method for the systematic measurement and improvement of various types of economic and organizational activities. For external benchmarking, products, services, production and logistical processes, operational and organizational procedures, and treatment algorithms or similar processes of one's own organization or institution are compared with those of outside organizations. Internal benchmarking reviews practices only within the respective organization, e.g., between different branches or business operations, and between teams or individual employees. Benchmarking can be carried out only once, periodically, or continuously.

The *quality indicators* and *key performance indicators* most amenable to measurement must be identified to ensure successful benchmarking. Once performance data have been collected and compared, the different results are analyzed. The findings can then be used to optimize workflows and resource utilization. Hence benchmarking is also aimed at the implementation of "best practice" and "learning from the best."

> **Note**
>
> Benchmarking is aimed at the implementation of "best practice" and "learning from the best."

The term *benchmarking* was first introduced in the early 1980s in business management theory and practice. At that time, Robert C. Camp gave a detailed account of the optimization of production processes, based on benchmarking, for the American photocopier manufacturer Xerox (Camp 1989). Following the expiry of patent protection, the company was facing stiff competition from suppliers from the Far East, and therefore initiated its first benchmarking process in order to be better able to estimate its relative competitive position versus its new opponents. A photocopy machine from a Japanese competitor was dismantled and compared with a similar Xerox model. This helped to identify, and eliminate, cost disadvantages in the production process. Later, benchmarking was used to analyze other areas of their business, such as logistics and sales, while comparing the operations of companies from different sectors of industry. What ultimately became part of the management culture in the Xerox Corporation was soon emulated by other enterprises, branches of the economy, and in the public administration sector.

Benchmarking in the Health Care Sector

As borne out by literature searches in PubMed (search strategy: "benchmarking"[MeSH Terms] OR "benchmarking"[All Fields]), the term *benchmarking* began to be used in the medical and health economics literature from around 1990. The method has been used ever since to compare the performances of hospitals, hospital departments, laboratories, and other service providers in the health care sector. Benchmarking data in the health care sector are analyzed to identify the potential for structural, technical, and educational improvements and to better allocate resources, thus leading to better overall medical and clinical services and better patient outcomes.

> **Note**
>
> Benchmarking in the health care sector involves the measurement of diagnostic, therapeutic, and other medical or clinical services in comparable institutions, or the measurement of comparable processes with regard to resource utilization and outcome. Analysis of the differences is the basis for optimizing the performance and, in particular, patient outcomes.

▶ **Diagnosis-related groups.** Patient groups are often defined using diagnosis-related groups (DRGs). Within DRGs, hospital managers are particularly interested in continuously benchmarking mortality, average length of stay, hospital-acquired complications, and hospital readmissions. Exchanging, analyzing, and discussing interhospital outcomes data per DRG can highlight areas for improvement in hospital efficiency and quality of care. This has become an important element of modern hospital management in Australia (www.healthroundtable.org). However, for benchmarking results to be meaningful to clinicians, adjustment for differences in the patient mix is essential. Although DRGs may go some way to explaining the patient type, further adjustment for potential confounders is recommended. For example, adjustment for patient age and important comorbidities will assist the physician who treats older, sicker patients. Moreover, benchmarking is not a substitute for clinical observational studies.

The term *benchmarking* with regard to transfusion has appeared only recently in the literature, whereas the term *transfusion variability* has been used since 1990 (Apelseth et al 2012).

1.6.2 Why Benchmarking is Indicated in the Transfusion Setting

Benchmarking of specific health care services for essentially comparable patients is indicated when they
- Have a high incidence and are affecting a large number of patients,
- Are macroeconomically relevant, and
- Have widespread variability in resource use and/ or outcome.

If all of these criteria are met, benchmarking can help to bring about structural improvements, and valuable resources can be wisely reallocated. The extent to which these criteria are met in the current transfusion setting is explained below.

Transfusion Incidence Rates

The administration of allogeneic blood components has been a common part of medical and surgical treatment for several decades. In the annual report of the WHO for the reporting period 2004–2005, the annual blood donation figure for 167 countries is given as just under 81 million (WHO 2008). In the 2011 report, that figure had risen to 92 million, involving around 8,000 blood donation services in 159 countries (WHO 2012). In most cases, around half a liter of blood is collected from each donor. This is then fractionated, using an automated technique, into its three principal components. Based on an estimated 7% wastage rate, it is thought that currently 85 million units of RBCs are transfused to an estimated 25 million patients. It is difficult to estimate the global volume of transfused platelet concentrates and FFP; however, some national consumption figures are available for the individual components. Based on surveys by the Paul Ehrlich Institute, 4.34 million RBC units, 0.52 million platelet units, and 1.47 million units of FFP are consumed in Germany alone. For the United States, the country with the highest consumption of blood components, these figures for 2011 were 13.78 million RBC and whole blood units, around 1.97 million apheresis platelets, 0.99 million whole-blood-derived platelets, and 3.88 million units of plasma (Whitaker and Hinkins 2011).

Note

Transfusions are used as supportive therapy in a broad range of patient populations in surgery and medicine. Some 85 million RBC units alone are administered each year to an estimated 25 million patients.

Cost Dimension of Transfusions

Process cost analyses in European and U.S. hospitals have revealed that the total costs incurred for the transfusion of RBCs are three to five times higher than the actual blood product costs, and that the total transfusion costs per transfused surgical patient, who in general receives 3–4 units of RBCs per hospital stay, are between $2,400 and $3,600 (Shander 2005, Shander et al 2007, Shander et al 2010). The average transfusion costs are likely to be even higher for hematology and oncology patients, who often receive transfusions in day-clinic infusion centers. This is due to the fact that a significant part of the infrastructure of such clinics is specifically designed for transfusion and infusion services, leading to higher overhead costs. Also, iron overload is often diagnosed in some of these patients because of transfusion dependency. This calls for chelation therapy, with attendant high costs (Payne et al 2007, Shander and Sazama 2010).

Moreover, a growing number of studies have identified a statistically significant association between the number of allogeneic RBC units administered and the rise in health care-associated (nosocomial) infections, ischemia, multiorgan failure, ARDS, SIRS, and relapses of malignant tumors (see Chapter 1.3). Since the evidence available from the literature is suggestive of a causal link between transfusion and these adverse outcomes, the costs incurred for the prolongation of ICU and hospital length of stay and for increased hospital readmission rates should be included in the transfusion-related costs (Isbister et al 2011, Hofmann et al 2012).

That transfusion-related costs constitute a macroeconomically relevant variable has been demonstrated by a retrospective study based on the 2004 Nationwide Inpatient Sample of the U.S. Agency for Healthcare Research and Quality. The Nationwide Inpatient Sample is a database developed for the Healthcare Cost and Utilization Project that contains information on more than 8 million discharges for around 20% of all hospitalized patients in the United States, enabling representative conclusions to be drawn for the entire U.S. health care system with an estimated 39 million discharges in 2004. According to these figures and after adjustment for age, sex, comorbidity as per Charlson Comorbidity Index, admission type, and DRG, the average hospital charges incurred for 2.33 million transfused patients were $17,194 higher (*p* < 0.0001) than those incurred for the nontransfused control group, and the average hospital stay was 2.5 days longer (Morton et al 2010). As such, the overall additional expenditure for the transfused cohorts amounted to $40.1 billion. In comparison, the total volume of prescription-only drugs for the same year in the United States was $192.2 billion (CMS 2013).

Note

Transfusion-related costs account for a significant portion of the overall costs incurred for hospitalized patients. In nonactively bleeding, relatively hemodynamically stable, anemic patients, studies increasingly suggest that transfusions are responsible for additional morbidity and an associated prolongation of hospital stay. Overall, in the more developed countries, transfusion-related costs have acquired a macroeconomically important dimension.

Variability in Transfusion Practices

There is widespread variability in transfusion practices at international, interinstitutional, and intrainstitutional levels.

▶ **International Level.** Based on surveys carried out by the European Commission, the variability in the use of RBC units is between 60/1,000 inhabitants in Denmark and 19.5/1,000 in Bulgaria. Even when comparing EU countries with a similarly high standard of care, there continues to be relatively widespread variability. Whereas the number of RBC units transfused per 1,000 inhabitants was 60.2 in Denmark and 57.3 in Germany, it was 36.1 in the United Kingdom and 35.4 in France (**Fig. 1.7**) (Eurostat 2015, van der Poel et al 2011).

▶ **Interinstitutional level.** The interinstitutional variability is significantly greater than the variability seen at the international level. The first studies on transfusion variability between different hospitals were conducted around 1990. Surgenor and colleagues (1991) observed the transfusion practices for a specific DRG of patients undergoing orthopaedic surgery in 151 U.S. hospitals. There was widespread variability in the number of transfused patients, but not in the mean number of units administered per transfused patient (Surgenor et al 1991). In 1994, the Sanguis study was commissioned by the European Commission (SSG 1994). This was the first study to systematically investigate the transfusion rates for six types of standardized surgical procedures in 43 large European teaching hospitals. Allogeneic transfusion rates of between 0 and 96% were identified for CABG surgery, and of between 0 and 100% for total hip replacement (SSG 1994). One study conducted in

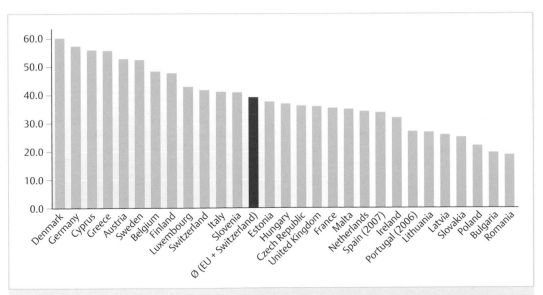

Fig. 1.7 Number of red blood cell transfusions per 1,000 inhabitants in EU countries and Switzerland in 2008.

five hospitals in the U.S. state of Massachusetts compared transfusions for 384 Medicare patients who had undergone an orthopaedic procedure. There were significant differences in both the percentage of transfused patients and in the number of RBC units transfused per patient. The variability could not be explained by differences between patients, but were attributed to failure to comply with relevant transfusion guidelines. The authors concluded that virtually half of all transfusions could have been avoided (Audet et al 1998). An observational study in the United States with 102,470 patients undergoing primary isolated CABG surgery with cardiopulmonary bypass during 2008 at 798 sites showed perioperative transfusion rates of 7.8–92.8% for RBCs, 0–97.5% for FFP, and 0.4–90.4% for platelets (Bennett-Guerrero et al 2010).

A number of studies have been conducted in Canada on the variability of allogeneic and, in some cases, autologous transfusions. A multicenter cohort study with 5,298 intensive care patients, conducted within the framework of the Canadian Critical Care Trials Group, revealed significant transfusion variability. Contributing to this was that—contrary to widely disseminated guidelines recommending RBC transfusions being given 1 unit at a time based on clinical judgment and not a predefined hemoglobin value—40% of the physicians administered transfusions 2 units at a time and at a high hemoglobin threshold. Compliance with these guidelines varied between institutions (Hébert et al 1999b).

In an observational study with 41,568 patients in 11 Canadian centers, the transfusion practices were studied in hip fracture repair and cardiac surgery procedures. Also included were surgical intensive care and polytrauma patients. Between 23.8 and 51.9% of the enrolled 7,552 patients received RBC transfusion. The adjusted OR of transfusion in relation to the median of an institution selected as reference center was 0.44–1.53 when taking account of all patients, 0.42–1.22 for patients with hip fracture, 0.72–3.17 for cardiac surgery patients, and 0.27–1.11 for intensive care and trauma patients. The mean adjusted nadir hemoglobin, which can be used as surrogate marker for the transfusion threshold, ranged from 71.2 ± 2.9 g/L to 82.8 ± 1.7 g/L for hip fracture patients, from 65.7 ± 1.1 g/L to 77.3 ± 1.0 g/L for cardiac surgery patients, and from 66.1 ± 3.04 g/L to 87.5 ± 2.5 g/L for intensive care and trauma patients (Hutton et al 2005).

Practicing Canadian anesthesiologists belonging to the Canadian Anesthesiologists' Society were surveyed to enquire about their transfusion practices. The survey depicted clinical scenarios of elective surgical procedures with different risks of bleeding. The respondents were requested to choose hemoglobin thresholds for which they would transfuse RBCs in each scenario. The response rate to the survey was 47% (719/1512). Of the respondents, 48% selected a hemoglobin threshold of 70 g/L for the general surgery setting outlined, 56% selected it for the orthopaedic surgery, and 79% selected it for the vascular surgery situation depicted ($p < 0.001$). For patients with a history of coronary artery disease, 31% chose a threshold of ≥ 100 g/L ($p < 0.001$) for the general surgery scenario, 20% chose it for the orthopaedic surgery, and 49% chose it for the vascular surgery setting. Conversely, if the patient age cited in the various scenarios was reduced from 60 to 20 years, the threshold selected by > 30% of participants in two of the three scenarios was ≤ 60 g/L. An interesting observation in terms of benchmarking was the strong correlation between the year of respondent graduation and the choice of thresholds (Turgeon et al 2006).

In 2008, Snyder-Ramos et al published a prospective investigation of transfusion practice in cardiac surgery patients. Seventy centers in 16 countries participated in the study, and a total of 5,065 cardiac surgery patients of the Multicenter Study of Perioperative Ischemia Epidemiology II (EPI II) were randomly selected and evaluated. The use of RBCs, FFP, and platelets was assessed daily, before, during, and after surgery until hospital discharge. The percentage of patients who received an intraoperative RBC transfusion varied from 9% to 100% among the 16 countries, whereas that of patients receiving a postoperative transfusion varied from 25% to 87%. Intraoperative transfusion of FFP varied from 0% to 98%, and postoperative transfusion from 3% to 95%. For platelet transfusion, the rates varied from 0% to 51% and 0% to 39%, respectively. Furthermore, there were major differences not only in transfusion rates between centers in different countries but also when comparing institutions within certain countries (Snyder-Ramos et al 2008).

> **Note**
>
> There is widespread variability in the number of RBC units transfused per 1000 inhabitants from one country to another. Likewise, there is marked variability in transfusion rates for comparable patients from one center to another. This can vary from 0% to 100%. Transfusion indices also vary greatly. Overall, these differences appear to be related to behavior, culture, and quality within the hospitals and medical teams.

The extreme variability in transfusion rates for similar patients, which in some cases can even reach the maximum range possible (0–100%), and the manifest failure of some centers to observe available transfusion guidelines, highlight that this inadequacy in patient care stems from behavioral, cultural, and quality-related issues rather than from patients' clinically indicated requirements. Apart from the ethical concerns and especially the legal consequences arising from such issues, the economic implications of such inappropriate practice variations must be borne in mind. The latter are thought to result in avoidable costs of several billion dollars each year in the United States and the European Union alone. It is only through wide-ranging and continuous benchmarking that clinicians can identify where they and their department or center are positioned versus others, and understand what improvements can be made.

> **Note**
>
> Benchmarking programs are urgently indicated to counter the extreme variability in transfusion practices. Doing so will not only improve outcomes but also achieve annual cost savings in the range of double-digit billions of U.S. dollars.

1.6.3 Examples of Effective Benchmarking in the Transfusion Setting

▶ **Belgium.** One example attesting to the benefits of benchmarking is the Biomed study conducted in 63 Belgian hospitals. While this revealed similarly widespread variability in transfusion rates as that seen in the case of the Sanguis study described

above (SSG 1994), two of the 63 hospitals in the Biomed study had already participated in the Sanguis study, following which they drastically reduced their transfusion rates. For colectomies, the rate dropped by a factor of 5. At the same time, the average hospital stay was shortened, against a background of unchanged morbidity and mortality (Baele et al 1998, Baele et al 1994a).

▶ **Canada.** Public authorities in Canada conducted successful benchmarking projects aimed at reducing the consumption of blood components. These included the Transfusion Ontario programs of the Ontario Ministry of Health and a study by the Ontario Blood System Reference Group. In addition to assuring continuing education and quality management in transfusion medicine, the projects were aimed at the continuous implementation of a blood conservation program for the entire province of Ontario. Twenty-three hospitals participated in one of these programs, the Ontario Transfusion Coordinators (ONTraC) program. During the first 12 months of continuous benchmarking, marked improvements were achieved by most hospitals. Overall, the transfusion rate declined by 24% for knee arthroplasty, 14% for aortic aneurysms, and 23% for CABG surgery. In quantitative terms, blood conservation was even higher because of the reduction in the transfusion index. A significantly lower postoperative infection rate and a shorter length of stay were also observed for those patients who did not receive allogeneic transfusions. After 6 months, a further reduction was observed in the transfusion rate and transfusion index (Freedman et al 2005).

1.6.4 Key Performance Indicators for Transfusion Benchmarking

For intercountry comparisons of RBC, platelet, or FFP transfusions, the performance indicator normally used is the number of transfused units per 1,000 of the population (van der Poel et al 2011). For interinstitutional, intrainstitutional, and interpersonal comparisons, the *transfusion rate* and, occasionally, the *transfusion index* are given.
- Transfusion rate: proportion of transfused patients within a defined patient population.
- Transfusion index: average number of blood components administered per patient of a defined patient population.

An expanded, combined key performance indicator composed of the transfusion rate and transfusion index, is the *total transfusion index* (TTI).
- TTI: product of transfusion rate and transfusion index.

The TTI can be used to draw up a ranking list showing blood component consumption within a benchmark cohort in descending order. Furthermore, the quotient of the highest and lowest TTI can be used as an overall measure of transfusion variability.

Fictitious Example of Interpersonal Transfusion Benchmarking

Table 1.6 illustrates fictitious, but realistic, results of the interpersonal transfusion benchmarking of six surgeons. Surgeon I has the second lowest transfusion rate at 18%, and the lowest transfusion index at 1.2 RBC units per transfused patient. Surgeon II has the lowest transfusion rate at 12%, but only the second lowest transfusion index with 1.8 RBC units. Nonetheless, they are equally successful because the TTI is equally low for both. Surgeon II has used four fewer RBC units than surgeon I only because he carried out fewer operations than Surgeon I. Surgeon III has the highest TTI at 2.4, which is 11.11 times higher than the TTI of surgeons I and II. This means that he used over 11 times more RBC units per patient or operation than his peers with the lowest consumption. If, in his 123 cases, he had the same TTI as surgeon I or II, who define the "best practice" for this cohort, he would have used only 26 instead of 295 RBC units, i.e., 269 fewer units. Using the same approach, to achieve the "best practice" benchmark, surgeons IV, V, and VI would need 29, 17, and 80 fewer RBC units, respectively.

This example shows that in total, there is the potential to reduce RBC units by 394, i.e., from 535 to 141, which is a 74% decrease. In theory, and assuming that patients can be compared, surgeons I and II can still learn from each other and jointly devise a new "best practice" strategy, since for surgeon I there is still potential for reducing the transfusion rate, and for surgeon II there is potential for reducing the transfusion index.

This example illustrates the key function of the TTI in benchmark analyses: variability of the transfusion rate is only around 1:7 and that of the transfusion index is 1:2.5, whereas variability of the TTI is 1:11, making it a better indicator of where potential reductions can be made. Surgeon III is responsible for just over 50% of all transfused RBC units, and for 68% of the potential to reduce the total consumption within the cohort of surgeons.

Fig. 1.8 shows how interpersonal benchmarking can be displayed for surgeons I to VI as per Table 1.6 using a color-coded presentation. For surgeons I and II, light blue spheres denote "best practice," whereas surgeon III is in the worst range, as denoted by the dark blue sphere, highlighting the need to improve practice and reduce both the transfusion rate and the transfusion index. The size of the spheres reflects the number of operations for each surgeon.

Table 1.6 and Fig. 1.8 are good examples that can be used as templates for the regular reporting on persons taking part in continuous transfusion benchmarking.

Table 1.6 Fictitious example of interpersonal transfusion benchmarking

Surgeon	TR	TI	TTI	Total number of operations	Total number of RBC units transfused	Number of units transfused unnecessarily based on "best practice"
Surgeon I	18%	1.2	0.216	200	43	0
Surgeon II	12%	1.8	0.216	172	39	0
Surgeon III	80%	3.0	2.400	123	295	269
Surgeon IV	55%	2.7	1.485	23	34	29
Surgeon V	26%	2.0	0.520	55	29	17
Surgeon VI	67%	2.0	1.340	71	95	80
Total	36%	2.3	0.835	644	535	395

Abbreviations: RBC, red blood cell; TI, transfusion index; TR, transfusion rate; TTI, total transfusion index.

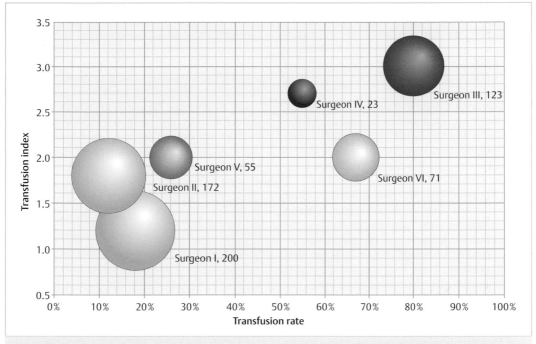

Fig. 1.8 Interpersonal transfusion benchmarking. The size of the spheres represents the number of operations.

Note ❗

The transfusion rate gives the proportion of transfused patients within a defined patient population, whereas the transfusion index gives the average number of blood components administered per transfused patient of a defined patient population. The TTI is calculated from the product of transfusion rate and transfusion index, giving the average number of blood components per patient across the whole cohort (transfused and nontransfused). The quotient of the highest and lowest TTIs shows the variability within the benchmarking cohort.

1.6.5 Benchmarking and PBM

As described in detail in Chapter 1.1.8, PBM goes well beyond the concept of Optimal Blood Use, because it entails a preemptive strategy aimed at the timely modification of risk factors that could result in a transfusion, e.g., preexisting anemia or bleeding. A pioneering role was played here by the First Austrian Benchmark Study on elective surgical procedures, published under the title "Blood use in elective surgery: the Austrian benchmark

study" (Gombotz et al 2007). This study did not only collect data on blood consumption and thresholds, but it also focused on other factors leading to transfusion. It was carried out in 2006 within the framework of a research project of the Austrian Federal Ministry of Health in 18 public hospitals to study the transfusion rates in 3,600 elective surgical procedures with comparable patients, and identify potential transfusion-related cost-saving mechanisms. The hospitals were randomly selected and stratified by region to obtain representative information for the whole of Austria. The aim was to collect data on high-volume surgical procedures known to be associated with a high consumption of allogeneic blood components that could be easily compared in terms of surgical technique. Data were collected on a total of 3,622 evaluable operations. These consisted of: 1,401 total hip replacements and 1,296 knee replacements in 16 centers; 777 CABG operations in 6 centers; and 148 hemicolectomies in 11 centers. The variability of the transfusion rates was highest for orthopaedic procedures at 13% to 84%, but no differences were noted in terms of 30-day postoperative morbidity and mortality. The transfusion rates for cardiovascular procedures ranged from 37% to 63%.

► **Causes of transfusion variability.** Unlike the studies published on transfusion variability rates up till then, the Austrian study was the first to investigate and quantify the potential causes of widespread variability. Accordingly, it noted that 97.4% of all transfusions could be predicted on the basis of three indicators:

- Prevalence and degree of preoperative anemia.
- Perioperative blood loss volume calculated according to the Mercuriali algorithm (Mercuriali and Inghilleri 1996).
- Hemoglobin-value transfusion threshold.

The authors of the Austrian Benchmark Study noted that the centers in which the following three measures were partially, or fully, implemented had the lowest blood consumption:

- Diagnosis and treatment of anemia before elective procedures.
- Minimization of perioperative blood loss through meticulous surgical technique, use of cell salvage and hemostatic agents, and other measures.
- Application of restrictive transfusion thresholds.

The authors also concluded: "Our main predictors for RBC transfusion support the concept of the three pillars of blood conservation: 1) augmentation of preoperative RBC mass, 2) reduction of surgical blood loss, and 3) acceptance of low Hb levels." This was the first study to demonstrate the substantial reductions in blood consumption that could be achieved by modifying these three risk factors through PBM (**Fig. 1.9**). (The three-pillar concept has since come to be known in the literature as the *Patient Blood Management* approach rather than simply a blood conservation concept.)

Note

The majority of transfusions are predicted by three modifiable risk factors: preoperative anemia, volume of perioperative blood loss, and the chosen hemoglobin-based transfusion threshold. Accordingly, future benchmark studies on PBM should not only measure the consumption of blood components but also review key performance indicators for the management of anemia and bleeding, which are key elements of PBM.

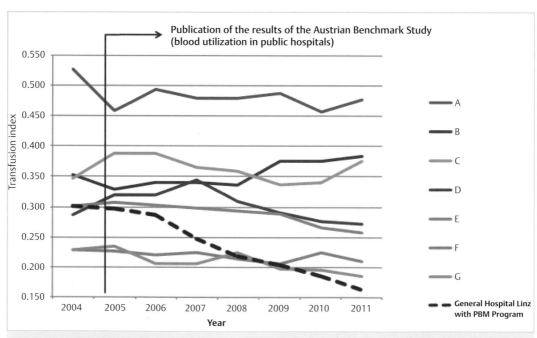

Fig. 1.9 Transfusion index for the eight largest public hospitals in Austria (average length of stay > 0 days). Adapted from Gombotz and Hofman (2013) with kind permission from Springer Science and Business Media.

▶ **Potential for reduction.** In the final report on the First Austrian Benchmark Study addressed to the Austrian Ministry of Health, it was pointed out that the overall blood consumption rate for the procedures of interest could have been reduced by well over 50 % if the mean blood (component) consumption rate achieved by the five centers with the lowest consumption had been emulated across the other centers (**Fig. 1.10a, b**). As illustrated by the numerical data from the Second Austrian Benchmark Study, it would appear that centers learnt lessons from the First Austrian Benchmark Study and subsequently achieved marked reductions (Gombotz et al 2012, Gombotz et al 2014). Since the data collected for the centers were anonymized and only accessible to the

study management, it is not possible to determine which of these centers used preoperative outpatient anemia treatment, perioperative management of anemia and bleeding, or more physiological and restrictive transfusion thresholds. However, each center was informed of its rank in the overall ratings, so that progress could be made in driving forward the benchmarking process.

▶ **Implications of the Austrian Benchmark Study.** Although the data collection was anonymized, the center with the highest transfusion rate voluntarily published its data and conducted an internal audit to verify its customary transfusion practices (**Table 1.7** and **Fig. 1.11**). In 2004, when baseline data began to be collected for the

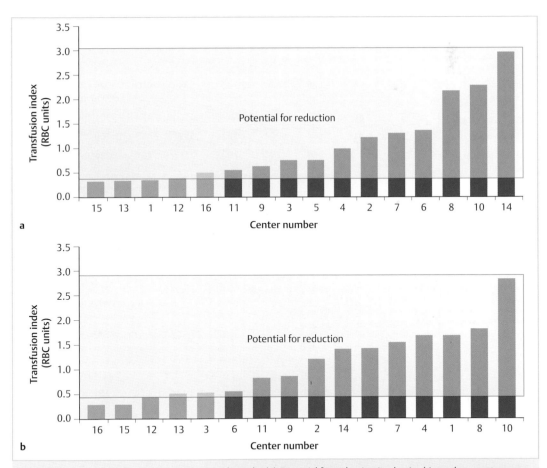

Fig. 1.10 Results of the First Austrian Benchmark Study. (a) Potential for reduction in elective hip replacement surgery. (b) Potential for reduction in elective knee replacement surgery. The line at the bottom of the box depicts the median of the five centers with the lowest RBC consumption, and the bar sections above this line show the potential for reduction. CI, confidence interval; RBC, red blood cell.

Table 1.7 Reduction of RBC transfusions in the center with the highest transfusion rate recorded in the First Austrian Benchmark Study

Year	2003	2004	2005	2006	2007	2008	2009	2010	2011	Decline 2004–2011
Number of transfusions per year										
Cardiac ICU	425	341	449	352	333	354	251	193	326	−4.4%
Internal Medicine I (Cardiology, Nephrology)	652	714	805	611	583	591	419	322	426	−40.3%
Internal Medicine II (Gastroenterology, Hepatology, Oncology)	1,345	1,335	1,246	1,165	1,298	1,198	1,316	1,437	1,287	−3.6%
Surgery	971	1,018	964	738	642	700	592	522	440	−56.8%
Gynecology and Obstetrics	232	265	105	126	97	87	101	169	146	−44.9%
Admission ward	730	855	733	686	626	753	593	610	624	−27.0%
ENT	85	97	84	20	39	51	41	47	19	−80.4%
Orthopaedics	1,007	1,146	812	384	274	322	332	451	260	−77.3%
Anesthesiology and Intensive Care Medicine	657	905	658	369	290	290	278	264	226	−75.0%
Urology	548	464	401	263	275	318	292	291	259	−44.2%
Trauma Surgery	1,300	1,325	1,120	867	930	1,141	1,047	909	885	−33.2%
Other	80	183	130	113	91	83	84	79	102	−44.3%
Total	**8,032**	**8,648**	**7,507**	**5,694**	**5,478**	**5,888**	**5,346**	**5,294**	**5,000**	**−42.2%**
Hospital admissions per year	27,618	28,633	29,202	29,583	29,748	30,169	29,593	28,749	27,843	−2.8%
Number of transfused patients per year	1,786	1,906	1,812	1,433	1,373	1,462	1,388	1,319	1,334	−30.0%
Transfusion rate (RBC concentrates)	6.5%	6.7%	6.2%	4.8%	4.6%	4.8%	4.7%	4.6%	4.8%	−28.0%

Continued ▶

Table 1.7 Continued

Year	2003	2004	2005	2006	2007	2008	2009	2010	2011	Decline 2004–2011
Transfusion index (RBC concentrates)	4.50	4.54	4.14	3.97	3.99	4.03	3.85	4.01	3.75	–17.4%
Transfusion global index (RBC concentrates)	0.29	0.30	0.26	0.19	0.18	0.20	0.18	0.18	0.18	–40.5%

Abbreviations: ENT, ear nose and throat; ICU, intensive care unit; RBC, red blood cell.

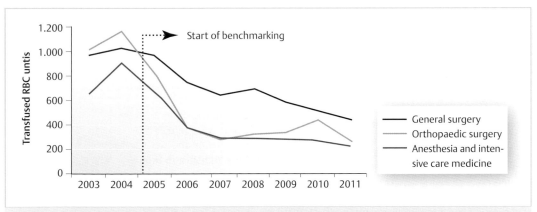

Fig. 1.11 Reduction in red blood cell (RBC) transfusions in selected departments in the center with the highest transfusion rate recorded in the First Austrian Benchmark Study. Data provided with kind permission by Dr Friedrich Marian, Landeskrankenhaus Gänserndorf-Mistelbach, Austria.

First Austrian Benchmark Study, that center had its highest annual consumption rate at 8,648 RBC units. When the benchmarking results were communicated to the various centers in the second quarter of 2005, the center immediately launched an internal audit and took remedial measures to reduce blood consumption. By 2006, despite an increase in hospital admissions, it drastically reduced its annual consumption to 5,694 units. By 2011, that figure had dropped to 5,000 RBC units, representing a 42.2% decline, albeit that was accompanied by a concurrent 2.8% reduction in admissions. Overall, between 2004 and 2011 the transfusion rate was reduced from 6.7% to 4.8%, and the transfusion index from 4.54 to 3.75 RBC units. The direct impact that benchmarking had on all surgery-related transfusions in this center was particularly salient because the benchmark study focused exclusively on the variability of elective surgical procedures. Between 2004 and 2011, RBC consumption in orthopaedic surgery declined by 77.3%, in general surgery by 56.8%, and in anesthesia by 75.0% in some centers (Friedrich Marian, personal communication, 2012).

Had the transfusion rate and transfusion index remained constant in this center since 2004—based on the number of cases in the following years 2005 to 2011—the total consumption would have been 61,882 RBC units. However, only 40,207 units were transfused representing 21,675 fewer units. This corresponds to a reduction of around €2.9 million in blood product costs, and around €7.9 million in the total process costs incurred for RBC transfusions (Shander et al 2010).

1.6.6 A Trendsetting PBM Benchmarking Program in Western Australia

A trendsetting benchmarking project—the PBM data system—is currently evolving within the framework of the PBM program run by the Department of Health in Western Australia (www. health.wa.gov.au/bloodmanagement) (Mukhtar et al 2013). Through data linkage of transfusion data and patient information from the hospital and laboratory information systems, patient outcomes in relation to the transfusion rate and transfusion index can be continually monitored.

Goals

The Western Australian PBM data system is a powerful benchmarking tool and helps to achieve the following:
• Implement PBM as a general standard of care.
• Audit, analyze, and change transfusion practices.
• Augment the clinical and pharmacoeconomic evidence for PBM and transfusion through corresponding research.
• Set a template for other jurisdictions, with the potential of establishing a national database that could be accessed at any time giving a comprehensive overview of transfusion use and costs.
• Improve blood product-use planning through the identification of demographic trends and epidemiological changes.
• Generate compelling evidence to integrate PBM into medical under- and postgraduate educational programs.
• Improve compliance with national PBM guidelines.
• Improve preconditions to attain hospital accreditation.
• Enable national and international benchmarking with PBM centers of excellence.

The data system contains the following reporting levels:
• Department of Health.
• Clinical directors and hospital administrators/ executives of all public hospitals.
• Heads of all departments with traditionally high transfusion volumes (selected according to the Pareto 80–20 rule).
• Individual clinicians responsible for transfusions within departments.

Data Collection

The following data will be collected (this is not an exhaustive list).

▶ **Demographic details of all patients (transfused and nontransfused):**
• Sex.
• Age.
• Ethnicity.
• Religion.
• Insurance status (private/public).

▶ **Data collected on blood components and blood products:**
• Number of RBC units.
• Number of platelet units.
• Number of FFP units.
• Number of cryoprecipitate units.
• Number of factor concentrates.
• Age/shelf life of RBCs.
• Age/shelf life of platelets.

▶ **Basic data:**
• Transfusion rate.
• Transfusion index.
• Total transfusion index.
• Number of components transfused per transfusion episode (monitoring of "single-unit transfusion policies").
• Location or department where transfusion administered.
• Time of transfusion.
• Actively bleeding (yes/no).
• Physician responsible for transfusion.

▶ **Indicators of the PBM three-pillar concept:**
• Pre- and postoperative hemoglobin.
• Pretransfusion hemoglobin.
• Perioperative blood loss calculated using the Mercuriali algorithm.
• Body weight.
• Height (not yet routinely collected in most hospital information systems).
• Perioperative blood loss, corrected for cell salvage volume, calculated using the Mercuriali algorithm (not yet routinely collected in most hospital information systems).

▶ **Epidemiology:**
• Major diagnostic category.
• DRG.
• Elective surgery.

- Nonelective surgery.
- Principal diagnosis (combined from admission and discharge diagnosis according to the ICD-10).
- Procedure according to ICD-10 (Principal Procedure).
- Anemia prevalence.
- Prevalence of iron deficiency.
- Coagulopathies.

▶ **Outcomes of transfusion recipients and nontransfused controls:**
- Average length of (hospital) stay.
- Average length of stay in ICU.
- Readmission rate.
- Reoperation rate.
- Infection rate.
- Other complications such as TRALI, ARDS, etc.
- Hospital mortality.
- 30-day mortality.
- 1-year mortality.
- 5-year mortality.

▶ **Economic data:**
- Product costs of transfused blood components.
- Product costs of discarded and expired blood components.
- Number of different tests or laboratory diagnostic processes.
- Process costs of transfusions.

> **Note**
>
> PBM benchmarking contains all elements of transfusion benchmarking, but is more comprehensive and outcome-focused.

Conclusion

The switch from traditional product-focused transfusion practices to PBM marks a paradigm shift (Thomson et al 2009, Farrugia 2011, Hofmann et al 2011, Vamvakas 2013). Evidence of the potential to save costs in the double-digit billions annually through PBM, while at the same time improving patient outcome, is already beginning to emerge in studies (Moskowitz et al 2010, Yoo et al 2011, Kotze et al 2012). Through its resolution, the World Health Assembly has created a collective awareness of PBM among national competent authorities, and in some countries transfusion guidelines are now supplemented with, or even replaced by, PBM guidelines. To ensure that PBM can be implemented at the clinical level, individual clinicians must know how their transfusion practices compare with those of their peers. Likewise, heads of department must know how the transfusion culture of their institution compares with that of other hospitals. Just how important this can be is illustrated by the fact that the transfusion variability observed for certain surgical procedures is between 0 and 100%. Fostering an awareness of these issues signals the first step toward successful change management, and can only be achieved through transfusion benchmarking. In a second step, transfusion benchmarking should evolve into PBM benchmarking, incorporating patient-centered outcome data. This will help to monitor the progress made in implementing the three-pillar strategy, identify where support, training, and equipment are needed, and determine the extent to which the most important outcome parameters are improved. The Australian model can serve as a template for this (Spahn et al 2008).

Chapter 2

Practical Aspects of Preoperative Patient Management

2.1 Role of the Preanesthesia Assessment Clinic in Patient Blood Management

G. Fritsch

2.1.1 Function of the Preanesthesia Clinic

The preanesthesia clinic is an integral part of modern anesthesia departments and hospitals. Its role is to provide information and to take charge of the medical optimization and risk stratification of patients undergoing a surgical procedure under anesthesia. This also explains its pivotal role in the perioperative sequence of events. Although reports on the first preanesthesia clinics date back considerably (Howland and Wang 1956), it was only in the 1990s that this approach was used on a broader scale (Fischer 1996). The perioperative medical optimization of patients in particular would be inconceivable without a well-functioning preanesthesia clinic. Only the preanesthesia clinic can guarantee the timely enrollment of patients in a PBM program, i.e., enrollment with a sufficient time reserve. This calls for close cooperation between diverse specialist disciplines, which is possible only when there is widespread acceptance of the preanesthesia clinic as an institution in its own right. The aims are to reduce the transfusion rates and to improve the general perioperative course of disease and the scheduling of operations.

2.1.2 Organization of a Preanesthesia Clinic

Patient Flow and Appointment Scheduling

Patient flow in the preanesthesia clinic is determined by several factors. These include the clinic times and the organizational procedures used by the referring departments on the one hand, and various circadian factors on the other. It is beneficial to assure a regular patient flow throughout the entire day. Patient satisfaction is closely linked to the amount of time—including waiting times—patients spend in the clinic. Therefore, the patient flow should be regulated such that waiting times are kept to the minimum, and that the ratio of contact time (consultation/treatment time) to waiting time is high (Edward et al 2008, Harnett et al 2010).

In principle, there are three models of appointment scheduling from which a preanesthesia clinic can choose:
- Appointments arranged in advance.
- No appointments, as in the case of a walk-in clinic.
- Combination of advance appointments and a system where a defined proportion of patients can present without an appointment.

▶ **Clinic with scheduled appointments.** In a clinic with scheduled appointments, patients are seen only if they have been given an appointment in advance. This helps to better allocate personnel resources and integrate services into the clinical pathways (e.g., management of admissions or diagnostic pathways for certain indications), and to reduce waiting times. However, it requires effective operational time management. Often, such a system will not have the flexibility to receive patients at short notice. Moreover, smooth functioning of a clinic with scheduled appointments depends on the contact time of the patients. The more variable these times are, the more difficult it will be to adhere to the scheduled appointments.

▶ **Walk-in clinic.** Compared with a clinic with scheduled appointments, a walk-in preanesthesia clinic that does not arrange appointments in advance faces certain drawbacks such as operational peaks and idle times when there is no patient contact, making it impossible to manage resources in a well-targeted and rational manner. Typically, peaks occur in the late mornings, when the highest patient throughput from referring clinics is expected. Naturally, these operational peaks mean increased patient waiting times and decreased patient satisfaction. The advantage conferred by a system that does not operate on the basis of fixed appointments is that it enables a certain amount of flexibility in scheduling appointments. This benefits patients who have to be integrated into the surgical schedule at short notice or because of an emergency.

▶ **Combination.** An appointment scheduling system that combines the two forms described above can offer the advantages inherent in both systems while minimizing the disadvantages. In particular, a certain amount of flexibility in arranging appointments increases acceptance among the referring parties. The proportion of clinic visits available without appointment should be tailored to the total proportion of acute operations in the operating room schedule.

Generally, organizational interventions can have a positive influence on waiting times and contact times in the preanesthesia clinic (Edward et al 2010).

> **Note** !
>
> Appointment scheduling is aimed at achieving patient satisfaction and optimizing resource utilization. Preference should be given to a combined system with a high proportion of fixed appointments and a certain number of freely available time slots.

Documentation and Administration

For administrative purposes, a preanesthesia clinic must be fully integrated into the hospital information technology system (HITS). This is essential because medical information, for example laboratory values and their progression over time, medical reports, and other medical history data, is required for the preoperative treatment of patients. Details of treatments received in, or suggested by, the preanesthesia clinic should be clearly documented in the HITS. Many of the current systems have facilities for the electronic allocation of appointments. This can greatly reduce the administrative effort.

A medical record must be maintained for each patient seen in the preanesthesia clinic. This should contain all the information needed for further preoperative measures, including any preoperative PBM optimization measures. The medical record should give a transparent overview of appointments, laboratory values, and treatment regimens (**Table 2.1**).

Human Resources Planning

▶ **Length of stay of patients.** Planning of human resources for a preanesthesia clinic should be tailored to the patient flow, patient group(s) (comorbidities, age) seen in the clinic, and services rendered. This plan should strike a balance between

Table 2.1 Content of medical records in the preanesthesia clinic

Administrative information	Medical information
• Admission date • Examiner • Patient name • Date of birth • Patient identification number • Address • Other appointments	• Diagnoses and secondary diagnoses • Surgical procedure (including classification) • Allergies • Medical history • Clinical examination • Respiratory tract evaluation • Weight, height, body mass index • Risk indices, e.g., ASA score, Lee index • Premedication • Transfusion threshold • Other treatments • Other diagnostic measures

Abbreviation: ASA, American Society of Anesthesiologists.

patient throughput, medical care, and personnel workload. For mixed patient groups, an effective length of stay of 20–30 minutes per patient can be assumed. This does not include the waiting time. The physician contact time should be estimated at 15 to 20 minutes. The given time frames must be viewed as a guide only, and can be shortened or prolonged if justified. Parameters that help to predict the length of stay in the preanesthesia clinic include the number of long-term medications, the patient's physical status according to the American Society of Anesthesiologists classification, and the patient's age (Dexter et al 2012).

▶ **Nursing personnel.** Assuming that 25 patients per physician can be seen per day, this amounts to a throughput of approximately 6,000 patients per year. To achieve these figures, it is imperative that administrative tasks and medical diagnostic procedures be delegated to secretaries and nurses, respectively. There are marked differences in the range of professional activities entrusted to nursing personnel in various countries. For example, nurses in Austria and Germany are not authorized to engage in independent professional practice, whereas graduate nurses in the United Kingdom, the Netherlands, France, and Switzerland have much greater competencies. Therefore, it is not possible to give general recommendations for preanesthesia clinics. It should, however, be possible to achieve an optimum division of the workload in accordance with the legal regulations.

▶ **Medical specialist personnel.** The qualifications required by the medical specialists who work in preanesthesia clinics are a matter of much debate in clinical practice. However, there is unanimous agreement that at least one anesthesiologist is required (ÖGARI 2012a). Important decisions such as the therapeutic measures to be taken for PBM should be left to the anesthesiologist. Besides, having an anesthesiologist on site has financial implications because the number of preoperative tests ordered depends on the medical specialty and qualification of the requesting physician (Vogt and Henson 1997, Katz et al 2011). The preanesthesia clinic is the ideal place for providing the patient with information in accordance with the guidelines. The financial benefits can be clearly calculated and documented (Flamm et al 2011). In-depth knowledge of the processes of PBM and preoperative evaluation can be imparted on a routine basis in a preanesthesia clinic.

Note

The documentation of activities in the preanesthesia clinic is intended as a means of assuring the highest possible standard of information provision and communication. The electronic documentation systems available in the hospital should be used.

2.1.3 Therapeutic Measures in the Preanesthesia Clinic

The preoperative optimization of patients scheduled to undergo a surgical procedure can dramatically influence the outcome. Medical interventions aimed at improving the physical state of preoperative patients are best undertaken at a site where medical information and competence are concentrated. Hence, a well-managed preanesthesia clinic is eminently suited to this task. The chief determinant of a successful outcome is the timely implementation of such optimization measures. If undertaken too close to the date of surgery, medical interventions may even present a danger to patients, or at best be ineffective. Often, a number of weeks are needed for the patient to respond to

preoperative optimization. Another benefit of the timely implementation of interventions is that they offer the chance to monitor and, if necessary, adjust or modify treatments. Cooperation with other specialist disciplines is advantageous in the case of PBM, especially if preoperative anemia is multifactorial or if the patient has a complex comorbidity. In this regard, hematology and nephrology play a key role.

▶ **Structural prerequisites.** As already mentioned, certain structural preconditions for therapeutic measures must be met:
- Swift and easily accessible diagnostic testing and contact with other specialist disciplines such as cardiology, hematology, nephrology, and neurology.
- A sufficient number of suitably equipped treatment rooms.
- Reimbursement guarantee for the therapeutic agents and their administration.

Medical competence is an indispensable prerequisite because of the complex nature of the problems associated with PBM. Training and provision of information to the entire medical personnel of a preanesthesia clinic underpins the quality of preoperative optimization strategies.

Note

The preanesthesia clinic is the ideal place to plan and implement measures aimed at optimizing the postoperative outcome.

2.1.4 Patient Blood Management in the Preanesthesia Clinic

General Aspects

Each preoperative optimization strategy must be organized in a stringent and reproducible manner. This includes allowing for a sufficiently long interval between therapeutic measures, such as preoperative iron therapy, and the operation date. It is unacceptable in the case of PBM that patients do not attend the preanesthesia clinic until the day before the scheduled operation. The ideal time for a preoperative patient consultation in the preanesthesia clinic is 4 to 6 weeks prior to the date set for surgery. In practice, PBM comprises a complex network of collaborations, and this should be made clear from the outset. The following disciplines are involved: surgical disciplines, anesthesia, hematology, and transfusion medicine.

Organization of PBM

It is generally advisable to draw up a plan for the introduction of PBM. The project management should be left to the management board of the preanesthesia clinic because of the integrative and multidisciplinary functions of the clinic. It is recommended that the details regarding planning, implementation, and audit of the PBM project are set out in writing in the form of a project plan.

Planning, Information, and Implementation

First of all, the potential medical partners in the hospital should be identified. Ideally, certain surgical disciplines and procedure types should be defined as suitable candidates for PBM on the basis of their associated transfusion rates. Once suitable patient groups and surgical disciplines have been identified, contact must be established and stringent agreement on the order of events must be reached. In a pilot phase, it must be determined which, and how many, patients are suitable candidates for PBM, and how they will benefit from PBM. Likewise, it must be established in advance whether, and to what extent, PBM patients will represent an additional burden to the preanesthesia clinic in terms of time and personnel resources.

The following organizational steps are advisable at the time of introducing a PBM project.

▶ **Planning phase.** Right at the start of the project, suitable patient groups should be identified and initial contact should be established with the respective surgical disciplines. Next, evaluation of patient throughput is recommended. The preoperative process will need to be modified if patients only present to the preanesthesia clinic on the day before surgery. It is important that certain parties are appointed to take responsibility on behalf of the clinic and of the surgical partners. This communication channel is essential throughout the entire project. Presentation of the financial aspects of the project is advisable because the need for any additional resources should be justified. One way to ensure financial evaluation of the project would

be to establish contact with the hospital's accounting department and to request supervision of the project.

▶ **Information and training of all participants.** After the planning phase, it is important to pass on information to all participants in a well-regulated, selective, comprehensive, and easily accessible manner:
- *Information seminars:* The aim of information seminars is to reach all participants, not forgetting any professional group, since hospital processes are often codetermined by administrative and nursing personnel.
- *Process description in the form of a manual or other information materials:* This manual should list all patient routes and the responsible personnel. It is also advisable to define algorithms and dosage regimens for preoperative treatment regimens such as iron and erythropoietin therapies.

▶ **Pilot phase.** In the pilot phase, a limited number of patients should be enrolled in the PBM project for a defined period of time (ideally only for a few months). The entire pilot phase should be evaluated in medical and financial terms.

▶ **Implementation phase.** Any weak links in the organization and implementation can be identified during the pilot phase. These should be documented during the implementation phase and appropriate remedial measures should be taken. It is recommended that the medical and financial performance of the project is evaluated at regular intervals. Often, the communication and information channels need to be improved. Naturally, PBM can only be effective if as many patients with preoperative anemia as possible are identified and appropriately treated.

Preoperative Examination and Clinical Aspects Specific to PBM

The preoperative evaluation should be based on the current guidelines and recommendations (Geldner et al 2010, De Hert et al 2011, ÖGARI 2012b). These guidelines are designed to help identify patients who can potentially be included in the PBM project. The criteria to consider when deciding whether PBM strategies are indicated are the type of surgery, the comorbidities associated with anemia, and the patient's age, sex, and body mass index.

Severity Classification of Surgical Procedures

During the preoperative evaluation, the type and invasiveness of a surgical procedure must be determined. The guidelines available use somewhat different classification systems.

▶ **American College of Cardiology/American Heart Association and European Society of Cardiology.** The tripartite classification employed in the guidelines of the American College of Cardiology/American Heart Association and the European Society of Cardiology is used on a broad scale (**Table 2.2**) (Fleisher et al 2009, Poldermans et al 2009). This categorization of surgical procedures determines the cardiac risk of a given operation. For patients undergoing a procedure belonging to the moderate- or high-risk category, it is necessary

to identify any existing anemia and to enroll patients for PBM if required.

▶ **Austrian Society for Anesthesiology, Resuscitation and Intensive Care (ÖGARI).** Another method of classifying procedures is that proposed by the Austrian Society for Anesthesiology, Resuscitation and Intensive Care (ÖGARI 2012b). Here operations are classified according to three criteria: duration of the operation, potential blood loss, and anatomical region (**Table 2.3**). All patients with a predicted intraoperative blood loss of more than 500 mL should be assigned to the PBM program. The volume of 500 mL is independent of the patient's weight or height and serves only as a guide value that was deliberately kept small. What is important is that no patient who might need a transfusion or is at risk of significant anemia is missed during preoperative diagnostic testing. The basic threshold for the need for transfusion is a blood loss of 10–15% of the calculated blood volume. The guideline algorithm stipulates the re-

Table 2.2 Classification of surgery as per American College of Cardiology/American Heart Association and European Society of Cardiology guidelines: classification based on cardiovascular risk (Fleisher et al 2009, Poldermans et al 2009)

High risk	Moderate risk	Low risk
• Aorta surgery • Procedures on the peripheral arterial system	• Abdominal procedures • Carotid artery surgery • Peripheral angioplasty • Endovascular aneurysm surgery • ENT surgery • Neurosurgery • Major orthopaedic surgery • Transplant surgery • Major urologic surgery	• Breast surgery • Dental surgery • Endocrinologic surgery • Ophthalmologic surgery • Gynecologic surgery • Plastic surgery • Minor orthopaedic surgery • Minor urologic surgery

Abbreviation: ENT, ear, nose, and throat.

Table 2.3 Classification of operations according to the Austrian Society for Anesthesiology, Resuscitation and Intensive Care (ÖGARI 2012b)

Criterion	Minor surgery	Major surgery
Duration	< 2 hours	≥ 2 hours
Blood loss	< 500 mL	≥ 500 mL
Anatomical region	• No procedures involving body cavities • Diagnostic endoscopic procedures, including laparoscopic cholecystectomy, laparoscopic hernia repair, and thoracoscopic procedures without resection	• Chest or abdominal procedures, including laparoscopic intestinal surgery (resection and anastomosis) and thoracoscopic lobectomy
Pathophysiological interactions	—	Hemodynamic, respiratory effects; major fluid shifts

quirement for a blood count during the initial series of tests.

Medical History

Each preoperative evaluation should start with a medical history. Further tests will only be performed in combination with clinical examination. The aim of taking the history is to obtain a comprehensive overview of the patient's entire state of health prior to surgery. Special attention must be paid to certain organ systems, such as the cardiovascular system, kidneys, liver, hematopoietic system, and coagulation system, in relation to PBM. It should be borne in mind that diseases of these organ systems are often associated with anemia and with unexpected intraoperative bleeding complications. Cancer patients who are scheduled to undergo neoadjuvant chemo- or radiation therapy need special attention.

It is recommended to use standardized medical history forms, focusing in particular on the cardiac history, the cardiac stress test results, and the coagulation history. In addition to the type of procedure, any abnormal findings in the medical history constitute risk factors for perioperative complications (Fritsch et al 2012).

▶ **Coagulation history.** Taking a detailed coagulation history is imperative to detect any existing coagulation disorders. This is of greater diagnostic relevance than conventional laboratory parameters such as prothrombin time, partial thromboplastin time, and platelet count (Pfanner et al 2007). Any measures designed to reduce blood transfusions must be viewed in the context of the functioning of the coagulation system. If coagulation abnormalities are suspected, further laboratory tests, such as prothrombin time, partial thromboplastin time, platelet count, and fibrinogen testing, are indicated. Special attention should be paid to platelet function.

▶ **Transfusion trigger.** A transfusion threshold must be defined for each patient in the preanesthesia clinic, based on a thorough understanding of the patient's underlying conditions and demographic characteristics. The guiding principle is that transfusion in the clinical setting should be tailored to the clinical symptoms. For example, typical lead symptoms are chest pain, orthostatic intolerance, and fluid-refractory tachycardia.

> **Conclusion**
>
> The preanesthesia clinic is the hub of PBM. Its most important prerequisite is the provision of high-quality administrative and medical services that are based on current guidelines.

2.2 Role of the General Practitioner

J. Steinhaeuser, T. Kuehlein

2.2.1 Health Care Sectors

The role of the general practitioner (GP) differs remarkably in the health care systems in Western countries. In Germany, for example, approximately 90% of the population have a GP, who is usually (but not necessarily) the first physician to consult in the ambulatory care sector. For most of their lifetime, patients will be cared for by their GP. Only 5% of a GP's patients are treated in a hospital. At the same time, some 50% of all physicians work in the inpatient sector (BAEK 2011b). The two sectors often come into contact with each other when patients are admitted to hospital, in particular during the preoperative preparation for an elective procedure. Chapter 2.1 describes the challenges faced when defining standards for the preoperative preparation of patients for elective procedures in general practice.

> **Note**
>
> In most countries, the majority of the population is cared for by GPs.

2.2.2 Role of the General Practitioner in Preoperative Assessment

To understand the role of the GP in preoperative assessment, understanding the status of primary care is of major importance. For example, in Germany current legislation makes a clear distinction between the inpatient and outpatient sectors. Office-based GPs are reimbursed through the National Association of Statutory Health Insurance Physicians (KBV) if they are involved in the preoperative assessment before procedures performed in the outpatient or GP-ward setting.

▶ **Prerequisites for outpatient operations.** Patients must meet certain medical and social prerequisites to be considered as suitable candidates for outpatient surgical procedures. In particular, such patients have no underlying general disease ("otherwise healthy patients") or, at most, only a mild form of a general disease. Based on the classification of the American Society of Anesthesiologists (ASA), these are patients belonging to ASA groups I and II. The social prerequisites include having someone available to care for the patient during the first 24 postoperative hours. The procedures that best lend themselves to the outpatient setting are operations involving a minimal risk of secondary bleeding or postoperative complications, and procedures that do not require any special postoperative care (DGAI 1999).

▶ **Responsibilities of the general practitioner.** For these types of procedures and patients, intensive preoperative diagnostic testing is only needed in exceptional cases. The GP's main task will be to ensure that only those patients undergo outpatient surgery who belong to ASA groups I and II and who also meet the other criteria mentioned above, rather than determining which additional diagnostic tests should be performed. As such, the treating GP plays a pivotal role in assuring the safety of an outpatient procedure. In addition to verifying the patient's suitability, the GP gives advice and discusses the pros and cons of outpatient surgery.

In Germany, preoperative assessment is reimbursed at €60 for patients aged 60 years or more. We mention this figure to clarify the scope of the preoperative workup expected from the GP. It includes medical history taking, a complete physical examination, and the preparation of a medical report that sets out all the information that is relevant for the anesthesiologist and the surgeon. The report should include a complete list of current medications, an overview of all relevant diagnoses, and warnings of allergies or intolerances. As an optional service, the GP may assess the patient's suitability for surgery, and perform a resting electrocardiogram or laboratory tests if this is warranted by findings from the medical history or physical examination. The results should not be older than 6 weeks.

2.2.3 Collaboration between Health Care Sectors

In line with the increasing population age in other developed countries, one-third of the German population will be aged 65 years or more by 2060. It is expected that population aging will be accompanied by rises in the number of chronic diseases and, accordingly, in the number of medications taken. In 2010, patients aged 65 years or more received an average of 3.6 daily doses of medication. Some 42% of this age group received five or more active ingredients, thus meeting the definition of polypharmacy (Thürmann et al 2012). In terms of patient safety, this opens up a number of prospects for cross-sector collaboration. In particular, the GP's knowledge about patients, their medical history, and their medication should not be lost at the interface between ambulatory and hospital care.

▶ **Information for the hospital clinician.** When being admitted to hospital, patients should receive a list of their current medications, including over-the-counter drugs. This applies even to patients who are not scheduled for surgery. Information about complications that occurred during previous procedures, and about intolerances or previous allergic reactions, can provide valuable insights to hospital clinicians. Measures to optimize the blood sugar metabolism should be taken prior to admission.

▶ **Information for the general practitioner.** In an age of increasingly shorter hospital stays and, accordingly, of discharge earlier during the postoperative period, hospital clinicians should ensure that the GP will receive any important information in a timely fashion to effect a smooth transition from the inpatient setting to ambulatory care. For example, the information provided by the discharging physician is essential for the organization of care at home or at a nursing home. Medication prescriptions at discharge should ideally reflect the main medications used in the outpatient sector (KBV 2011).

> **Note**
>
> In the interest of patient safety, both hospital clinicians and GPs should be provided with comprehensive information at an early stage.

2.2.4 Preoperative Diagnostic Testing

▶ **Recommendations.** Several guidelines advise against the preoperative measurement of standard laboratory values without a specific indication (DGAI 2010, Card et al 2014). However, for some clinical scenarios there is not enough scientific evidence available.

▶ **False-positive results.** As early as in 1993, a meta-analysis of routine preoperative chest X-rays noted that these investigations were more likely to lead to false-positive results than to procedural changes. One outcome of false-positive results is that they give rise to more-invasive testing with associated risks, anxiety, and costs (Archer et al 1993).

The following examples are intended to explain why the routine ordering of preoperative diagnostic tests tends to lead to false-positive results, especially in a low-prevalence setting such as general practice, and can therefore not be recommended. A routine approach to preoperative diagnostic testing does not only run the risk of conferring no benefit but—in the worst case—it can even harm the patient. We will try to demonstrate this using the three most common preoperative tests—electrocardiography, chest X-rays, and blood count—as examples. Similar limitations are associated with other preoperative tests that are carried out without a clear indication, such as lung function tests and blood tests to determine the level of thyroid-stimulating hormone.

Electrocardiography

The sensitivity of electrocardiography (ECG) for detecting coronary heart disease (CHD) is approximately 50% and the specificity is 90% (Abholz and Donner-Banzhoff 2006). As our first example, we take the case of a 55-year-old asymptomatic female patient who has no significant underlying conditions. The pretest probability (i.e., the prevalence) of CHD in this age group is approximately 8%. A positive ECG result has a positive predictive value of approximately 3% to detect hitherto undiagnosed CHD. This low positive predictive value, i.e., the low probability that a patient with a positive ECG result does indeed have CHD, is attributable to the low prevalence of this disease among patients in general practice.

If the patient for whom the ECG was performed had been a 65-year-old male smoker with a high blood pressure and chest pain on exertion, the prevalence would have been 94% and the positive predictive value would have been approximately 90%.

The calculation of the positive predictive value is based on the Bayes theorem, which will be explained below using a 2×2 contingency table and the example of a preoperative chest X-ray.

Chest X-ray

Example from a Low-prevalence Setting

Let us assume that 1,000 patients are scheduled to undergo surgery. A routine chest X-ray is carried out for each patient. If the prevalence of a disease of interest "XY" were 0.5%, the ratio of patients with and without the disease would be 5:995. At an assumed sensitivity of 80%, a chest X-ray would identify four of five patients with the disease. With a specificity of 65%, 647 of these patients would have a true-negative result, but 348 would have a false-positive result. This would therefore produce a total of $4 + 348 = 352$ positive chest X-ray results despite the fact that only four patients really have the disease. The probability of each of them actually having the disease would be just over 1% (**Table 2.4**).

- Sensitivity (ability of a test to detect a disease when it is indeed present): $a / (a + c) = 4 / (4 + 1)$ = 80%.
- Specificity (ability of a test to indicate the absence of a disease when no disease is present): $d / (b + d) = 647 / (348 + 647) = 65\%$.
- Positive predictive value (the probability that a patient with a positive test result does indeed have the disease): $a / (a + b) = 4 / (4 + 348) = 1\%$.
- Negative predictive value (the probability that a patient with a negative test result does not have the disease: $d / (c + d) = 647 / (1 + 647) =$ almost 100%.

For a patient with a normal chest X-ray result, the presence of the disease of interest can be ruled out with almost 100% certainty. However, even for a patient with a positive result, the probability of the disease being present is extremely low.

For almost 99% of patients with a positive chest X-ray result for the disease of interest "XY," the

Table 2.4 Chest X-ray examination in a low-prevalence setting

X-ray result	Disease of interest is present	Disease of interest is not present	Total
Positive	4 (a)	348 (b)	352
Negative	1 (c)	647 (d)	648
Total	5	995	1,000

Table 2.5 Chest X-ray examination in a high-prevalence setting

X-ray result	Disease of interest is present	Disease of interest is not present	Total
Positive	160 (a)	280 (b)	440
Negative	40 (c)	520 (d)	560
Total	200	800	1,000

result would trigger a cascade of further diagnostic tests. This would not only delay the scheduled operation and result in unnecessary additional costs, but it would also cause anxiety to the patient, often for no reason. This phenomenon is sometimes called the *cascade effect in medicine* (Kuehlein et al 2010). In addition to the false-positive results for the disease of interest, an X-ray can "generate" a plethora of other signs of diseases with an even lower prevalence, with even lower positive predictive values.

Example from a High-prevalence Setting

Let us now assume that 1,000 patients who are scheduled to undergo surgery come from a setting with a different prevalence, for example a hospital with a 20% prevalence of the disease of interest "XY." Once again, a routine chest X-ray is carried out for each patient. If the prevalence is 20%, the expected ratio of patients with and without the disease will be 200:800. If the sensitivity is 80% (as before), the chest X-ray will detect 160 of 200 patients who have the disease. If the specificity is again assumed to be 65%, 520 patients will have a true-negative X-ray result, but 280 patients will have a false-positive result. This will produce a total of 160 + 280 = 440 positive X-ray results, despite the fact that only 200 of these patients do indeed have the disease. The probability of each of them actually having the disease will thus be 36%. However, the percentage of patients with a false-positive X-ray result will still be as high as 64%. It will depend on the threat posed by the disease and on its impact on the risks associated with anesthesia and surgery whether the consequences of a false-positive result will offset the gains in safety for the 36% of patients who have a true-positive result (**Table 2.5**).

- Sensitivity (ability of a test to detect a disease when it is indeed present): a / (a + c) = 160 / (160 + 40) = 80%.
- Specificity (ability of a test to indicate the absence of a disease when no disease is present): d / (b + d) = 520 / (280 + 520) = 65%.
- Positive predictive value (the probability that a patient with a positive test result does indeed have the disease): a / (a + b) = 160 / (160 + 280) = 36%.
- Negative predictive value (the probability that a patient with a negative test result does not have the disease: d / (c + d) = 520 / (40 + 520) = 93%.

These examples illustrate the consequences of engaging in diagnostic testing for diseases where the clinical probability is low because neither the patient's medical history nor the physical examination show any evidence of the disease being present. Since such evidence would increase the pretest probability for this disease and thus also the positive predictive value, this attests to the paramount importance of taking an in-depth preoperative medical history, followed by a thorough physical examination.

Blood Count

Matters are somewhat different when it comes to performing a blood count to rule out anemia. The blood count does not simply provide a diagnostic hint—it is the standard diagnostic test for anemia. The prevalence of anemia is very high for certain diseases, and this should also be taken into consideration (see **Table 3.1**, Chapter 3.1.1). There are no false-positive or false-negative results depending on the interpretation of the findings, as seen in the case of X-rays. False-positive or false-negative results can only occur because of measurement errors in the laboratory or a mix-up of blood samples.

CONTENT is a project at Heidelberg University Hospital (Laux et al 2005). The acronym stands for CONTinuous Morbidity Registration Epidemiologic NeTwork. It entails the establishment of a morbidity registry in primary care to answer questions about the morbidity in this health care sector. With the help of documentation according to the International Classification of Primary Care (ICPC-2), and by taking treatment episodes into account, a database was set up using a modified practice management software package. This enables the demonstration of relationships between the reasons for a consultation, the medical procedures, and the outcomes of the consultation. To date, the registry contains data on more than 130,670 patients. Based on data from the CONTENT project, the total prevalence of anemia among patients in primary care is 1.8%. For patients aged 50 years and older, it is 2.8%. For patients aged 50 years and older who belong to ASA groups I and II, it is presumably somewhat lower, whereas it will be somewhat higher for ASA groups III and IV. There is therefore a marked difference between the prevalence of anemia in primary care versus hospitals. The positive predictive value for preoperative outpatients should always be interpreted in light of the prevalence of the disease of interest in the outpatient setting. All physicians involved in the care of these patients should bear this in mind when analyzing the test results, because the power of these tests is largely dependent on the prevalence in the respective setting.

2.2.5 Summary of Recommendations

Preoperative diagnostic testing must take account of the special characteristics of the low-prevalence setting in which the GP works. Routine measurement of laboratory parameters is not recommended. An in-depth diagnostic workup is advisable in certain patient groups or if there is clinical evidence to warrant this approach, especially prior to high-risk operations.

The GP's primary task is to present as comprehensive a picture as possible of the patient's medical history and comorbidities. On the part of the hospital, good discharge management is desirable.

Conclusion

Any diagnostic testing in a low-prevalence setting that is not warranted by findings from the medical history or clinical examination will cause unnecessary anxiety to the patient, while achieving limited or no benefit in terms of anesthesia and surgical safety.

2.3 Calculation of the Transfusion Probability—the Mercuriali Algorithm

P. H. Rehak

2.3.1 Significance of the Perioperative Transfusion Probability

Knowledge of the perioperative transfusion probability, or rather of the likely number of perioperative units of red blood cell (RBC) concentrate required, will help to make exact provision for the blood products needed and, accordingly, to avoid an unnecessary supply.

The perioperative need for RBC concentrates can be estimated using the Mercuriali algorithm (Mercuriali and Inghilleri 1996).

2.3.2 Circulating Blood Volume

All subsequent calculations are based on an estimate of the circulating blood volume. The blood volume is calculated according to the following equation (Nadler et al 1962):

$$BV = a \times H^3 + b \times W + c \qquad (1)$$

where BV = blood volume (L), H = height (m), and W = weight (kg). The constants a, b, and c are gender-specific (**Table 2.6**).

Table 2.6 Constants used for calculating the blood volume

Constant	Women	Men
a	0.3561	0.3669
b	0.03308	0.03219
c	0.1833	0.6041

The following equations for the gender-specific calculation of the blood volume can be derived from equation 1:

Formula

Blood volume

Women: $BV = 0.3561 \times H^3 + 0.03308 \times W + 0.1833$ (2)

Men: $BV = 0.3669 \times H^3 + 0.03219 \times W + 0.6041$ (3)

BV = blood volume (L), H = height (m), W = weight (kg).

▶ **Example.** A woman, height = 170 cm (1.7 m), weight = 65 kg:

$BV = 0.3561 \times 1.7^3 + 0.03308 \times 65 + 0.1833 = 4.083\,L = 4,083\,mL$

Alternatively, the blood volume can be determined without any calculation on the basis of the nomogram illustrated in **Fig. 2.1**.

> **Note** ❗
>
> The circulating blood volume is calculated based on the height and weight, adjusted for gender.

2.3.3 Circulating Red Blood Cell Volume

The circulating RBC volume can now be calculated easily from the blood volume and whole body hematocrit:

$RCV = BV \times Hctb$ (4)

where RCV = RBC volume (L), BV = blood volume based on equation 2 or 3 (L), Hctb = whole body hematocrit (L/L); hematocrit values expressed in % have to be divided by 100.

The whole body hematocrit represents an average hematocrit value that lies between the lower arterial hematocrit and the higher venous hematocrit. The whole body hematocrit is obtained by multiplying the measured venous hematocrit (Hctv) with the empirically determined correction factor 0.91 (Chaplin et al 1953):

$Hctb = Hctv \times 0.91$ (5)

If one inserts equation 5 into equation 4, one obtains the RBC volume calculated on the basis of the venous hematocrit value:

Formula

RBC volume

$RCV = BV \times Hctv \times 0.91$ (6)

RCV = RBC volume (L), BV = blood volume based on equation 2 or 3 (L), Hctv = venous hematocrit (L/L).

Since the hematocrit is a dimensionless variable (L/L), the blood volume can also be expressed in milliliters rather than in liters, which gives the RBC volume in milliliters, too.

> **Note** ❗
>
> The circulating RBC volume is calculated from the blood volume and the whole body hematocrit.

2.3.4 Tolerated Red Blood Cell Loss

To calculate the tolerated RBC loss, the minimally acceptable hematocrit must be estimated for the individual patient based on clinical assessment.

It is calculated from the difference between the preoperative RBC volume and the tolerated (i.e., minimally acceptable) postoperative RBC volume:

$tlRCV = RCV_{preop} - RCV_{min\ acceptable}$ (7)

where tlRCV = tolerated RBC loss (L), RCV_{preop} = preoperative RBC volume (L), $RCV_{min\ acceptable}$ = minimally acceptable postoperative RBC volume.

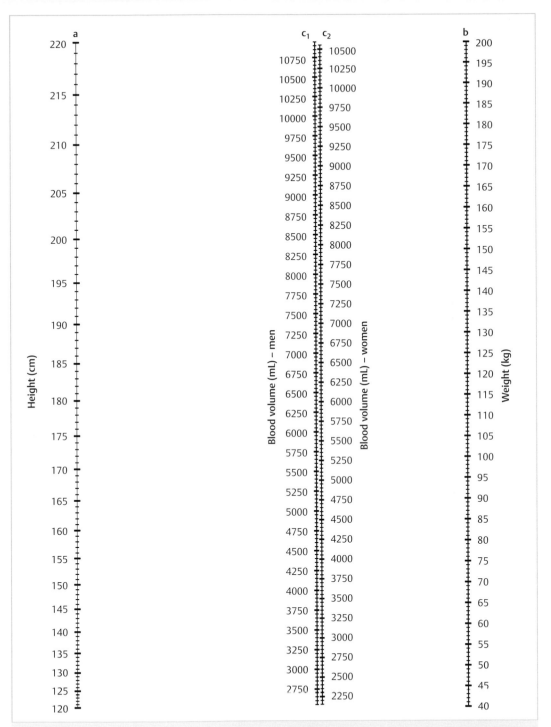

Fig. 2.1 Nomogram to determine the blood volume (in mL). Instructions: Mark the height on axis a and the weight on axis b. Join the two marks with a straight line. The point of intersection between this straight line and the relevant middle axis (c_1 for men, c_2 for women) gives the blood volume in mL.

The preoperative and minimally acceptable postoperative RBC volumes are calculated using equation 6:

$$RCV_{preop} = BV \times Hctv_{preop} \times 0.91 \qquad (8)$$

$$RCV_{min\ acceptable} = BV \times Hctv_{min\ acceptable} \times 0.91 \qquad (9)$$

The values for Hctv must be given in L/L or mL/mL.

Equations 8 and 9 can now be inserted into equation 7, giving the tolerated RBC loss:

$$tlRCV = BV \times Hctv_{preop} \times 0.91 - BV \times Hctv_{min\ acceptable} \times 0.91 \qquad (10)$$

which can be simplified further:

Formula

Tolerated RBC loss

$$tlRCV = BV \times (Hctv_{preop} - Hctv_{min\ acceptable}) \times 0.91 \qquad (11)$$

tlRCV = tolerated RBC loss (L), BV = blood volume based on equation 2 or 3 (L), Hctv$_{preop}$ = preoperative venous hematocrit (L/L), Hctv$_{min\ acceptable}$ = minimally acceptable postoperative venous hematocrit (L/L).

Here, too, the values can be entered in milliliters instead of in liters.

▶ **Example.** The woman from the example given in Chapter 2.3.2; BV = 4.083 L, Hctv$_{preop}$ = 0.36 L/L, Hctv$_{min\ acceptable}$ = 0.22 L/L:

$$tlRCV = 4.083 \times (0.36 - 0.22) \times 0.91 = 0.5202\ mL$$

The tolerated RBC loss is thus approximately 520 mL.

Note

The tolerated RBC loss is calculated from the blood volume and the difference between the preoperative and minimally acceptable hematocrit values.

2.3.5 Predicted Perioperative Red Blood Cell Loss

To estimate the predicted perioperative RBC loss as recommended by Mercuriali, the perioperative RBC loss is to be calculated for all operations of the same type (e.g., all primary unilateral total hip replacements) carried out in the respective center over the previous 6–12 months (Mercuriali and Inghilleri 1996). The perioperative period is defined as the interval from the start of the operation until day 5 after surgery.

In analogy to the calculation of the tolerated RBC loss (see Chapter 2.3.4), the perioperative RBC loss can be calculated from the difference between the preoperative RBC volume and the RBC volume on day 5 after surgery, adding the RBC volume of any RBC concentrates transfused perioperatively (the compensated RBC loss) (Mercuriali and Inghilleri 1996):

$$plRCV = RCV_{preop} - RCV_{5d\ postop} + tRCV \qquad (12)$$

where plRCV = perioperative RBC loss (L), RCV$_{preop}$ = preoperative RBC volume (L), RCV$_{5d\ postop}$ = RBC volume on day 5 after surgery (L), tRCV = transfused RBC volume (L).

The pre- and postoperative RBC volumes are calculated using equation 6:

$$RCV_{preop} = BV \times Hctv_{preop} \times 0.91 \qquad (13)$$

$$RCV_{5d\ postop} = BV \times Hctv_{5d\ postop} \times 0.91 \qquad (14)$$

The transfused RBC volume is calculated from the number, volume, and hematocrit of the transfused RBC concentrates:

$$tRCV = n_{RCC} \times V_{RCC} \times Hct_{RCC} \qquad (15)$$

where tRCV = transfused RBC volume (L), n$_{RCC}$ = number of transfused RBC concentrates, V$_{RCV}$ = volume of the transfused RBC concentrates (L), and Hct$_{RCC}$ = hematocrit of the transfused RBC concentrates (L/L).

Equations 13, 14, and 15 can now be inserted into equation 12 and simplified as seen in Chapter 2.3.4:

Formula

Perioperative RBC loss

$$plRCV = BV \times (Hctv_{preop} - Hctv_{5d\ postop}) \times 0.91 + n_{RCC} \times V_{RCC} \times Hct_{RCC} \qquad (16)$$

plRCV = perioperative RBC loss (L), BV = blood volume based on equation 2 or 3 (L), Hctv$_{preop}$ = preoperative venous hematocrit (L/L), Hctv$_{5d\ postop}$ = venous hematocrit on day 5 after surgery (L/L), n$_{RCC}$ = number of perioperatively transfused RBC concentrates, V$_{RCC}$ = volume of the perioperatively transfused RBC concentrates (L), and Hct$_{RCC}$ = hematocrit of the perioperatively transfused RBC concentrates (L/L).

Here, too, the volumes can be expressed either in liters or in milliliters.

▶ **Example.** The woman from the example in Chapter 2.3.2; BV = 4.083 L, $Hctv_{preop}$ = 0.36 L/L, $Hctv_{5d\ postop}$ = 0.27 L/L; perioperative transfusion of 3 units of RBC concentrates with a volume of 300 mL (V_{RCC} = 0.3 L) and a hematocrit of 60% (Hct_{RCC} = 0.6 L/L):

plRCV = 4.083 × (0.36 – 0.27) × 0.91 + 3 × 0. 3 × 0.6 = 0.3344 + 0.54 = 0.8744 L = 874.4 mL.

The perioperative RBC loss in this operation is therefore approximately 875 mL

Note

The perioperative RBC loss is calculated from the blood volume and the difference between the preoperative and postoperative hematocrit values. If RBC concentrates have been transfused, their RBC volume must be added.

This calculation must now be carried out for all operations of the same type that have been performed over the past 6 to 12 months. If the algorithm is to be routinely used, it is advisable to carry this calculation out prospectively for all operations in which RBC concentrates are used, and to integrate it into the clinical documentation.

From the distribution of the values calculated above for the RBC loss, Mercuriali recommends using the 80th percentile as the predicted perioperative RBC loss for the respective type of operation. The 80th percentile is the RBC loss value that is higher than 80% of all the calculated values.

▶ **Example.** "Unilateral total hip replacement" is considered as the type of surgery; N = 250 such operations were performed over the previous 12 months in a given institution. If the 80th percentile of the RBC loss is 915 mL, this means that the RBC loss for 80% of the operations (200 operations) was less than or equal to 915 mL, and it was higher for the remaining 20% (50 operations).

The 80th percentile can be calculated using statistics software or table calculation software. In the latter case, the values denoting RBC loss are entered into one column and sorted in ascending order. The 80th percentile will be the value given in line N × 0.8; in the example this is the value in line 200 (N = 250 operations, N × 0.8 = 200).

2.3.6 Predicted Transfusion Requirement

The predicted transfusion requirement—the RBC volume that will most likely be needed—can now be calculated from the difference between the anticipated RBC loss according to Chapter 2.3.5 and the tolerated RBC loss according to Chapter 2.3.4 (Inghilleri 2010):

Formula

Mercuriali algorithm

$$rRCV = alRCV - tlRCV \qquad (17)$$

where rRCV = required RBC volume (L), alRCV = anticipated RBC loss (L), tlRCV = tolerated RBC loss (L).

The anticipated RBC loss is calculated according to Chapter 2.3.5, the tolerated RBC loss according to equation 11. Insertion of equation 11 in equation 17 gives:

Formula

Predicted volume of red blood cells required

$$rRCV = alRCV - BV \times (Hctv_{preop} - Hctv_{min\ acceptable}) \times 0.91 \qquad (18)$$

rRCV = predicted volume of RBC concentrates required (L), alRCV = anticipated RBC loss (L), BV = blood volume based on equation 2 or 3 (L), $Hctv_{preop}$ = preoperative venous hematocrit (L/L), $Hctv_{min\ acceptable}$ = minimally acceptable postoperative venous hematocrit (L/L).

If a negative number is obtained for rRCV, the tolerated RBC loss is greater than the predicted loss. In such a case, no RBC concentrates will be required.

Note

The predicted transfusion requirement is calculated from the difference between the predicted and the tolerated RBC loss. A negative transfusion requirement indicates that no transfusion will be required.

The predicted number of RBC concentrates required is obtained by dividing the predicted volume of RBC concentrates required by the volume of RBC concentrates transfused:

Formula

Number of red blood cell concentrates required

$$rn_{RCC} = rRCV / (V_{RCC} \times Hct_{RCC}) \tag{19}$$

rn_{RCC} = predicted number of RBC concentrates required, $rRCV$ = predicted volume of RBC concentrates required (L), V_{RCC} = volume of RBC concentrates used (L), Hct_{RCC} = hematocrit of RBC concentrates used (L/L).

▶ **Example.** The woman from the example in Chapter 2.3.2; BV = 4.083 L, $Hctv_{preop}$ = 0.36 L/L, $Hctv_{min\ acceptable}$ = 0.22 L/L, alRCV = 0.915 L (from the example in Chapter 2.3.5), v_{RCC} = 0.3 L, Hct_{RCC} = 0.6 L/L:

rRCV = 0.915 – 4.083 × (0.36 – 0.22) × 0.91 = 0.915 – 0.5202 = 0.3948 L = 394.8 mL

The predicted volume of RBC concentrates required is therefore approximately 395 mL.

rn_{RCC} = 0.3948 / (0.3 × 0.6) = 2.193

The predicted transfusion requirement is 2.2 units of RBC concentrates.

Postoperative Hematocrit

The predicted postoperative hematocrit—with or without the transfusion of RBC concentrates—can also be calculated from the predicted perioperative RBC loss. To do this, the perioperative RBC loss (plRCV) in equation 16 is replaced with the anticipated RBC loss (alRCV):

$$alRCV = BV \times (Hctv_{preop} - Hctv_{5d\ postop}) \times 0.91 + n_{RCC} \times V_{RCC} \times Hct_{RCC} \tag{20}$$

Solving this equation for the postoperative hematocrit gives:

Formula

Postoperative hematocrit

$$Hctv_{5d\ postop} = Hctv_{preop} - (alRCV - n_{RCC} \times V_{RCC} \times Hct_{RCC}) / (BV \times 0.91) \tag{21}$$

$Hctv_{5d\ postop}$ = venous hematocrit on day 5 after surgery (L/L), $Hctv_{preop}$ = preoperative venous hematocrit (L/L), alRCV = anticipated RBC loss (L), n_{RCC} = number of perioperatively transfused RBC concentrates, V_{RCC} = volume of perioperatively transfused RBC concentrates (L), Hct_{RCC} = hematocrit of perioperatively transfused RBC concentrates (L/L), BV = blood volume based on equation 2 or 3 (L).

▶ **Example.** The woman from the example given in Chapter 2.3.2; BV = 4.083 L, $Hctv_{preop}$ = 0.36 L/L, alRCV = 0.915 L (from the example in Chapter 2.3.5), V_{RCC} = 0.3 L, Hct_{RCC} = 0.6 L/L:

$Hctv_{5d\ postop}$ = 0.36 – (0.915 – n_{RCC} × 0.3 × 0.6) / (4.083 × 0.91)

The results for n_{RCC} = 0 (no transfusion) to n_{RCC} = 4 are given in **Table 2.7**. Hemoglobin was calculated as described in Chapter 2.3.7, with a mean corpuscular hemoglobin concentration (MCHC) of 34 g/dL.

Note

The anticipated RBC loss can also be used to calculate the predicted postoperative hematocrit, rather than the predicted transfusion requirement, for various scenarios (no transfusion, transfusion of various numbers of RBC units).

Table 2.7 Predicted postoperative hematocrit and hemoglobin values

n_{RCC}	$Hctv_{5d\ postop}$ (L/L)	$Hb_{5d\ postop}$ (g/dL)
0	0.114	3.9
1	0.162	5.5
2	0.211	7.2
3	0.259	8.8
4	0.308	10.5

Abbreviations: $Hb_{5d\ postop}$ = hemoglobin value on day 5 after surgery; $Hctv_{5d\ postop}$ = venous hematocrit on day 5 after surgery; nRCC, number of red blood cell concentrates transfused.

2.3.7 Conversion between Hematocrit and Hemoglobin

The required hematocrit can also be calculated from the corresponding hemoglobin concentration. The two values are linked through the MCHC:

$$Hct = Hb / MCHC \qquad (22)$$

where Hct = hematocrit (L/L), Hb = hemoglobin concentration (g/dL), MCHC = mean corpuscular hemoglobin concentration (g/dL).

The hemoglobin concentration is calculated from the hematocrit:

$$Hb = Hct \times MCHC \qquad (23)$$

The MCHC is calculated from the mean corpuscular hemoglobin and the mean corpuscular volume:

$$MCHC = 100 \times MCH / MCV \qquad (24)$$

where MCHC = mean corpuscular hemoglobin concentration (g/dL), MCH = mean corpuscular hemoglobin (picogram, pg), MCV = mean corpuscular volume (femtoliter, fL).

The factor 100 is obtained from conversion to the customary unit of g/dL (pg/fL is the same as g/mL). If the MCH and MCV are not available, an MCHC value of 34 g/dL can be assumed (reference range, 33–36 g/dL).

> **Note**
>
> The MCHC can be used for conversion between the hematocrit and hemoglobin values. Normally, an MCHC value of 34 g/dL can be assumed.

2.3.8 Discussion and Summary

Correction Factor to Obtain the Whole Body Hematocrit

In the original study by Mercuriali and Inghilleri (1996), the correction factor 0.91 was not used to obtain the whole body hematocrit from the peripheral venous hematocrit measured, as per Chaplin and colleagues (1953). This factor was only used in later studies (e.g., Sonzogni et al 2001).

Omission of this correction has a direct impact on the value calculated for the tolerated RBC loss—the estimate will be approximately 10% higher. When estimating the perioperative RBC loss and

the predicted volume of RBC concentrates required, the effect is reduced because the difference between two hematocrit values is being calculated. In the cited examples, omission of the correction factor would result in an estimated perioperative RBC loss that is approximately 4% higher, whereas the predicted volume of RBC concentrates required would be approximately 3.5% lower.

As such, the error caused by omission of the correction is relatively small, especially since all calculations are estimates. Therefore, useful results can also be obtained without using the factor of 0.91.

80th Percentile

The 80th percentile for the anticipated RBC loss is a cutoff that has been chosen arbitrarily and it should be considered as a suggestion. Naturally, other cutoffs for the distribution of the perioperative RBC loss can also be used, e.g., the 90th percentile or the upper limit of the 80%, 90%, or 95% confidence interval.

If the 80th percentile is used to estimate the transfusion requirement, it can be assumed—provided that the data from previous operations are representative—that the actual transfusion requirement will be equivalent to, or less than, the estimated requirement in 80% of all operations, and it will be higher in only 20% of all operations. If a negative value is obtained for the predicted transfusion requirement, there is an 80% probability that no transfusion will be needed.

Conclusion

Based on the Mercuriali algorithm and data from previous operations of the same type, it can be estimated whether any—and how many—RBC units will be needed for a scheduled surgery. This will enable a targeted supply and administration of blood products.

If the algorithm is to be used routinely, it is advisable to integrate the perioperative RBC loss into the routine documentation. This will provide the basis for calculating the transfusion requirement for individual patients. In addition, it enables quality control through monitoring of the perioperative RBC loss.

2.4 Ordering Procedures for Blood Products

A. Weigl

2.4.1 Importance of the Procedures Used to Order and Issue Blood Products

When following the principles of PBM, blood products are only needed if there is a transfusion requirement despite application of the three pillars of PBM. However, if blood products are indeed needed, their prompt availability is vital, and the procedures used to order blood products are thus a component of a successful patient management strategy in hospitals.

The costs incurred for ordering and issuing blood products are an important component of the transfusion-related process costs (Shander et al 2010). Efficient and economical ordering procedures are particularly important for RBC concentrates, since these account for the largest and most cost-intensive proportion of blood products transfused in the hospital setting (**Table 2.8**).

Note

The procedures used to order and issue blood products are an important factor to be considered when calculating process costs.

2.4.2 Prerequisites for Transfusion

Economical ordering procedures are designed to assure the availability of serologically compatible blood products for the individual patient, with the lowest wastage rate possible. Serology testing for blood supply purposes involves determination of the blood group antigens (ABO system), including

screening for relevant antibodies to prevent immune-mediated hemolytic transfusion reactions. The greatest immunogenicity, i.e., the ability to induce antibody formation, is generated by the RBC antigens. Immunocompetent individuals form IgM antibodies against A and B antigens as early as during the first year of life. In addition to the A and B antigens, the Rhesus D factor on RBCs is highly immunogenic. Even small numbers of RBCs with the Rhesus D factor are able to induce the formation of anti-D antibodies. A single RBC has more than 500 RBC antigens, which have been serologically defined on the basis of their corresponding antibodies and integrated into the ABO system. In transfusion practice, consideration of the ABO properties and the Rhesus D factor is therefore a top priority.

Note

Ordering procedures should include extensive testing of antigenic properties to assure optimum serological compatibility between donor and recipient.

2.4.3 Red Blood Cell Concentrates

Medical Emergencies

A medical emergency arising because of an emergency admission or bleeding complications may result in an emergency transfusion or a massive transfusion. Because of the enormous time pressure faced when administering an emergency transfusion, uncrossmatched blood (compatible ABO group or blood group 0) will be used (**Table 2.9**). The only safety measure taken is an ABO bedside test of the patient's blood before the transfusion. For forensic reasons, compatibility testing must be carried out at a later stage.

Table 2.8 Consumption of blood products

Blood products	% Number	% Costs
RBC concentrates	73%	56%
Platelet concentrates	6%	34%
Fresh frozen plasma	21%	10%

Abbreviations: RBC, red blood cell.
Note: General hospital in Linz, Austria; the consumption in 2011 is projected for 1,000 beds.

Table 2.9 Compatible transfusion of blood components

Recipient blood group	RBC concentrate blood group	FFP blood group	Platelet concentrate blood group
0	0	0, A, B, AB	0, A, B, AB
A	A, 0	A, AB	A, 0, B, AB
B	B, 0	B, AB	B, 0, A, AB
AB	AB, A, B, 0	AB	AB, A, B, 0

Abbreviations: FFP, fresh frozen plasma; RBC, red blood cell.
Source: Kretschmer et al 2008.

Elective Procedures

The procedures used to order blood components for elective surgical procedures have important financial implications. The costs for testing and issuing blood components account for up to 30% of the total costs incurred for blood products (Shander et al 2010). Hence, for financial reasons alone, it is important to keep the ratio of ordered to transfused blood components as small as possible without jeopardizing patient care. The proportion of crossmatched blood held in reserve and the proportion of blood units ordered but not used should be kept as small as possible (**Fig. 2.2**).

▸ **Crossmatch-to-transfusion ratio.** Ideally, the ratio of tested serologically compatible RBC concentrates to RBC concentrates actually transfused (*crossmatch-to-transfusion ratio* or CTR) should be 1.0; however, it is only in the outpatient setting that this value can be achieved to any extent. The CTR is a key performance indicator that is easy to calculate and serves as a measure of the effectiveness of ordering procedures. In practice this value varies between 2.0 and 5.0 depending on the department and the surgical speciality; a value of 1.7 is an achievable quality target for the surgical setting (**Table 2.10**). A reduction in the mean CTR from 3.0 to 2.0 corresponds to a 33% decline in the number of unnecessary RBC units that have undergone full serological testing. Achievement of the potential CTR target value of 1.7 means a 56% decline in the number of RBC units ordered.

> **Note**
>
> The CTR is the ratio of crossmatched to actually transfused RBC units. For surgical procedures the CTR target value is 1.7.

▸ **Ordering systems.** The number of RBC units to be ordered for an elective procedure depends on several factors and should be jointly agreed by the

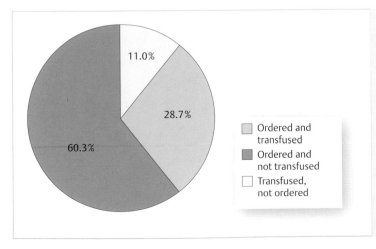

Fig. 2.2 Ratio of ordered to actually transfused RBC concentrates in Austrian hospitals (Gombotz et al 2011b).

11.0%
28.7%
60.3%

Ordered and transfused
Ordered and not transfused
Transfused, not ordered

Table 2.10 Improvement of the ordering procedure

Authors	Type of surgery	Ordered:transfused	
		Before the intervention	After the intervention
Rogers et al 2006	Orthopaedic surgery	3.21:1	1.62:1
Mehra et al 2004	Knee joint replacement	4.90:1	1.70:1
Foley et al 2003	Gynecology	2.25:1	1.71:1
Source: Gombotz et al 2011b.			

surgeon and anesthesiologist. For standard operations, hospitals normally have an ordering catalog based on longstanding experience. This approach corresponds to the Maximum Surgical Blood Ordering Schedule described in the literature (Palmer et al 2003). In general, blood products are ordered largely independently of patient-specific factors. The advantage of such a system is that it is so easy to manage; good results can only be achieved for operations where blood loss is primarily dependent on the surgeons involved.

Various parameters can be used to predict the need for RBC transfusion. In addition to the obvious factors, such as baseline hemoglobin, predicted blood loss, and the transfusion threshold, parameters that are specific to the respective center, such as the type of procedure, surgical technique, duration of the operation, treating surgeon, and distance between blood bank and operating room, also play a role (Gombotz et al 2007). A patient-specific blood ordering system that is tailored to the characteristics of the individual patient can thus further optimize the ordering process (Palmer et al 2003).

▶ **The most important predictive factors.** The parameters of practical relevance in predicting the transfusion requirement with high reliability are the preoperative hemoglobin value, the retrospectively calculated perioperative blood loss, and the transfusion trigger (three-pillar strategy) (**Fig. 2.3**).

By using the Mercuriali algorithm, which was formulated on the basis of these parameters and also includes the blood loss tolerated by the individual patient, the transfusion requirement can be calculated for the individual patient (Mercuriali and Inghilleri 1996) (see Chapter 2.3). Mathematical algorithms are better able to calculate the transfusion probability than other prediction

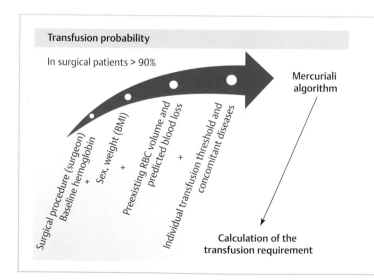

Fig. 2.3 Predictors of the probability of RBC transfusion (Gombotz et al 2011b). BMI, body mass index.

models, in particular for specific patient groups (e.g., children or overweight patients).

Note

The Mercuriali algorithm enables a patient-specific calculation of the predicted transfusion requirement before elective procedures.

Ordering based on the Predicted Transfusion Requirement

▶ **Transfusion probability.** Based on the calculation of the predicted transfusion requirement, the required number of RBC units are ordered from the blood bank. In practice, it is advisable to combine the various systems available for predicting the transfusion probability. This will give a sufficiently accurate estimate within a justifiable amount of time and diagnostic effort. In **Fig. 2.4**

an example of an ordering algorithm is shown, based on previous anemia treatment.

In light of the legal regulations on quality control in transfusion medicine, it is advisable to compare the calculated and ordered number of RBC units with the number that has actually been used, and to analyze these data for each indication. A 2 × 2 table can be used to verify the validity of the calculated transfusion probability (**Table 2.11**). The statistical parameters of sensitivity, specificity, positive predictive value, negative predictive value, and the efficacy can be calculated from the table using the corresponding patient data.

▶ **Specificity.** The specificity (a measure of the probability of correctly calculating unnecessary blood in advance) is an important key performance indicator of an ordering algorithm. In practice, a high specificity means that the conclusion of "no predicted transfusion requirement" has high reliability. In financial terms, this statement

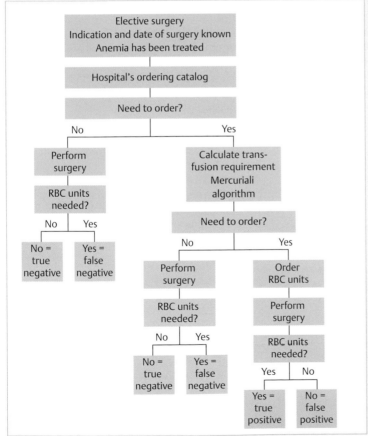

Fig. 2.4 Decision-making tree for ordering procedures.

Table 2.11 2 × 2 table for the calculation of statistical parameters

Predicted transfusion requirement	Patient transfused	Patient not transfused
Yes	True positive	False positive
No	False negative	True negative

means that no costs will be incurred for ordering blood products for patients in this segment.

▶ **Positive predictive value.** Costs are incurred when ordering blood products for patients with a predicted transfusion requirement. The positive predictive value is a measure of the probability that the blood products ordered are actually needed. For a CTR of 2, the positive predictive value is 50%, whereas a targeted CTR of 1.7 leads to a positive predictive value that is close to 59%!

▶ **Statistical verification.** Regardless of the model chosen by a center to predict the transfusion requirement, it is advisable—and indeed imperative—that this method is statistically evaluated at regular intervals and that the reasons for any false-positive and false-negative predictions are identified. This should be a collaborative endeavor between the transfusion director, the patient blood manager, and the teams in the respective departments. The conclusions drawn can be applied to future ordering procedures.

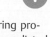

> **Note**
>
> Regular statistical verification of ordering procedures improves the accuracy of the predicted transfusion requirement.

▶ **Financial and legal consequences.** This also has clear financial implications for ordering procedures. If the percentage of transfused patients among those with a given indication is less than 5%, a type-and-screen order can be used instead of routinely ordering RBC units (Gombotz et al 2007). Crossmatching of RBC concentrates despite a low transfusion probability is only advisable in patients with a positive antibody screening test, to counter any unforeseen eventualities in the operating room. The practice of routinely ordering RBC concentrates can be fully dispensed with for elective procedures that have been carried out without

transfusions over a longer period of time (6 months).

In addition, precise prediction of the transfusion probability must be viewed against the legal background. For example, the legally binding hemotherapy guidelines in Germany stipulate that patients must be informed about the risk of allogeneic RBC transfusion if the transfusion probability is greater than 10% (Lauscher et al 2012).

2.4.4 Platelet Concentrates

In general, platelet concentrates, which are particularly expensive, are not ordered in advance—they are requested when needed and transfused immediately after their release from the blood bank because of their special storage requirements (continuous agitation at +22 ± 2°C) and short shelf life (5 days maximum). The number of RBCs contained in 1 unit of platelet concentrate is generally not enough to trigger a major hemolytic transfusion reaction due to ABO antibodies. Normally only ABO and Rhesus D factor are taken into account for platelet transfusions. However, transfusion of the identical blood group improves the clinical course and should be preferred (Sadani et al 2006). Additional testing for human leukocyte antigens (HLA) and/or human platelet antigens (HPA) is carried out only if the platelet count increment is less than 50% of that expected. Such a patient is considered to be treatment-refractory.

> **Note**
>
> Platelet concentrates must be stored at room temperature and transfused as soon as possible after release from the blood bank.

2.4.5 Fresh Frozen Plasma

A similar approach must be used for fresh frozen plasma (FFP), which should ideally be administered to patients immediately after it has thawed. If it is not immediately administered, thawed FFP in an intact bag can be stored in the drugs refrigerator for up to 1 week. The thawing process will destroy any residues of RBCs, platelets, and leukocytes, and hence there is a marked decline in the immunogenicity of the FFP cellular components. The use of lyophilized plasma obviates the need for thawing, but the plasma must then be transfused immediately after it has dissolved (Van et al 2011). Transfusions are administered between patients of the same ABO blood group or of compatible ABO blood groups, and serology compatibility testing can be omitted. For details on the compatibility of blood products see **Table 2.9**.

>
>
> **Note**
>
> Only the ABO blood group system needs to be borne in mind for the transfusion of FFP.

2.4.6 Ordering Blood Products

Blood products are prescription-only medicines. As such, the name and signature of the requesting physician must appear on the prescription. Thanks to extensive investment in diagnostic tests to detect pathogens, blood products have become very safe in recent years. The adverse reactions that do occur are more often attributable to mistakes made when requesting or administering the blood products.

▶ **Blood sampling.** The blood ordering process begins on the ward when blood is drawn for blood typing, crossmatching, and antibody screening. The samples must be labeled and the information on the blood tube checked against that on the order form. Asking patients to confirm their identity and comparing the details on the blood tube with those on the order form after drawing blood can help to avoid mistakes.

▶ **Order form.** The order form must also list certain drugs administered to the recipient (e.g., plasma expanders, medications that affect coagulation). Details of any current or recent (received during the previous 3 months) RBC transfusions and of any pregnancy must be forwarded to the test laboratory. This information has important implications for the validity of the antibody screening test, which is generally valid for up to 1 week, but its validity is restricted to 4 days

(blood draw day + 3 days) if the above conditions apply.

It is also important to specify if the request is urgent. The laboratory must be able to identify emergency requests since this information will determine the scope of the parameters to be tested.

▶ **Tests.** In general, when RBC concentrates are ordered, the blood group (ABO and Rhesus D) is determined and antibody screening and crossmatching tests are performed. In emergencies, one can deviate from this rule if this is necessary to ward off danger to life or serious damage to the recipient. If warranted by time constraints, one should not wait for the result of the serological compatibility test (crossmatch test), and in life-threatening situations one should not wait for the ABO test result either. The test results must be added to the patient documentation at a later stage.

In patients without antibodies whose ABO blood group has been assessed at least twice, electronic crossmatching may be performed (provided the transfusion service has a corresponding validated computer system). This is substantially faster than serologic crossmatching and can therefore be performed directly before transfusion (Frank et al 2014a).

Single-unit Strategy

The indication for transfusion is based on the clinical picture and the transfusion threshold. In the past, it was customary practice to transfuse 2 units (a double unit), or a multiple of 2 units, of RBCs. There is absolutely no rational explanation for such an approach, which only serves to increase the transfusion risks and costs. Gradual and controlled replacement of the deficient RBC volume until the recommended transfusion threshold is reached is an effective method for avoiding unnecessary transfusions in nonbleeding patients. Working groups that have implemented a single-unit strategy in the hematology/oncology setting have reported a reduction in the use of RBC concentrates by around 25 % (Berger et al 2012).

A single-unit strategy is relatively easily to implement for nonbleeding patients by using a computerized ordering system, and it has a direct impact on blood product consumption in the participating departments.

Note

The single-unit ordering strategy for nonbleeding patients reduces blood consumption and costs.

Conclusion

Blood ordering is an important component of transfusion practice and requires considerable logistical effort. Optimum ordering and issuing procedures based on the actual consumption and the needs of the patient guarantee a reliable supply and the best utilization of the available resources.

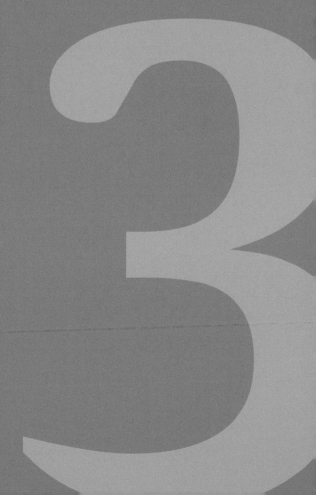

Chapter 3

First Pillar of PBM—Optimization of the Red Blood Cell Volume

3.1 Definition, Diagnosis, and Consequences of Preoperative Anemia

G. Lanzer

3.1.1 Definition, Causes, and Prevalence of Anemia

The term *anemia* is derived from the ancient Greek (αναιμος [*anaimos*]) and means "bloodless" (αν [*an*] "without," αιμα [*haima*] "blood"). As the red blood cell (RBC) mass is very difficult to measure—it requires the use of radioisotopes (Fairbanks et al 1996)—the quantitative deficiency in the oxygen carrier molecule hemoglobin, stored in RBCs, is used instead.

▶ **Hemoglobin thresholds.** In the majority of cases, the thresholds published in a WHO report on nutritional anemia in 1968 continue to be valid: < 13 g/dL for men, < 12 g/dL for menstruating women, and < 11 g/dL for pregnant women. These thresholds were calculated based on average values in the normal population at sea level and have no pathophysiological relevance (WHO 1968). Other authors have suggested a lower

limit of normal of 13.7 g/dL for men younger than 60 years, 13.2 g/dL for men aged 60 years and older, and 12.2 g/dL for women (Beutler and Waalen 2006). Additional adjustments must be made for children, adults aged 65 years and older, and people of different races. Further details on the distribution of hemoglobin concentrations are given in **Fig. 3.1**.

▶ **Causes.** Anemia can be congenital (e.g., in hemoglobinopathy) or acquired. The possible causes include blood loss, malnutrition, hemolysis, autoimmune diseases, hematopoietic disorders, kidney and liver diseases, hormone imbalances, toxins and drugs, parasites, and chronic inflammatory diseases, including various malignancies.

Anemia is rarely a single disease entity. It is predominantly the result of an iron-deficiency state, in particular in the preoperative setting. However, it can also be of multifactorial etiopathogenesis, and there are "idiopathic" forms of anemia, especially among elderly people, e.g., anemia due to age-mediated changes in stem cell physiology, diminished erythropoietin reactivity, or senescent hormonal changes (Guralnik et al 2004).

▶ **Prevalence.** A WHO report states that 1.62 billion people worldwide have anemia of various eti-

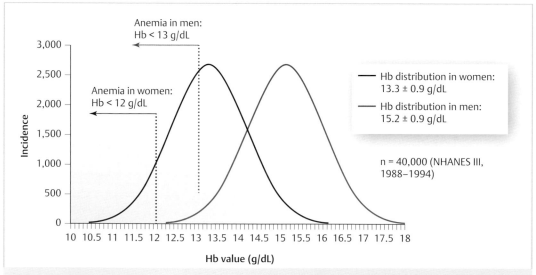

Fig. 3.1 Distribution of hemoglobin concentrations in the general Caucasian population and their relationship to the WHO definition of anemia (Dallman et al 1996). Hb, hemoglobin; NHANES III, National Health and Nutrition Examination Survey III.

ologies. Those affected include, in particular, children of preschool age (prevalence: 47.4%) and women of reproductive age (prevalence among pregnant women: 30.2%). This underestimated health problem is not confined to developing countries; it is also widespread in industrialized countries (McLean et al 2009).

In light of the current demographic trends—in particular in industrialized countries and in preoperative settings—the clinical picture of multifactorial "anemia" is now mainly identified in a multimorbid, previously treated population aged 65 years and older (Patel 2008, Tettamanti et al 2010) (**Table 3.1**). The high prevalence of preoperative anemia (Patel and Carson 2009, Gombotz et al 2011b) must be taken into account in diagnostic and treatment algorithms and must have consequences for preoperative medical management approaches.

Table 3.1 Prevalence of preoperative anemia (Source: Gombotz et al 2011a)

Preoperative anemia	Prevalence (%)
Based on underlying disease	
Diabetes	14–15
Heart failure	10–80
Acute myocardial infarction	6–18
Infections	up to 95
Malignancies	up to 77
Autoimmune disease	up to 71
Kidney disease	up to 50
Chronic obstructive lung disease	23
Preoperative	
ASA I und ASA II	1
Knee and hip operations	20–35
General surgical procedures	up to 40
Colon surgery	25–70
Cardiovascular operations	16–40

Abbreviation: ASA, American Society of Anesthesiologists.

3.1.2 Diagnosis of Anemia

For the diagnosis of anemia, the medical history, clinical picture, clinical examination, and laboratory tests go hand in hand.

Medical History and Clinical Examination

The clinical picture of anemia often goes unnoticed by those affected—depending on the underlying disease—or it is ignored or perceived only after a long delay.

> **Note**
>
> Anemia is often an incidental finding (e.g., it is diagnosed during a routine test or during preoperative assessment).

▶ **Medical history.** Conventional medical history taking is of paramount importance for the (differential) diagnosis, and should be used to classify the multifaceted symptoms on the basis of the subjective complaints (**Table 3.2**).

Next, concurrent issues should be clarified; this goes well beyond the determination of hemoglobin values:
• Preexisting illnesses: kidneys, liver, endocrinopathies, infections; treatment requirements (e.g., because of bleeding), operations, malignancies.
• Bleeding: abnormal menstruation, melena, hematemesis, hemoptysis, hematuria.
• Dietary abnormalities, exposure to toxins, alcohol abuse, medications, drug abuse.
• Previous diagnostic results (e.g., blood count), blood donations, RBC transfusions.
• Unintentional and unexplained weight loss.

▶ **Physical examination.** The accompanying physical examination should focus on:
• Skin/mucosal paleness?
• Signs of cardiorespiratory decompensation?
• Heart murmurs (changes to blood flow and blood viscosity)?
• Bleeding signs (purpura, petechiae)?
• Icteric skin?
• Impaired metabolism (thyroid gland)?
• Hepatomegaly, splenomegaly, lymphadenopathy?
• Reflexes, deep sensibility?

Table 3.2 Multifaceted symptoms in patients with iron deficiency or resultant anemia

Organ systems and symptoms
General symptoms
• Fatigue, exhaustion, weakness, sensitivity to cold
Immune system
• Infection susceptibility due to impaired functioning of the cells of the immune system
Gastrointestinal tract
• Loss of appetite, nausea
Cardiorespiratory system
• Shortness of breath, exertional dyspnea • Tachycardia • Palpitations • Arrhythmias • Stenocardia, dyscardia
Vascular system
• Low skin temperature • Paleness • Vertigo, tendency to collapse
Central nervous system
• Impaired cognitive function, lack of concentration • Absentmindedness • Despondency, depression

Lastly, urine and stool tests should be performed.

Any diagnostic measures aimed at identifying the cause of pathologic blood loss must take account of any iatrogenic blood loss (blood donor?) and interventional blood loss (e.g., due to routine blood draws in intensive care units or cardiac catheter examination).

Laboratory tests

Laboratory tests are an important adjunct to medical history taking and meticulously recorded clinical findings. In addition to obtaining a full blood count and iron metabolism parameters, the stepwise diagnostic workup may include the determination of biochemical parameters, relevant vitamin levels, and/or immunohematology parameters (e.g., antibody screening), and—as a last resort—a bone marrow biopsy.

The full blood count includes the RBC count, RBC indices, reticulocyte parameters, white blood cell count, platelet count, and differential blood count.

Red Blood Cell Count and Indices

The RBC count is measured in accordance with the principles of light scatter or impedance. The hematology analyzer also measures the RBC volume and the hemoglobin concentration (based on the hemoglobincyanide method), and calculates other RBC indices from the results obtained (Thomas 2008):

• *MCV*: mean corpuscular volume (Hct/RBC count) in femtoliters (fL, 10^{-15} L); reference range in adults: 80–96 fL (an MCV-based algorithm for the evaluation of anemia is illustrated in **Fig. 3.2**).

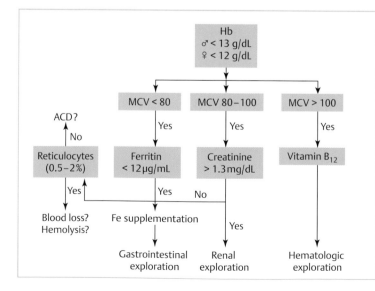

Fig. 3.2 Diagnostic algorithm based on MCV. ACD, anemia of chronic disease; Hb, hemoglobin; MCV, mean corpuscular volume.

- *RDW*: RBC distribution width, MCV distribution, a measure of anisocytosis (RDW = [standard deviation of MCV/mean MCV] × 100); reference range: < 15%.
- *MCH*: mean corpuscular hemoglobin (Hb/RBC count) in picograms (10^{-12} g)/cell; reference range: 28–33 pg.
- *MCHC*: mean corpuscular hemoglobin concentration, a measure of the hemoglobin concentration of the circulating RBC mass (MCH/MCV = Hb/Hct); reference range: 33–36 g/dL.
- *Hct*: hematocrit, packed cell volume in % (RBC count × MCV); reference range in Caucasians: men 36% to 48%, women 40% to 53%.

▶ **Additional information.** Some hematology analyzers can also measure the proportions of hypochromic, microcytic, and macrocytic RBCs:
- *%HYPO*: proportion of hypochromic RBCs (RBCs with hemoglobin < 28 pg); reference range: 1–5%; used for the assessment of a potential iron deficiency—it is an earlier indicator of iron deficiency than the MCV.
- *%MICRO*: proportion of microcytic RBCs; the quotient of %MICRO/%HYPO is used in the diagnosis of β-thalassemia.
- *%MACRO*: proportion of macrocytic RBCs; used to test for vitamin-B_{12} or folic-acid deficiency anemia and for alcohol abuse.

Table 3.3 shows the classification of anemia based on the RBC indices MCV, MCH, and MCHC.

▶ **Causes.** In detail, the findings may indicate the following.
- Normocytic normochromic anemia (a more detailed diagnostic algorithm used to test for this includes the reticulocyte production index [see below]):
  - Hyporegenerative anemia occurring in the presence of chronic or malignant diseases, inflammation, or renal changes.
- Normocytic hypochromic anemia:
  - Early iron deficiency anemia (additional indicators include the RDW, %HYPO, and CHr [see below]).
- Normocytic hyperchromic anemia:
  - Intravascular hemolysis.
  - Incorrect determination of hemoglobin in hyperlipidemia.
  - Heinz bodies in toxic anemia.
- Microcytic hypochromic anemia:
  - Classic iron deficiency anemia.
  - Anemia of chronic disease with functional iron deficiency.
- Macrocytic normochromic anemia:
  - Folic-acid or vitamin-B_{12} deficiency anemia.
  - Alcohol abuse.
  - Cirrhosis of the liver.
  - Myelodysplastic syndrome.
- Macrocytic hypochromic anemia:
  - Regenerative anemia (indicating treatment response).
- Macrocytic hyperchromic anemia:
  - Possibly an incorrect result because of RBC agglutination, e.g., if cold agglutinins are present (RBC count calculated too low, MCV calculated too high).

Reticulocytes

The diagnostic tests involving RBCs—in particular those for the differential diagnosis of anemia—

Table 3.3 Classification of anemia on the basis of the RBC indices MCV, MCH, and MCHC

Anemia	MCV (fL)	MCH (pg)	MCHC (g/dL)
Normocytic normochromic anemia	80–96	28–33	33–36
Normocytic hypochromic anemia	Normal	< 28	Normal
Normocytic hyperchromic anemia	Normal	> 33	> 36
Microcytic hypochromic anemia	< 80	< 28	< 33
Macrocytic normochromic anemia	> 96	Normal	Normal
Macrocytic hypochromic anemia	> 96	< 28	< 33
Macrocytic hyperchromic anemia	> 96	> 28	> 36

Abbreviations: MCH, mean corpuscular hemoglobin; MCHC, mean corpuscular hemoglobin concentration; MCV, mean corpuscular volume.

must be complemented by the additional assessment of reticulocytes.

▶ **Reticulocyte count.** The reticulocyte count gives insights into bone marrow activity, impaired erythropoiesis, and response to treatment, e.g., erythropoietin therapy. The reticulocyte count is provided as the proportion of RBCs that are reticulocytes (reticulocytes/100 mature RBCs; reference range: 5–15%) or expressed as an absolute value (reticulocytes/μL = [% reticulocytes × RBC count/μL]/100; reference range: 50,000–100,000 reticulocytes/μL) (Wick et al 2011).

▶ **Reticulocyte index.** If the reticulocyte count is elevated or the RBC count decreased, the reticulocyte index is calculated to adjust for the altered proportions and for a normal hematocrit (= 45%):

Formula

Reticulocyte index (%) =
[% reticulocytes × Hct %] / 45

This correction is recommended for the assessment of patients with anemia, and a hematologist must be consulted if there are any issues to be clarified.

▶ **Reticulocyte production index.** The reticulocyte production index (RPI) is used to gain additional information, e.g., about the proliferative activity of bone marrow (Patel and Carson 2009). It takes the current hematocrit value of the patient into account:

Formula

RPI = % reticulocytes × [patient Hct/normal Hct (= 45)] × [1 / shift correction factor (= 1–2.5)]

The correction factor is 1.0 if Hct = 36–45%; 1.5 if Hct = 26–35%; 2.0 if Hct = 16–25%; and 2.5 if Hct ≤ 15%.

The term *shift* is used to denote the relationship between the hematocrit and the reticulocyte retention time in peripheral blood (it refers to the shift in the maturation or retention time of reticulocytes upon their release from the bone marrow into the peripheral blood). The physiological maturation time of reticulocytes is approximately 3 days in bone marrow and 1 day in peripheral blood. If the RBC production is accelerated, the retention and maturation time of reticulocytes in bone marrow will be shorter because of their accelerated release. Depending on the respective hematocrit, this will lead to a relative increase in the reticulocyte count in peripheral blood because of the shift in the maturation time and the associated prolonged retention time. Therefore, the relationship between the hematocrit and the retention time (see the shift correction factors given above) is taken into account when calculating the RPI (alternative formula: RPI = [reticulocyte count % / retention time in blood] × [patient Hct / 45] (Wick et al 2011). The RPI thus corresponds to the reticulocyte count adjusted for the maturation time and maturation site of the cells.

▶ **Hypo- and hyperproliferative anemia.** The RPI is an integral part of the diagnostic algorithm in the case of normochromic normocytic (normal MCH and MCV) anemia.

A "hypoproliferative" (RPI < 2) finding calls for the additional testing of haptoglobin, creatinine, ferritin, C-reactive protein (CRP), soluble transferrin receptor (sTfR), erythropoietin, and bilirubin, from which the differential diagnoses can be inferred (**Table 3.4**):
• Impaired erythropoiesis → next step: bone marrow biopsy.
• Kidney failure.
• Anemia of chronic disease.

In the event of RPI > 2 ("hyperproliferative" anemia), lactate hydrogenase (LDH) is measured additionally. The combination of a low haptoglobin level and elevated levels of LDH, bilirubin, and sTfR is suggestive of hemolytic activity. This indicates the need for a blood smear (assessment of RBC morphology) and a direct and indirect Coombs test (assessment of noncorpuscular hemolysis secondary to antibody formation against RBC surface antigens).

▶ **Other reticulocyte indices.** Additional parameters give qualitative information about the cell volume of reticulocytes and their hemoglobin load (Thomas 2008):
• *MCVr*: mean corpuscular reticulocyte volume; the volume of reticulocytes (reference range in adults: 92–120 fL) is around 20% greater than that of RBCs, and the average MCVr is 106 fL

Table 3.4 Additional parameters needed to diagnose a "hypoproliferative" disorder (reticulocyte production index < 2)

Haptoglobin	Creatinine	Ferritin	CRP	sTfR	Erythropoietin	Bilirubin	Disorder
Normal	Normal					Normal	Impaired erythropoiesis
	Elevated	Normal			Decreased		Kidney failure
		Elevated	Elevated	Low	Decreased		Anemia of chronic disease

Abbreviations: CRP, C-reactive protein; sTfR, soluble transferrin receptor

(compared with 88 fL for RBCs). Macroreticulocytes (> 120 fL), known as *stress reticulocytes*, are a sign of accelerated hematopoiesis (e.g., after hemolysis or hyperstimulation with erythropoietin). Elevated MCVr values are found in folic-acid and vitamin-B_{12} deficiency anemia. Decreased MCVr values are an early indicator of iron deficiency.

- *CHCMr*: mean corpuscular hemoglobin concentration of reticulocytes (reference range: 27–33 g/dL) (Thomas and Thomas 2002); it is measured by suitably equipped hematology analyzers as the hemoglobin concentration in the reticulocyte fraction and is used for the calculation of the reticulocyte hemoglobin content (CHr, see next bullet point).
- *CHr, Ret-Hb*: reticulocyte hemoglobin content; the CHr is the mathematical product of the MCVr and the CHCMr (MCVr × CHCMr) and hence a measure of reticulocyte hemoglobinization. It is expressed in picograms (pg, 10^{-12} g) and is a marker used in the differential diagnosis of anemia to identify changes in iron metabolism, e.g., to monitor treatment with erythropoietin. In adults it has a reference range of 8–35 pg (Thomas 2008).

> **!**
>
> **Note**
>
> The insights gained from the evaluation of reticulocyte parameters expand the scope of the differential diagnosis of anemia through the addition of categories such as hypo-, normo-, and hyper-regenerative anemia and hypo-, normo-, and hyperproliferative anemia.

Blood smear

Occasionally, additional information can be gained from the morphology of RBCs—e.g., information about target cells, schistocytes (fragmented cells), and spherocytes—and from the differential blood count (e.g., information about granulocytes, platelets).

Iron Parameters

Iron metabolism is highly complex (**Fig. 3.3a–d**) and is often difficult to evaluate in clinical practice.

Just under 80% of all anemia cases are caused by absolute or relative iron deficiency. The WHO states that > 30% of the world's population have iron deficiency anemia (WHO 1968). Iron deficiency anemia means that an iron deficiency state has already progressed to an advanced stage. This condition is preceded by ferritin (stored iron) deficiency (prelatent if ferritin is in the range of 35–12 μg/L; latent if ferritin < 12 μg/L) and functional iron deficiency. The latter two states are mostly clinically silent, but nonetheless of paramount importance in the postoperative phase.

The diagnosis of anemia and the closely related iron deficiencies is based on the medical history, the clinical picture, and any additional diagnostic measures needed, and rests on four pillars: the blood count and related blood cell diagnostic tests as described above, the measurement of ferritin (and CRP, to rule out inflammation), the calculation of the "ferritin index," and possibly—depending on the laboratory equipment available—the determination of transferrin saturation.

▶ **Ferritin and C-reactive protein.** The serum *ferritin concentration* is a measure of the amount of stored iron. It should not be used as a sole diagnostic indicator because ferritin is not only an acute-phase protein but is also released during

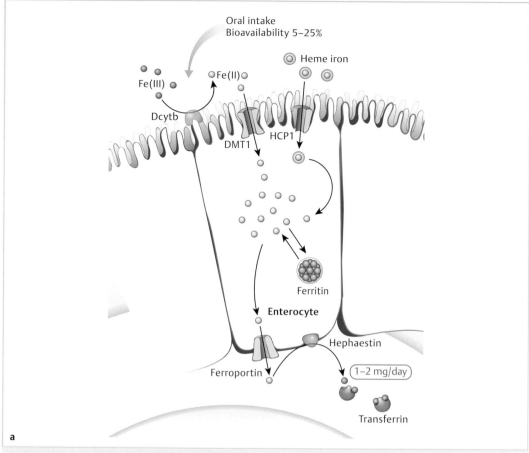

a

Fig. 3.3 Iron metabolism. (Reproduced with kind permission of Vifor Pharma. Illustrations: Descience, A. Ulrich & N. Stadelmann). **(a)** Iron is absorbed in the duodenum and upper jejunum in the form of reduced Fe^{2+} only. To that effect, the iron salts must be soluble in the acidic pH of the stomach. Iron ions are transported across the cells lining the duodenum by a series of carrier proteins: apical absorption after reduction by ferrireductase (duodenal cytochrome b, $Fe^{3+} \rightarrow Fe^{2+}$), then cell-membrane passage of Fe^{2+} via DMT 1 and shuttle transport via mobilferrin (not illustrated here), with possible iron transfer to ferritin. This is followed by the basolateral release by ferroportin and the transfer to ferroxidase (hephaestin, $Fe^{2+} \rightarrow Fe^{3+}$), with subsequent binding of Fe^{3+} to transferrin. The nutritive iron in hemoglobin enters the enterocytes via HCP1 as an intact metalloporphyrin; from there, it is either transported further in the manner described, or transferred via the heme exporter protein (HEP, not illustrated here) to transferrin in the blood circulation. Transferrin is a bilobed molecule that can be present in di-, mono-, or apoferric (without a load) form; when loaded with Fe^{3+}, it binds to the ubiquitously distributed transferrin receptors. Dcytb, duodenal cytochrome b; DMT 1, divalent metal transporter 1; HCP1, heme carrier protein 1.

Continued ▶

cell disintegration (e.g., in inflammation or malignancies). Therefore, to clarify any issues relating to iron metabolism, the CRP concentration must also be measured.

CRP is synthesized in the liver and released in response to inflammatory cytokines such as interleukin-6. It is the most suitable and most commonly used acute-phase protein for the diagnosis of infection. Against that background, it has broad clinical application and its role in the diagnosis of anemia is restricted to interpreting elevated levels of acute-phase ferritin. The CRP reference value is < 0.5 mg/dL.

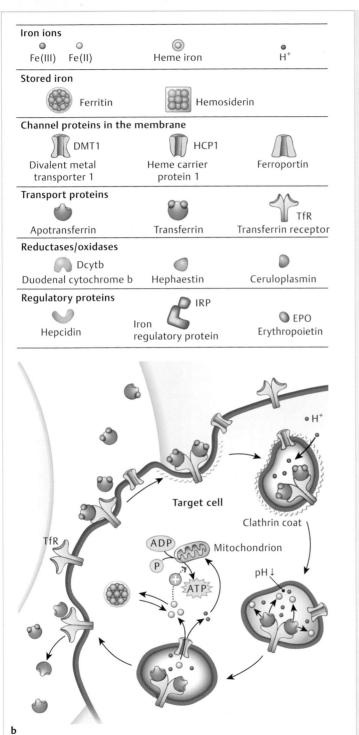

Iron ions

Fe(III)   Fe(II)   Heme iron H^+

Stored iron

Ferritin   Hemosiderin

Channel proteins in the membrane

DMT1   HCP1   Ferroportin
Divalent metal   Heme carrier
transporter 1   protein 1

Transport proteins

Apotransferrin   Transferrin   TfR
                                                Transferrin receptor

Reductases/oxidases

Dcytb
Duodenal cytochrome b   Hephaestin   Ceruloplasmin

Regulatory proteins

                                    IRP
                        Iron   EPO
Hepcidin   regulatory protein   Erythropoietin

TfR

ADP

P

Target cell

Clathrin coat

Mitochondrion

pH↓

ATP

H^+

b

Fig. 3.3 Continued.
(b) The TfR–transferrin complex enters the target cells via endosomes; in the endosomes, Fe^{3+} is reduced to Fe^{2+}; via DMT 1 and the cytosolic iron store, it reaches its main site of use, the mitochondria (e.g., production of the iron-sulfur clusters in enzymes of the electron transport chain)—unless it is stored in ferritin. Other target sites of cytoplasmic iron are heme and nonheme proteins (enzymes) as well as iron receptor proteins, which are important in iron hemostasis. The soluble TfR (TfR portion after cleavage from the intracellular part of the TfR) and apoferritin (the protein component of ferritin) are removed from the cell and enter the bloodstream. DMT 1, divalent metal transporter 1; TfR, transferrin receptor.

Continued ▶

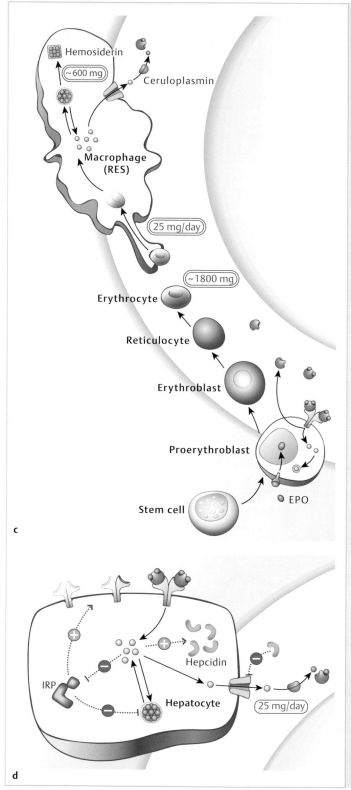

Fig. 3.3 Continued.

(c) Erythropoiesis (iron absorption and EPO-mediated stimulation of proerythroblasts; hemoglobin synthesis in erythroblasts) and RBC breakdown in the RES. At the end of their lifespan, RBCs undergo phagocytosis by RES macrophages, and their iron is stored in ferritin or hemosiderin (a heterogeneous group of ferritin breakdown products). To recycle the iron taken up by macrophages, its release via ferroportin is inhibited by hepcidin. EPO, erythropoietin; RES, reticuloendothelial system.

(d) During inflammatory processes, interleukin-6 stimulates the synthesis of hepcidin (hepatic bactericidal protein) in the liver. Hepcidin inactivates ferroportin in enterocytes (no release of iron), macrophages, and the liver (intracellular iron blockade), resulting in impaired iron distribution, as seen for example in anemia of chronic disease. IRP, iron regulatory protein.

▶ **Soluble transferrin receptor.** Iron deficiency triggers an increased synthesis of the transferrin receptor, which in turn leads to an increase in soluble transferrin receptor (sTfR)—a cleaved portion of the transferrin receptor—in the patient's serum. Elevated levels of sTfR are suggestive of a hyperproliferative form of anemia (expansion of erythropoiesis, e.g., after a hemolytic event).

▶ **Ferritin index.** The quotient of sTfR (mg/L) divided by the logarithm of serum ferritin (μg/L) has proved to be a useful anchor point in the diagnosis of iron metabolism disorders. The higher this index, the greater the functional iron deficiency!

▶ **Transferrin saturation.** The transferrin saturation (in %) is the quotient of serum iron (μg/dL) divided by transferrin (mg/dL) multiplied by the factor 70.9.

A summary of iron metabolism parameters indicative of anemia is given in **Table 3.5**.

▶ **Additional tests.** Other biochemical tests that can support the diagnosis of anemia include:
- Kidney, liver, thyroid parameters.
- Direct and indirect bilirubin.
- LDH.
- Haptoglobin.

Folic Acid and Vitamin B$_{12}$

Anemia may also be the result of impairments at the hematopoietic stem cell level, e.g., because of exposure to noxious substances or deficiencies in compounds that are essential for cell metabolism. Such impairments are often not confined to erythropoiesis, but may also affect myelopoiesis and thrombocytopoiesis. The causes can be autoantibodies, infections, toxins, or ionizing radiation. A bone marrow biopsy may be needed to make a conclusive diagnosis.

▶ **Macrocytic anemia.** Vitamin deficiency-induced disturbances of the proliferation and maturation of erythropoietic cells, as seen in macrocytic anemia, can be diagnosed more easily through determination of the serum levels of folic acid and vitamin B$_{12}$. Both parameters must be measured since they complement each other: folic acid can be converted into its active form only in the presence of vitamin B$_{12}$. Besides, myelodysplastic syndrome must be ruled out. The reference range for folic acid is > 4.4 ng/mL, and that for vitamin B$_{12}$ is > 300 ng/L.

Macrocytic anemia—resulting from impaired DNA synthesis attributable to absence of the C 1 transport molecule—is mainly caused by a deficiency of folic acid or vitamin B$_{12}$. It can also be caused by intoxication or medications.

▶ **Causes.** An elevated LDH level with concomitant reticulocytosis and hyperbilirubinemia can serve as an additional diagnostic tool. It is primarily suggestive of a vitamin B$_{12}$ deficiency, or it could be due to a folic acid deficiency (in pregnancy or linked to alcohol abuse). Other possible causes to be explored include a radical vegetarian diet, gastric resection, chronic atrophic gastritis, intrinsic factor antibodies, and intestinal diseases (including infection caused by the fish tapeworm). The most common causes of vitamin B$_{12}$ deficiency are pernicious anemia (triggered by an autoimmune process directed against the parietal cells of the stomach), and total gastrectomy.

Patients with folic acid deficiency—apart from elderly persons and rapidly growing adolescents—are often characterized by a poor nutritional status and a whole range of gastrointestinal symptoms. These are both triggers (e.g., celiac disease) and sequelae of the deficiency. In general, there are no neurologic manifestations; in particular, there is no disturbance of deep sensibility as seen in vitamin B$_{12}$ deficiency.

Erythropoietin

Erythropoietin levels are measured if renal anemia is suspected, at the beginning of anemia treatment with recombinant human erythropoietin (rHuEPO), and—at the other end of the disease spectrum—in cases of erythrocytosis.

The results obtained can be evaluated only in relation to the hematocrit or the hemoglobin concentration. The reference values vary widely

Table 3.5 Iron metabolism parameters indicative of anemia

Parameter	Suggestion of anemia
Ferritin	< 12 μg/L
Soluble transferrin receptor	> 5 mg/L (method-dependent)
Ferritin index	> 3.2 (method-dependent)
Transferrin saturation	< 15 %

between 5 and 25 IU/L, and are independent of age and gender (Wick et al 2011).

Coombs Tests and Bone Marrow Biopsy

In the agglutination test—at least when using the gel method—immunohematology testing is carried out to screen for antibodies against RBC surface antigens using anti-immunoglobulins (Coombs serum) and cell panels.

Bone marrow biopsy is the diagnostic measure of last resort. If it is needed, the patient has in all probability disease manifestations that cannot be addressed through surgical intervention alone.

3.1.3 Consequences of Anemia

There are myriad reports in the literature on the consequences of preoperative anemia, which include severe complications necessitating hospital admission as well as increases in morbidity and mortality (Patel and Carson 2009, Musallam et al 2011). The vicious circle implicated here is illustrated in **Fig. 3.4**. Therefore, a diagnosis of anemia is not a trivial matter, even though it is often seen this way; rather, it encompasses a broad spectrum of disease entities ranging from iron deficiency (the most common and most easily remedied ane-

mia-related condition) to life-threatening, severe, and treatment-refractory malignancies.

▶ **Scheduling.** In view of the additional surgical risks faced by anemic patients, when scheduling elective surgical procedures it is therefore of paramount importance to provide a sufficiently long time period for preoperative diagnostic tests and for any treatment interventions needed, e.g., treatment of iron deficiency anemia (Gombotz et al 2011a). On occasion, certain preoperative diagnostic investigations will also impact on the indication for elective procedures.

▶ **Therapeutic consequences.** An example for the possible therapeutic consequences that is based exclusively on the evaluation of laboratory results and has proved to be very effective involves the CHr and ferritin index (Thomas 2008). A 2 × 2 table is drawn up for the diagnostic evaluation of these laboratory parameters in anemic patients: CHr is entered as the column variable, and the ferritin index as the row variable. The cutoff for CHr is 28 pg, the cutoff for the ferritin index is 1.5. The four cells thus comprise the following: CHr > 28 pg, ferritin index < 1.5 (cell 1); CHr > 28 pg, ferritin index > 1.5 (cell 2); CHr < 28 pg, ferritin index > 1.5 (cell 3); and CHr < 28 pg, ferritin index < 1.5 (cell 4). The therapeutic consequence for cell 1

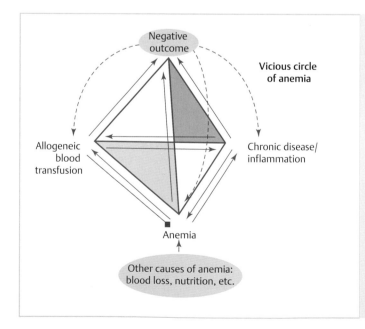

Fig. 3.4 Consequences of anemia. (Source: Shander et al 2011b.)

—iron stores and erythropoiesis normal—is erythropoietin; for cell 2—iron stores diminished—it is (oral) iron therapy; for cell 3—iron stores greatly diminished—it is (intravenous) iron therapy; and for cell 4—iron stores normal, functional iron deficiency—it is (intravenous) iron therapy plus rHuEPO. An elevated CHr is indicative of a high level of functional iron (cutoff 28 pg), and a high ferritin index (cutoff 3.2) is indicative of low levels of stored iron.

Preoperative anemia is not appropriately treated in the everyday clinical setting to the detriment of the patients affected (**Fig. 3.5**). Instead, such patients often receive RBC transfusions on the basis of inappropriate indications (**Fig. 3.6**).

Conclusion

The consequences of anemia, in particular preoperative anemia, are a higher morbidity and mortality, together with the complications of RBC transfusion, because anemic patients receive disproportionately more transfusions in the perioperative setting.

However, RBC transfusion is just one of the treatment options available to correct anemia— and should only be used as a last resort. It must be administered only subject to a strict indication and after stringent risk assessment, and has no justification in the preoperative time window before elective procedures, especially if transfusion only serves to secure the slot reserved in the surgical schedule.

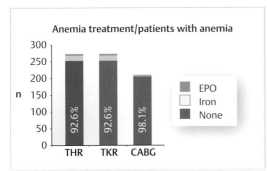

Fig. 3.5 Patients with preoperative anemia are rarely treated prior to elective surgical procedures. CABG, coronary artery bypass graft; EPO, erythropoietin; THR, total hip replacement; TKR, total knee replacement. Findings from the Second Austrian Benchmark Study (Gombotz et al 2011a).

3.2 Pros and Cons of Preoperative Anemia Treatment

P. Meybohm, K. Zacharowski

3.2.1 The Importance of Preoperative Anemia Treatment

Preoperative anemia is one of the strongest predictors of RBC transfusions during or after an operation (Gombotz et al 2007). In addition, preoperative anemia is an independent risk factor for postoperative complications and postoperative mortality (Musallam et al 2011). Since the transfusion of allogeneic blood, in particular for an

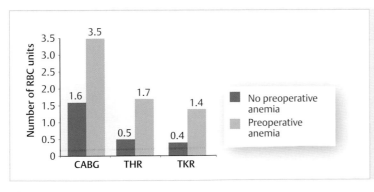

Fig. 3.6 Red blood cell transfusions in patients with preoperative anemia compared with patients without anemia. CABG, coronary artery bypass graft; RBC, red blood cell; THR, total hip replacement; TKR, total knee replacement. (Source: Gombotz et al 2011a.)

incorrect indication, is also an independent and additional risk factor for a poorer outcome (Westenbrink et al 2011), the primary correction and optimization of preoperative anemia must be an integral part of a holistic therapy concept.

▶ **Diagnosis and treatment.** Hence, any form of preoperative anemia—unless it is related to the surgical indication—should be clarified and non-emergency procedures should be postponed until appropriate anemia treatment has been completed. This is particularly important if the anticipated blood loss is more than 500 to 1,000 mL and the preoperative RBC volume in all probability no longer suffices for a transfusion-free perioperative management.

▶ **Prerequisites.** The general prerequisites for the preoperative treatment of anemia are as follows.
• The surgical procedure is elective.
• Any potential need to postpone the operation has been agreed with the surgeon.
• Cure of the underlying disease is not adversely affected.
• An adequate increase in hemoglobin can be achieved to obviate the need for allogeneic RBC concentrates.

In principle, the potential side effects and risks associated with anemia treatment must be acceptable in relation to the expected benefits.

Fig. 3.7 shows an exemplary algorithm for the differential diagnosis of preoperative anemia and for the therapeutic approaches tailored to the respective diagnoses.

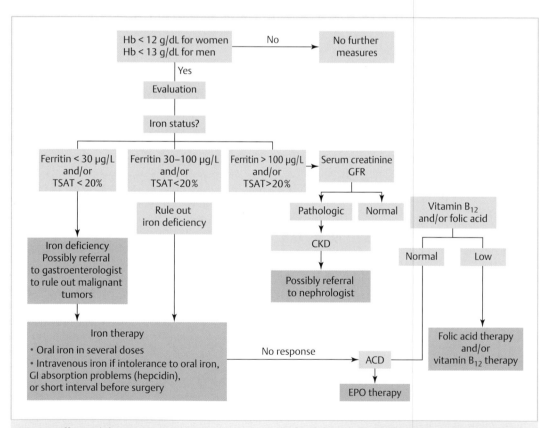

Fig. 3.7 Differential diagnosis and optimization of preoperative anemia. Note: if erythropoietin is administered, the hemoglobin target range should not exceed 10–11 g/dL. ACD, anemia of chronic disease; CKD, chronic kidney disease; EPO, epoetin; GFR, glomerular filtration rate; GI, gastrointestinal; Hb, hemoglobin; TSAT, transferrin saturation. (Source: Goodnough et al 2011.)

3.2.2 Iron Therapy

Pathophysiology

The total amount of iron in the human body is between 2,500 and 4,000 mg. Iron is stored in ferritin, especially in the liver and spleen. Iron deficiency can give rise to an impaired hematopoiesis, and thus to anemia. Even in the absence of disturbed erythropoiesis, depleted iron stores can have serious clinical consequences and reduce the quality of life. Therefore, a low hemoglobin value should be viewed as the final stage of a process that began with the gradual depletion of iron stores.

Often, iron deficiency is the sole cause of anemia, but anemia can also occur in the context of a chronic disease (anemia of chronic disease) and should always constitute a strict indication for iron supplementation.

Causes of Iron Deficiency Anemia

Absolute iron deficiency may be imputed to one of the following:
- Too little iron intake.
- Reduced bioavailability of iron from the diet.
- Increased iron consumption.
- Chronic blood loss.

If iron deficiency persists over a long period of time, it will result in iron deficiency anemia, i.e., microcytic hypochromic anemia. Conversely, a *functional* iron deficiency is found in particular in patients with a chronic inflammatory or malignant disease. Iron mobilization from the iron stores in the liver and spleen and iron absorption from the gastrointestinal tract are blocked because of active inflammation. A pivotal role is played here by hepcidin, which is produced in the liver and is stimulated by interleukin-6 during an infection. Hepcidin binds to the iron export protein ferroportin in enterocytes, preventing the release of iron into the bloodstream and its transfer to transferrin. In addition, hepcidin inhibits the mobilization of iron from reticuloendothelial macrophages and other stores.

Iron Requirement

Using the Ganzoni formula, the amount of iron to be administered can be estimated from the body weight and the desired target value of hemoglobin (Ganzoni 1970):

Formula

Total iron deficit (mg) = Weight × (Target Hb – Actual Hb) × 2.4 + Iron stores (500 mg)

Example: a 70-year-old man with a weight of 80 kg and a measured actual Hb of 9 g/dL (target Hb 11 g/dL).

Total iron deficit = $80 \times 2 \times 2.4 + 500 = 884$ mg

The amount of iron to be administered is often between 500 and 1,000 mg.

Oral Iron Therapy

For the treatment of iron deficiency and iron deficiency anemia, oral iron and intravenous iron complexes are available. However, the efficacy of oral iron therapy is limited as maximum duodenal absorption is limited to 10 mg iron daily—for a total amount of around 1,200 mg, approximately 120 days would be needed. In addition, several circumstances must be considered that can additionally curtail enteral iron absorption, e.g., hepcidin-mediated malabsorption, *Helicobacter pylori* infection, and comedication with antibiotics or antacids. Anemia correction through oral iron therapy can take weeks to months even if optimal compliance is assured, and even then the iron stores may still not be replete. In principle, oral iron therapy was proven to be successful in the management of preoperative anemia in patients undergoing orthopaedic or colorectal surgery (Lidder et al 2007). However, long-term treatment is restricted in particular by gastrointestinal side effects (nausea, flatulence, diarrhea or constipation, and dark stools).

Intravenous Iron Therapy

Because of the aforementioned side effects, and not least because of the low absorption rate associated with oral administration, iron should generally be administered intravenously during the preoperative phase (Beris et al 2008). Only if the preoperative waiting time is more than 2 to 3 months can oral iron therapy be initiated, with a switch to intravenous iron supplementation if there is no response to treatment. Intravenous iron therapy assures the rapid repletion of iron stores by circumventing the hepcidin-mediated blockade of iron absorption and the blockade of iron release from the liver's reticuloendothelial system into the bloodstream and bone marrow.

> **Note**
>
> Iron deficiency anemia should always be a clear indication for iron supplementation. Iron supplements are available as oral and intravenous compounds. Because of the gastrointestinal side effects, and not least because of the low absorption rate associated with oral administration, iron should generally be administered intravenously during the preoperative phase.

▶ **Iron formulations.** A number of intravenous iron formulations are available, but their approval status varies widely from country to country. To give an example, four intravenous iron formulations (ferrous gluconate, iron sucrose, iron dextran, and ferric carboxymaltose) are available in Germany; these formulations differ in their pharmacological properties, stability, maximum infusion duration, maximum single dose, and incidence of anaphylactoid reactions. Intravenous iron complexes are taken up by the macrophages of the reticuloendothelial system in the liver and spleen. Ferric carboxymaltose and iron dextran are the most stable complexes. Ferrous gluconate represents the least stable iron–ligand complex; hence Fe^{3+} is already released in the bloodstream, where it binds to transferrin. The more unstable the complex, the greater the amount of iron that will be released into the bloodstream, where it can cause acute toxicity with oxidative stress, endothelial damage, and a drop in blood pressure. The clinical consequences can in turn include cardiovascular complications and a deterioration of kidney function.

Conversely, ferric carboxymaltose and iron dextran have a high complex stability; therefore, hardly any iron is released into the bloodstream. For that reason iron, ferric carboxymaltose can be infused at a higher dose of up to 15 mg/kg (maximum 1,000 mg once weekly) over at least 15 minutes.

Iron dextran is typically associated with a high risk of anaphylactoid reactions with nausea, vertigo, hypotension, and tachycardia. Following a recent warning by the European Medicines Agency, the use of iron dextran is not recommended.

Other Side Effects

Other potential side effects of iron include in particular its impact on tumor growth and infections. However, these effects are still under investigation. The iron deficiency seen in chronic inflammation is also viewed as a "protective mechanism" against tumor or bacterial growth.

No evidence of these theoretical disadvantages of iron therapy has been found in clinical studies to date. However, parenteral iron supplementation should not exceed the normal range.

▶ **Acute infections.** Special attention must be paid to the interaction between iron supplements and acute systemic infection involving oxidative stress. In terms of pathophysiology, iron is a potent growth factor for bacteria. Bacteria express receptors that are similar to ferritin, and therefore iron supplementation might expedite bacterial growth and infection. Although no clinical studies have been carried out so far to investigate this hypothesis, intravenous iron supplements should be avoided for safety reasons in patients with acute infection and bacteremia.

Clinical Studies on Iron Therapy

▶ **Patients in internal medicine.** The benefits of intravenous iron therapy have been demonstrated primarily for patients in internal medicine: among patients with chronic heart failure (New York Heart Association II and III), the correction of iron deficiency with intravenous ferric carboxymaltose improved the patients' physical activity and quality of life without causing severe side effects (Anker et al 2009). Among patients with compensated renal failure with renal anemia, intravenous iron therapy based on 2400 mg of iron sucrose corrected previously low hemoglobin levels without the need for erythropoietin therapy (Mircescu et al 2006).

Anemia is often seen as a concomitant manifestation in patients with malignancies. The postulated causes include damage inflicted on the erythropoietic system by cytostatic agents and/or radiation-mediated destruction of the RBC precursor cells, as well as functional iron deficiency resulting from increased cytokine release and hepcidin synthesis.

▶ **Perioperative setting.** In 2008, a review article in the perioperative setting was published by the Network for Advancement of Transfusion Alternatives. However, out of eight studies reporting on short-term preoperative intravenous iron therapy, only two observational studies on orthopaedic patients identified a benefit in terms of a lower transfusion risk. Hardly any or no benefit was detected if iron was administered only at a late intraoperative stage, or indeed postoperatively (Beris et al 2008). However, the study group also emphasized that for elective patients at high risk for postoperative anemia, the hemoglobin value and iron status (serum iron, ferritin, transferrin saturation, C-reactive protein) should be determined well in advance—ideally at least 30 days before the planned procedure. For patients aged 60 years or more, the vitamin B_{12} and folic acid levels should be determined additionally.

One feature common to all clinical studies conducted to date in the perioperative setting is that they did not enroll enough patients to permit insights into the typical side effects of oral/intravenous iron.

The U.S. Food and Drug Administration (FDA) estimated the incidence of life-threatening events linked to intravenous iron therapy (ferrous gluconate, iron sucrose, iron dextran) at 2.2 per million, and the incidence of death at 0.4 per million. As such, the risks are much lower than those posed by transfusion-associated events (10 and 4 per million) (Muñoz et al 2012).

The Place of Intravenous Iron Therapy

The place of intravenous iron therapy in the treatment of preoperative anemia has not been conclusively determined. Because of potential safety implications, the FDA has not yet licensed ferric carboxymaltose for routine use in the correction of preoperative iron deficiency anemia. Besides, no large comparative study or unequivocal cost–benefit analysis has been conducted to date.

> **Note**
>
> Of the four intravenous formulations discussed above, preference should be given to ferric carboxymaltose because of its high complex stability and the absence of anaphylactoid effects (dose 15 mg/kg, maximum 1,000 mg once weekly). Since iron is a potent growth factor for bacteria, intravenous iron supplementation should be avoided for safety reasons in patients with acute infection and bacteremia.

Recommendations to Manage the Risk of Allergic Reactions

The Committee for Medicinal Products for Human Use (CHMP) of the European Medicines Agency has reviewed intravenous iron-containing medicines used to treat iron deficiency anemia (EMA 2013), and concluded that the benefits of these medicines are greater than their risks.

However, measures should be put in place to ensure the early detection and effective management of any allergic reactions that may occur. Iron preparations should only be given in an environment where resuscitation facilities are available, so that patients who develop an allergic reaction can be treated immediately. In addition, the CHMP considered that the current practice of first giving the patient a small test dose is not a reliable way to predict how the patient will respond when the full dose is given. A test dose is therefore no longer recommended; instead, caution is warranted with every dose of intravenous iron that is given, even if previous administrations have been well tolerated. Importantly, recent warning messages were the consequence of allergic reactions mostly documented in patients receiving iron dextran. Therefore, dextran solutions should no longer be used. Other intravenous formulations, e.g., ferric carboxymaltose, do not contain any dextran.

3.2.3 Vitamin B₁₂ and Folic Acid

Pathophysiology

Vitamin B_{12} (cyanocobalamin) and folic acid have essential functions in DNA synthesis, cell formation, and cell regeneration. Any deficiency is therefore first manifested in cells with a high division rate and leads to megaloblastic anemia. In anemia resulting from vitamin B_{12} deficiency (pernicious anemia), symptoms related to the stomach and the nervous system (paralysis, unsteady gait, and impaired sensory perceptions) occur in addition to the characteristic anemia complaints.

The daily requirement for vitamin B_{12} is 2 to 6 µg, and that for folic acid is 400 µg. Vitamin B_{12} is absorbed from the diet in the gut by means of a special protein (intrinsic factor), which is secreted into the stomach and binds to the vitamin, protecting it from destruction.

Vitamin B₁₂ and Folic Acid Deficiency and Supplementation

A deficiency can be caused by a reduced content in the diet, e.g., in the case of unbalanced vegetarian diets or alcoholism, or by malabsorption because of a lack of intrinsic factor (as seen in chronic inflammation of the gastric mucosa), autoimmune disease, gastrectomy, and the intensive use of antacids.

▶ **Vitamin B₁₂ supplementation.** The recommendations for baseline supplementation of a conclusively diagnosed vitamin B_{12} deficiency vary greatly, but the initial dose should be determined by the severity of the clinical symptoms (range 150–1,000 µg/day). Around 15% of each 1,000-µg injection remains in the body, and 85% is excreted again in the urine. Oral vitamin B_{12} supplementation can also be used, but this is advisable only if adequate intrinsic factor and a healthy ileum are assured.

▶ **Folic acid supplementation.** Before initiating folic acid therapy, tests must be carried out to establish whether there is a deficiency in vitamin B_{12}. Treatment of folic acid deficiency consists of the daily intake of folic acid tablets or folic acid injections. Since the human liver can only store small amounts of folic acid, folic acid deficiency leading to anemia can occur within the space of a few months if the diet is low in folic acid. For rapid repletion of the folic acid store, daily doses of up to 5 to 15 mg should be taken initially.

▶ **Response to treatment.** A response to vitamin B_{12}/folic acid supplementation is indicated through an increase in the reticulocyte count after 3 to 4 days, reaching a peak after 7 to 10 days. The rise in the reticulocyte count induced by folic acid can mask any vitamin B_{12} deficiency that may be present. Because of the risk of irreversible neurologic disorders, it must be ensured that megaloblastic anemia is not caused by a vitamin B_{12} deficiency before initiating treatment.

▶ **Interactions.** It should be noted that high doses of folic acid can negate the action of antiepileptic drugs such as phenytoin and barbiturates. If there is no response to folic acid supplementation, this could be due to the concomitant use of folic acid antagonists, e.g., antibiotics (trimethoprim), cytostatics (methotrexate), or diuretics (triamterene); it could also be explained by the reduced intestinal absorption of folic acid because of concurrent alcohol consumption.

> **Note** ❗
>
> Both vitamin B_{12} deficiency and folic acid deficiency can cause anemia. If this is the case, supplementation with vitamin B_{12} (up to 1,000 µg/day) or folic acid (5–15 mg/day) is the cornerstone of anemia treatment. The treatment success is manifested in a rising reticulocyte count after 3 to 4 days, reaching its peak after 7 to 10 days.

3.2.4 Erythropoiesis-stimulating Agents

Pathophysiology

Erythropoietin is an endogenous glycoprotein hormone that acts as a growth factor, stimulating the production of RBCs. When blood oxygen levels are low, erythropoietin is produced in the kidneys; this response is mediated by hypoxia-inducible factor 1α (HIF1α). Binding of erythropoietin to specific erythropoietin receptors on erythropoiesis precursor cells stimulates the proliferation and differentiation of these cells, and their survival is prolonged mainly because of an inhibition of programmed cell death (apoptosis). Accordingly, acute and chronic renal failure results in reduced erythropoietin production and hence in renal anemia. Apart from its principal hematopoietic function, erythropoietin appears to play a role in chemotaxis, angiogenesis, inhibition of apoptosis, and cell protection (Sargin et al 2010).

Indications

The use of erythropoiesis-stimulating drugs (epoetins; epoetin α, β, θ, and ζ, methoxy polyethylene glycol-epoetin β, and the epoetin analogue darbepoetin α) is restricted to the following scenarios:
- To treat symptomatic anemia in chronic renal failure.
- To treat symptomatic anemia in cancer patients undergoing chemotherapy.
- To increase the RBC volume in patients with moderate anemia and normal blood iron levels who are going to have an operation and donate their own blood before surgery (autologous RBC transfusion).
- To reduce the need for RBC transfusions in adults with moderate anemia who are about to undergo major orthopaedic (bone) surgery, such as hip surgery.

The main goal of treatment is to increase the hemoglobin value and to reduce, or avoid, the need for RBC transfusion. Based on the studies conducted so far, there is no evidence of a substantial improvement in the quality of life of patients receiving erythropoiesis-stimulating drugs.

Restrictions on Use

The European Medicines Agency issued use restrictions in 2008. Since then, epoetins may only be prescribed for patients with symptomatic anemia. Their use is no longer permitted for the correction of the hemoglobin concentration alone. Epoetins should be dosed such that a hemoglobin concentration of 10 to 12 g/dL can be reached. This target range should not be exceeded.

The FDA has repeatedly recommended the restrictive use of erythropoiesis-stimulating agents and has issued conservative dosing guidelines (FDA 2011).

Note

To date, erythropoiesis-stimulating drugs are licensed only to treat symptomatic anemia in patients with chronic renal failure or in patients with cancer undergoing chemotherapy. Their use is no longer permitted for the correction of the hemoglobin concentration alone. Epoetins should be dosed such that a hemoglobin concentration of 10 to 12 g/dL can be reached.

Side Effects and Contraindications

The typical *side effects* of epoetins are as follows:
- Flulike symptoms (headache, joint pains, fatigue, feeling of weakness).
- Critical rise in blood pressure, possibly with encephalopathy-like symptoms (e.g., headache and confusion).
- Thromboembolic complications such as deep vein thrombosis, pulmonary artery embolism, impaired cerebrovascular perfusion, and myocardial infarction, in particular if a hemoglobin value > 12 g/dL is being targeted.

Paradoxically, if epoetins are used over several months, severe anemia (erythroblastopenia) can develop in isolated cases because of the generation of anti-erythropoietin antibodies.

The following *contraindications* must be noted when using epoetins:
- Severe arterial hypertension.
- Surgical patients who do not receive thrombosis prophylaxis.
- Severe coronary heart disease, peripheral arterial occlusive disease, carotid artery vascular disease, or cerebrovascular disease.

Tumor Patients

Because of their low safety profile, the pros and cons of using epoetins must be evaluated on an individual basis. This applies particularly to tumor patients with anemia because erythropoietin receptors are expressed not only on erythropoiesis precursor cells but also on the surface of various tumor cells. Besides, since epoetins are growth factors, they can stimulate not only the production of RBCs but also the growth of tumors. For chemotherapy-associated anemia, the results of randomized controlled clinical trials, meta-analyses, and a Cochrane review have pointed to an increased mortality and a shorter progression-free survival after epoetin use, in particular if a hemoglobin value > 12 g/dL was targeted (Bohlius et al 2009a).

For this reason, the current guidelines recommend a lower target hemoglobin value in the range of 11–12 g/dL for patients with chronic renal failure or tumor-associated anemia (Rizzo et al 2008, Rizzo et al 2010). Whether this also applies to patients with normal renal function or with only minor renal impairment, or to the short-term use before surgery, has not been investigated to date.

Epoetins in the Preoperative Treatment of Anemia

The aforementioned indications aside, epoetin supplementation could also become of interest in the perioperative setting, to treat patients scheduled to undergo an elective surgical procedure who have been diagnosed with preoperative anemia but iron deficiency has already been ruled out or treated. However, so far only tenuous clinical evidence is available to support such an approach.

▶ **Orthopaedic surgery.** Epoetin α is licensed for the treatment of preoperative anemia prior to a major orthopaedic operation, to reduce the need for allogeneic blood in adult patients with no iron deficiency who are at high risk for transfusion complications and with an anticipated blood loss of 900 to 1,800 mL. In a multicenter study conducted in six European countries, the use of epoetin α in 460 patients undergoing hip, knee, or back surgery increased the hemoglobin value on the day of surgery from 12 g/dL to 14 g/dL; the number of patients requiring transfusion was reduced from 46% to 12% (Weber et al 2005).

▶ **Colorectal surgery.** By contrast, contradictory findings were obtained for colorectal surgery. A Cochrane review did not identify any effect of epoetin on the number of RBC transfusions administered, the number of transfused patients, or the survival probability (Devon and McLeod 2009). Whether a higher epoetin dose or a longer duration of preoperative use would have generated a greater effect is a matter of conjecture.

▶ **Cardiac surgery.** Contrary to current recommendations for the use of epoetin α, an interna-

tional review article has suggested an expansion of the indication spectrum to include anemic patients undergoing cardiac surgery: in the review article, the short-term use (a few days before surgery) of epoetins in combination with iron in these patients is classified as a Class IIa recommendation (evidence B) (Ferraris et al 2011a).

In the randomized clinical trials published to date for the cardiac surgery setting, the use of epoetins varies greatly in terms of optimum dose (100–600 IU/kg), optimum time point (0–30 days before the procedure), and mode of administration (subcutaneous or intravenous). In view of the aforementioned side effects of epoetins, the number of patients in virtually all studies on the short-term use of epoetin was too small to enable valid insights into the safety profile.

In the event of preoperative anemia, an elective procedure should generally be postponed by 4 to 8 weeks to allow time for an optimal management of anemia. However, this is often not possible in cardiac surgery. Noteworthy is also the finding that a single dose of epoetin on the day before heart surgery appears to reduce the risk of allogeneic blood transfusion in the immediate postoperative period, without any direct impact on the preoperative hemoglobin value (Yoo et al 2011).

However, the use of epoetin in nonorthopaedic patients constitutes off-label use.

Risk–Benefit Assessment

It is important to conduct a risk–benefit assessment when consulting a patient prior to any preoperative use of epoetin. This should focus on, among other things, the following: severity of anemia, clinical situation (e.g., concomitant cardiovascular or pulmonary diseases), and the patient's treatment preference. Patients must be thoroughly informed about the risks associated with the use of epoetins (higher mortality risk in patients with an increased hemoglobin level, thromboembolic complications, higher risk of stroke, and possible stimulation of tumor growth).

> **Note** ❗
>
> A risk–benefit assessment must be carried out when consulting a patient prior to any preoperative use of epoetins because of the risks associated with the use of epoetins, such as a higher mortality among patients with an in-

creased hemoglobin level, thromboembolic complications (deep vein thrombosis, pulmonary artery embolism, myocardial infarction, stroke), and the potential stimulation of tumor growth. Epoetin α is currently licensed for the treatment of preoperative anemia prior to a major orthopaedic operation, to reduce the need for allogeneic blood in adult patients with no iron deficiency who are at high risk for transfusion complications and an anticipated blood loss of 900 to 1800 mL. The use of epoetins for the preoperative treatment of anemia in nonorthopaedic patients is probably also beneficial, but this would be classified as off-label use.

3.2.5 Does Preoperative Anemia Treatment Pay?

To date, no controlled studies have been carried out to identify whether the treatment of preoperative anemia is cost-effective compared with allogeneic therapy, or whether it could even reduce costs. In particular, the costs incurred for epoetin

therapy are often put forward as an argument against the preoperative treatment of anemia.

However, in view of the scientific evidence supporting the efficacy of low-dose pre- and/or intraoperative epoetin therapy, the financial benefits of this treatment option should be reevaluated (**Table 3.6**). Cost and budgetary aspects aside, the preoperative treatment of anemia, when compared with allogeneic RBC transfusion, could pay off for the patients themselves (fewer transfusion-associated risks and side effects), for the hospital (patient recruitment and marketing), and for the general public (scarcity of blood products).

▶ **Multifactorial treatment approach.** A retrospective single-center study carried out in the United Kingdom demonstrated that the correction of preoperative anemia can be successfully integrated into a multifactorial treatment approach (Kotze et al 2012). In close cooperation with the respective general practitioner, elective procedures for anemic patients were postponed by around 4 weeks to begin with, in order to use this interval to treat the patients. Patients with a

Table 3.6 Estimated treatment costs for allogeneic RBC transfusion versus preoperative anemia treatment with iron and/or epoetin

Blood (2 RBC units)		Iron		Epoetin	
RBC unit ("purchase price")	€80–100	Iron(II) sulfate, iron(III) sucrose, or iron (III) carboxymaltose	€10–380	Darbepoetin α or epoetin α	€100–370
Materials/laboratory (blood group determination, crossmatch test, bedside test, transfusion system)	€80–100	Materials/laboratory (ferritin, Hb, CRP, transferrin saturation, creatinine)	Σ €50	Materials/laboratory (ferritin, Hb, CRP, transferrin saturation, creatinine)	Σ €50
		Laboratory (vitamin B_{12} level, folic acid level)	Σ €30	Laboratory (vitamin B_{12} level, folic acid level)	Σ €30
Personnel (physicians, nurses, blood bank, transport), ~ 60–90 min	€80–120	Personnel (physicians, nurses), ~ 15 min	€20	Personnel (physicians, nurses), ~ 15 min	€20
Complications	??	Complications	??	Complications	??
Total costs	~ €240–320	**Total costs**	~ €80–480	**Total costs**	~ €170–470

Abbreviations: CRP, C-reactive protein; Hb, hemoglobin.

ferritin value < 100 ng/mL received oral iron (operation postponed by more than 4 weeks) or intravenous iron (operation scheduled within 4 weeks), whereas those with ferritin value > 100 ng/mL received a combination of 300–600 IU/kg subcutaneous epoetin α (once weekly for 4 weeks) plus oral iron. Just by optimizing the hemoglobin value preoperatively, it was possible to achieve more than 50% reductions in the incidence of preoperative anemia on the day of surgery and in the risk of intraoperative allogeneic RBC transfusion (Kotze et al 2012).

Note

The preoperative treatment of anemia, compared with allogeneic RBC transfusion, is worth it in terms of cost and budgetary aspects, and pays off for the patients themselves (fewer transfusion-associated risks), for the hospital (patient recruitment), and for the general public (scarcity of blood products).

Conclusion

To date, no international guidelines exist on the preoperative treatment of anemia or on measures to be taken to avoid the need for allogeneic RBC transfusion.

The authors recommend for elective patients with preoperative anemia and an anticipated intraoperative blood loss of more than 500 to 1,000 mL that the waiting time should be used, or the operation should be postponed by 2 to 8 weeks if this can be medically justified. During this time period, the differential diagnosis of preoperative anemia can be established and anemia can be optimally treated. Because of the potential risks and side effects, a risk–benefit assessment must be conducted in consultation with the individual patient.

No large prospective randomized clinical studies with relevant endpoints have been published so far on the preoperative treatment of anemia. The authors believe that such studies are urgently needed.

Chapter 4

Second Pillar of PBM—Minimization of Bleeding and Blood Loss

4.1 Reduction of Diagnostic and Interventional Blood Loss

H. Gombotz

4.1.1 Iatrogenic Blood Loss

Diagnostic blood tests and interventional blood loss play an important role in the development of iatrogenic anemia among hospitalized patients (Rennke and Fang 2011, Fischer et al 2014). Like all other forms of anemia, hospital-acquired anemia is a risk factor for an unfavorable disease course (Thavendiranathan et al 2005, Musallam et al 2011). It is particularly pronounced among children, the elderly (because they often have preexisting anemia), and patients with a low body weight, and it increases in line with the severity of the underlying disease (Thavendiranathan et al 2005, Madsen et al 2000, Salisbury et al 2011). Among patients undergoing cardiac surgery, 37% had preoperative anemia, and anemia was more severe if coronary angiography was performed prior to surgery (Karski et al 1999). Furthermore, unnecessary blood draws are a major burden on a hospital's health care budget (Vegting et al 2012). Laboratory tests should only be performed if their results will have therapeutic consequences. However, in reality, laboratory tests are often ordered on a routine basis, without any evidence to support their usefulness and without any treatment implications (Sood et al 2007).

▶ **Distribution of laboratory tests.** Blood draws are more frequent when the patient is first admitted to hospital, and their frequency declines progressively in line with the length of hospital stay, and especially when the patient is admitted to the intensive care unit (ICU). This decrease in frequency is noted most commonly among patients undergoing cardiac surgery, patients receiving long-term respiratory ventilation, patients with coagulation disorders, and patients undergoing multiple surgical procedures. Hospital laboratories play a part in over 60% of all medical diagnoses. Outside ICUs, 50% of blood draws are for blood chemistry investigations, 32% for hematologic tests, and 18% for coagulation tests. By contrast, blood gas analysis accounts for the majority (63%) of all blood draws in ICUs (**Fig. 4.1**).

▶ **Study findings.** A comparison of trauma patients with a historical control group showed a marked and costly rise in the number of laboratory tests, without any impact on the outcome variables studied (Branco et al 2012). A study involving a pediatric ICU revealed that the blood volume drawn was around twice that needed for the respective laboratory test; the reasons for the blood tests were not investigated (Valentine and Bateman 2012). For premature neonates, the sampled blood volume correlated with the transfused blood volume (Obladen et al 1988). By contrast, the WHO recommends a safe blood sample volume limit of up to 3 mL/kg/day for pediatric patients involved in clinical research (Howie 2011).

▶ **Variability in the frequency of blood tests.** As with allogeneic blood consumption, the frequency of diagnostic blood tests, and accordingly the amount of blood drawn, varies widely between

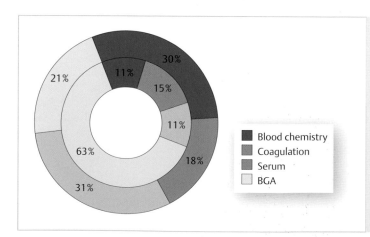

Fig. 4.1 Comparison of the distribution of laboratory analyses in a hospital with 1,000 beds and intensive care units. Inner circle: intensive care units, outer ring: remainder of hospital. BGA, blood gas analysis.

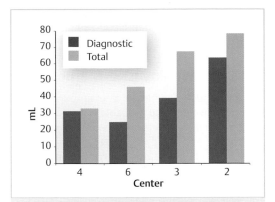

Fig. 4.2 Mean daily interventional and diagnostic blood loss in four comparable ICUs (results of the Second Austrian Benchmark Study). (Source: Gombotz et al 2007.)

different physicians, wards, and hospitals. However, it is not always possible to identify a plausible link between this frequency and therapeutic measures, let alone therapeutic consequences (Katz et al 2011). A pilot study carried out within the framework of the Second Austrian Benchmark Study revealed that there was enormous variability in the volume of diagnostic and interventional blood loss (25–75 mL per day and patient) in four comparable ICUs (**Fig. 4.2**). This variability could not be explained on the basis of the patients' conditions. The hemoglobin values of the patients became more similar over the course of their ICU stay. Patients whose baseline hemoglobin value was high saw their value decline because of frequent blood draws or because of their illness, whereas those with a low baseline hemoglobin were maintained at an acceptable level or their values were increased mainly through allogeneic red blood cell (RBC) transfusions (Vincent et al 2002).

> **Note**
>
> Frequent blood tests cause iatrogenic anemia, which can have a negative effect on the disease course.
>
> Overall, the diagnostic blood loss volume in routine practice is probably much too high and may have negative implications for the patients concerned. In general, a balance should be struck between the blood volume drawn and the potential risk to the patient (Raheman 2009).

4.1.2 Strategies to Avoid Diagnostic Blood Loss

A number of strategies can help to reduce diagnostic blood loss. However, the use of a single method alone is unlikely to prove successful. Only by combining several methods will it be possible to reduce the blood volume drawn by 50% or more, depending on the baseline value. In addition to reducing the rate of hospital-acquired anemia, this will lead to considerable cost savings.

Evaluation of Blood Draw Volume and Test Frequency

The volume of blood drawn as per current practice must first of all be identified to be able to optimize blood sampling (minimizing the blood draw volume without putting the patient at risk) (Mukhopadhyay et al 2010, Valentine and Bateman 2012, Page et al 2013). Simply being aware of this issue can already bring about a considerable reduction in the blood draw volume and the transfusion requirement (Fowler and Berenson 2003). Likewise, the purpose of laboratory tests should be considered. In ICUs, physician-requested, symptom-based laboratory testing is generally superior to routine testing, since routine tests are often continued for longer than needed. The blood volume drawn is also strongly correlated with the number and functional design of indwelling arterial and venous lines. The more lines there are and the easier it is to draw blood (e.g., if the lines are large), the more blood will be withdrawn.

Other interventions include the restriction of laboratory tests to those medically indicated (avoidance of requests that cannot be medically justified), identification and discussion of inappropriate blood tests and their implications for the patient, and feedback on the impact of newly introduced measures (audits, amended request forms, etc.) (Calderon-Margalit et al 2005, May et al 2006). It has been possible to reduce the number of ordered laboratory tests by half through the implementation of lectures and supervision (Attali et al 2006). Likewise, generous type-and-screen testing and blood product ordering practices should be scrutinized. After all, around two-thirds of all RBC concentrates issued for elective surgery are not transfused (Attali et al 2006, Gombotz et al 2007).

Reduction of the Blood Draw Volume

The blood draw volume can be reduced by half or more simply by switching from large-volume to pediatric blood sample tubes (Gleason et al 1992, Jung and Ahn 2013). Adult tubes can hold up to 7.5 mL of blood, but this amount is not always needed for a blood test. It is also unclear how much blood has to be discarded, for example from a heparinized line, to obtain reliable laboratory results. The recommendations differ, ranging from the system's dead-space volume plus 2 mL to 2.5 times the dead space. This means that around 2.5 mL have to be discarded for arterial lines. The use of smaller syringes (1 mL) also precludes the sampling of larger blood volumes. It may also be necessary to manually fill sampling tubes with a smaller volume. A further subject of debate is whether the blood drawn before sampling should be retransfused rather than discarded. Counter-arguments include the risks of infection, activation of blood coagulation, and hemolysis.

Evaluation of the Need for a Laboratory Test

This is an important point since unnecessary laboratory tests are often continued for days simply as a matter of routine. Based on a conservative estimate, up to 50% of all laboratory results are not taken into account in routine clinical practice. A regular review does not only help to reduce diagnostic blood loss, but it might also result in considerable savings. The argument that several tests can be performed from a single blood sample and that the cost for additional tests is then negligible only holds true if the request does not include expensive, usually modern, parameters (e.g., procalcitonin, troponin).

Point-of-care Testing

Point-of-care methods such as thromboelastography generally call for specific experience and knowledge, but confer a number of advantages over routine laboratory tests (Weber and Zacharowski 2012). They are timely, carried out on site, and paid more attention thanks to their immediacy; they permit quick decision-making but are generally associated with considerably higher reagent and material costs. For methodological reasons,

their analytical sensitivity and specificity are also lower. Besides, a greater blood volume may be needed than in the case of routine laboratory tests.

Switch to Noninvasive Methods

A large number of noninvasive, mainly continuous, methods have become available for the measurement of vital parameters. After initial alignment with their standard laboratory counterparts, these methods can be used for continuous routine monitoring. They include the assessment of blood sugar, hemoglobin, oxygen, and carbon dioxide. The benefit of continuous monitoring is that it provides for an earlier detection of pathologic fluctuations, and accordingly for earlier intervention. However, only a guess can be ventured at present as to what extent such noninvasive methods are able to reduce, or even replace, diagnostic blood tests.

> **Note**
>
> A marked reduction in the volume of diagnostic blood loss can only be achieved by combining several methods. These include reducing the blood draw volume and the frequency of blood tests, point-of-care testing, and using modern noninvasive diagnostic procedures instead of blood tests.

4.1.3 Strategies to Avoid Interventional Blood Loss

Blood loss during interventional investigations plays an additional role in hospital-acquired anemia. It is one of the reasons why preoperative anemia is more common among patients who have recently undergone coronary angiography than among those who have undergone orthopaedic surgery (Gombotz et al 2007). The volume of interventional blood loss is also strongly correlated with the duration of the investigation.

Since interventional blood loss can occur in many medical disciplines, multidisciplinary cooperation is often needed to reduce such blood loss. This is particularly the case when frequent and different interventions are prescribed by different medical specialists. Even if the blood loss associated with an individual intervention appears to be negligible, the total blood loss from several interventions can be of clinical importance. Therefore, a single multidisciplinary approach to PBM must be formulated for all specialisms involved. This includes—whenever possible—the timely discontinuation of anticoagulants and platelet aggregation inhibitors. However, the frequent practice of routinely increasing the anticoagulation parameters in ICU patients is pointless, at least in the case of nonbleeding patients, and only results in increased costs (Gajic et al 2006). In such patients, any invasive investigations should be carried out by experienced physicians.

Note

Interventional blood loss can only be reduced using a multidisciplinary approach.

Conclusion

Diagnostic and interventional blood loss can be reduced using a multidisciplinary combination of different approaches. These include evaluation of the need for individual laboratory tests, restriction of laboratory diagnostic tests to those medically indicated, reduction of the blood draw volume, point-of-care testing, and use of modern noninvasive diagnostic procedures instead of blood tests.

4.2 Coagulation Management

C. F. Weber, K. Zacharowski

4.2.1 Introduction

Interdisciplinary cooperation is needed in the event of perioperative bleeding complications to limit blood loss, reduce the transfusion rate of allogeneic blood products through effective coagulation management, reduce the incidence of thromboembolic complications, and—equally important—curtail the primary and secondary costs of hemotherapy.

By taking a standardized coagulation history, it will be possible to identify existing preoperative coagulation disorders and to draw up an individual bleeding risk profile tailored to the planned surgical procedure. Coagulation management should be based on hemotherapy algorithms that take account of both the individual bleeding risks (e.g., medication containing acetylsalicylic acid or antiplatelet agents) and the causes of bleeding specific

to a given patient group (e.g., anticoagulation for procedures involving extracorporeal circulation).

The key elements of modern coagulation management are the timely and comprehensive analysis of any underlying coagulation disorder, followed by its targeted treatment. Compared with conventional laboratory tests, point-of-care coagulation testing enables a more rapid and comprehensive analysis of the causes of an existing coagulopathy. The incorporation of point-of-care coagulation testing into hemotherapy algorithms can help to reduce perioperative blood loss and transfusion of allogeneic blood products.

4.2.2 Successive Escalation of Treatment for Coagulation Disorders

Surgical Hemostasis/Permissive Hypotension

Any initial surgery-induced bleeding can lead to coagulopathic bleeding in the ensuing course. If there is loss of volume, the infusion of crystalloids and/or colloids needed for the maintenance of normovolemia can induce dilutional coagulopathy. Therefore, surgical/interventional hemostasis is a fundamental prerequisite and an important key element for the prophylaxis and effective treatment of perioperative blood coagulation disorders. Provided that there are no contraindications, restrictive volume therapy and permissive hypotension (mean arterial blood pressure 60–65 mmHg) are temporary treatment options to reduce blood loss until surgical hemostasis is achieved.

Note

Effective hemotherapy is impossible without surgical/interventional hemostasis.

Maintenance of an Optimal Physiological Environment for Hemostasis

pH Value

Acidosis affects primary hemostasis and can reduce the adhesion and aggregation of platelets. It also restricts plasma coagulation, thus reducing the speed at which thrombin—a key enzyme in the coagulation cascade that is essential for the formation of blood clots—is formed. As buffering can only partially reverse an acidosis-induced coagulation disorder, the prevention of acidosis should have top priority in everyday clinical practice.

Temperature

Hypothermia (body temperature < 35 °C) reduces the hemostatic potential of primary hemostasis and the plasma coagulation system. Coagulation disorders resulting from hypothermia-induced thrombocytopathy can be aggravated by platelet sequestration in the spleen and liver.

Calcium

Calcium is an essential cofactor in all phases of blood coagulation. Among other things, it mediates complex formation between the negatively charged phospholipids on the surface of wounds and the likewise negatively charged coagulation factors II, VII, IX, and X, thus promoting the accumulation and activation of coagulation factors at the site of vascular injury. As there is an inverse relationship between lactate and calcium, metabolic acidosis can give rise to clinically relevant hypocalcemia. Besides, the free calcium concentration can be reduced through chelate formation with the citrate that is contained in allogeneic blood products for anticoagulation purposes. Hypocalcemia secondary to major blood loss and massive transfusion must be treated in a timely fashion. The plasma concentration of ionized calcium should be > 1 mmol/L.

Hematocrit

RBCs have multiple effects on blood coagulation. They circulate in the middle of blood vessels, pushing the smaller platelets toward the vessel wall and thus toward the site of injury. Besides, RBCs have a role in providing phospholipids, ADP, and thromboxane A2, and they are catalysts in the process of blood clotting. As oxygen carriers, RBCs help to maintain tissue oxygenation and prevent acidosis. It is recommended that the hematocrit should not drop below around 25% if there is acute bleeding.

Note

Continuous correction of the basic physiological parameters required for hemostasis is the first treatment step.

Treatment Step: Antifibrinolytic Therapy

▶ **Hyperfibrinolysis.** The systemic activation of fibrinolysis (hyperfibrinolysis) can lead to life-threatening bleeding through the dissolution of blood clots and the consumption of circulating fibrinogen. Polytrauma patients, patients undergoing extracorporeal circulation, and those undergoing surgery of organs that are rich in tissue plasminogen activator, such as the lungs, adrenal glands, prostate gland, or uterus, are at higher risk for the development of hyperfibrinolysis. Hyperfibrinolysis can also be associated with a tumor, caused by hyperthermia or hypothermia, or induced by medication. Classic laboratory parameters, such as D-dimer, are not suitable for the diagnosis of hyperfibrinolysis or the monitoring of its treatment; rather, viscoelastic methods such as thromboelastography or thromboelastometry represent the gold standard for the diagnosis of hyperfibrinolysis (Luddington 2005).

▶ **Tranexamic acid.** Since the restriction of aprotinin use in 2008, the lysine analogue tranexamic acid has become the most commonly used antifibrinolytic drug. Its early administration in trauma patients reduced the mortality without increasing the risk of undesirable side effects such as thrombosis (Shakur et al 2010). Any hyperfibrinolysis must be treated before the transfusion of fresh frozen plasma (FFP) or the administration of another form of hemotherapy; otherwise the administered factors will immediately be consumed. A clinical suspicion of hyperfibrinolysis—even without viscoelastic confirmation—is sufficient to justify early treatment with tranexamic acid, especially in trauma patients. The dosing recommendations vary, ranging from a single bolus dose to continuous administration.

> **Note** !
>
> If there is diffuse bleeding, the early adminis-
> tration of tranexamic acid is recommended
> even without thromboelastographic confirma-
> tion of hyperfibrinolysis.

Treatment Step: Replacement of Deficient Coagulation Factors

The infusion of crystalloids or colloids for the maintenance of normovolemia can induce dilutional coagulopathy. Besides, coagulation factors are activated and consumed in a bleeding situation. Factor concentrates and FFP are available to treat coagulation factor deficiencies.

Fibrinogen Concentrates

Fibrinogen—a ligand of the platelet glycoprotein IIb/IIIa receptor—promotes blood clotting and determines the mechanical stability of the clot (Levy et al 2012). The average plasma concentration of the acute-phase protein fibrinogen is around 150 to 300 mg/dL; it can rise to 400–600 mg/dL toward the end of pregnancy. Although fibrinogen accounts for 85% to 90% of the total mass of plasma coagulation factors, it reaches its critical concentration sooner than most other coagulation factors in a bleeding or dilutional situation (Hiippala et al 1995). The target value (measured for example with the Clauss method or with a viscoelastic method, e.g., the FIBTEM test) in bleeding situations has not been clearly defined. Studies have demonstrated that the propensity for bleeding is greater at a plasma concentration of < 150–200 mg/dL or with maximum clot firmness of < 8 mm according to the FIBTEM test.

German and European guidelines recommend that the plasma fibrinogen concentration should not drop below 150–200 mg/dL in massive bleeding situations (Rossaint et al 2010). The fibrinogen concentration can generally be increased through the transfusion of FFP or the administration of fibrinogen concentrates. The administration of fibrinogen concentrates to increase the fibrinogen concentration has proved to be a rapid, safe, and effective measure. This is particularly true for the treatment of bleeding at the end of pregnancy, because the required fibrinogen concentration cannot be achieved with FFP.

Prothrombin Complex Concentrates

Prothrombin complex concentrate (PCC) is a factor concentrate containing the coagulation factors II, VII, IX, and X (the prothrombin complex); depending on the manufacturer, PCC also contains varying concentrations of proteins C and S as well as small amounts of antithrombin and heparin. PCC is licensed for the treatment and prophylaxis of bleeding caused by hereditary or acquired factor deficiency. This applies for instance to patients with a low prothrombin time, for example because of cirrhosis of the liver, treatment with coumarin derivatives, or acute blood loss. Administration of 1 IU/kg PCC raises the coagulation factor concentration by around 1%. For diffuse bleeding, PCC should be given at a dose of at least 25 IU/kg. The combination of PCC with antithrombin III, which was standard practice a few years ago, is no longer recommended.

Factor XIII

Factor XIII stabilizes blood clots through the cross-linking of fibrin and the integration of proteins with antifibrinolytic activity (e.g., α_2-antiplasmin) into the clot. There is no clearly defined lower reference range. However, it is recommended that the factor XIII concentration should not drop below 60–70% in bleeding situations (Gerlach et al 2002). The factor XIII concentration can be increased with FFP or factor concentrate. Since neither conventional laboratory analysis nor thromboelastometry are suitable for the diagnostic evaluation of a potential factor XIII deficiency, specific factor analysis should be carried out in cases of doubt.

Fresh Frozen Plasma

In the majority of cases, the administration of fibrinogen concentrate and PCC is sufficient to assure adequate clot formation in patients with coagulopathy. However, if there is major blood loss and a massive transfusion is required, a deficiency of factors V, VIII, and XI can occur, which cannot be treated with concentrates. In such cases, FFP transfusion appears to be indicated. FFP should be transfused only at a dose with hemostatic efficacy (at least > 15 mL/kg) (BAEK 2011a). The indication for FFP transfusion should be based on strict criteria, since FFP transfusion is associated with a significant rise in the incidence of acute respiratory failure, nosocomial infections, sepsis, and multiple organ failure (Watson et al 2009).

Coagulation Therapy Based on Factor Concentrates versus Fresh Frozen Plasma

A number of retro- and prospective studies, predominantly among patients undergoing cardiac surgery or general surgery, have shown that selective coagulation therapy with coagulation factor concentrates is superior to the nonspecific treatment with FFP, with the exception of situations involving massive transfusion.

> **Note**
>
> Coagulation factor deficiencies can be treated with factor concentrates or FFP. With the exception of situations involving massive transfusion, selective coagulation therapy with coagulation factor concentrates appears to be superior to nonspecific therapy with FFP.

Treatment Step: Optimization of Primary Hemostasis

In bleeding situations, platelets tend to reach their critical limit of 50,000–100,000/μL only at a late stage (Hiippala et al 1995). However, the hemostatic potential of primary hemostasis can be reduced even before the onset of thrombocytopenia. The presence of impaired platelet function and a patient's individual bleeding dynamics can necessitate the optimization of primary hemostasis, regardless of the current platelet count.

Desmopressin

Administration of the vasopressin analogue 1-deamino-8-D-arginine vasopressin (desmopressin; dose: 0.3 μg/kg) leads to a threefold increase in the concentrations of von Willebrand factor and factor VIII (Cattaneo 2002), and can improve platelet adhesion and aggregation. As such, desmopressin represents a drug-based treatment option for the optimization of primary hemostasis. It has relatively few side effects and is more cost-effective than the transfusion of platelet concentrates. Since desmopressin can induce fibrinolysis, it is often used in combination with tranexamic acid.

Transfusion of Platelet Concentrates

The transfusion of platelet concentrates is often inevitable if there is major blood loss and thrombocytopenia. A rise in the platelet count by 20,000–30,000/μL can be expected following the transfusion of platelet concentrate. When transfusing platelet concentrates, particular attention should be paid to the legal restrictions on the shelf life, since the infection risk rises proportionally to the shelf life and the hemostatic potential of platelets declines from the time of harvesting (Cauwenberghs et al 2007).

> **Note**
>
> In addition to the transfusion of platelet concentrates, a drug-based treatment option (administration of desmopressin) is available for the optimization of primary hemostasis.

Treatment Step: Ultima Ratio

If life-threatening coagulopathy persists after the implementation of surgical or interventional hemostatic measures, the optimization of primary hemostasis, and adequate substrate replacement (fibrinogen > 200 mg/dL, platelet count > 100,000/μL), the administration of recombinant activated factor VII (rVIIa; NovoSeven, Novo Nordisk; dose: 90 μg/kg) constitutes the treatment option of last resort (Vincent et al 2006). However, meta-analyses of prospective randomized studies did not find any evidence for a positive effect on the rate of allogeneic blood transfusion or the perioperative mortality. They did, however, identify a higher incidence of severe thromboembolic events following rVIIa administration (Lin et al 2011). For this reason, rVIIa should only be administered in life-threatening situations.

> **Note**
>
> The administration of rVIIa represents the treatment option of last resort and should be governed by particularly stringent criteria.

4.2.3 Diagnosis of Coagulopathy: Conventional Laboratory Analysis versus Point-of-care Methods

The standard laboratory tests used for the diagnosis of coagulation disorders (activated partial thromboplastin time, international normalized ratio, platelet count, fibrinogen concentration) have several diagnostic shortcomings. Cell–cell interactions, the effects of hypothermia and acidosis, and fibrin polymerization disorders are not sufficiently captured in vitro. It is also impossible to gain insights into the clot stability. The positive predictive value and the specificity are low with regard to the diagnosis of perioperative bleeding. The time delay between a blood draw and the availability of the results can mean that inadequate hemostatic treatment is initiated (Toulon et al 2009).

National and international guidelines therefore state that conventional laboratory analysis is not adequate for the diagnosis of acute bleeding or the monitoring of its treatment (Lier et al 2011), and they point out that the treatment algorithms for blood coagulation disorders should include point-of-care coagulation testing. Several prospective randomized studies concluded that the incorporation of point-of-care methods in hemotherapy algorithms led to a reduction in the rate of allogeneic blood transfusion (in particular the transfusion of FFP and RBC concentrates). A prospective randomized trial of cardiac surgery patients with a coagulation disorder demonstrated that hemotherapy based on point-of-care testing compared with hemotherapy based on conventional coagulation laboratory analysis led to a reduction in the RBC transfusion rate (Weber et al 2012). Analysis of the secondary outcome parameters revealed that the transfusion rate for FFP and platelet concentrates was significantly lower in the point-of-care group. Furthermore, the duration of postoperative ventilation and the duration of intensive care treatment were significantly shorter in the point-of-care group. The postoperative blood loss, incidence of postoperative kidney failure, 6-month mortality, and costs incurred for hemotherapy were lower in the point-of-care group (Weber et al 2012).

Point-of-care Methods

A broad spectrum of different methods are available for point-of-care coagulation testing. These range from simple strip tests to procedures of such complexity that their performance, and the interpretation of the results, should be entrusted only to experienced and trained personnel. These methods can be implemented in patient care at the pre-, intra-, or postoperative stage (Fig. 4.3). In addition, the complex process of blood coagulation cannot be reproduced by a single point-of-care device. A combination of several methods is often needed for a comprehensive diagnosis of complex coagulation disorders.

Thromboelastometry and viscoelastic methods are based on the technique of thromboelastography presented by Hartert (1951). Following activation of the coagulation cascade in vitro, parameters such as the time to onset of clot formation, the clotting speed, and the clot firmness and stability in relation to time are analyzed (Fig. 4.4). Aggregometry methods are used for the point-of-care analysis of primary hemostasis, especially for the evaluation of platelet function. By combining aggregometry and viscoelastic methods, it is possible to obtain a diagnostic spectrum that greatly surpasses that of conventional laboratory coagulation tests.

General Advantages of Point-of-care Testing

Only small quantities of whole blood are needed to perform point-of-care diagnostic tests (1–5 mL). Whereas conventional coagulation analysis delivers only quantitative information (e.g., platelet count or fibrinogen concentration), thromboelastometry or aggregometry methods can also provide functional information. Among other things, this enables the diagnosis of, and treatment monitoring in, fibrin polymerization disorders (e.g., caused by colloid infusion or [hyper]fibrinolysis) and thrombocytopathy. An early detection of hypercoagulopathic states can help to reduce the incidence of thromboembolic complications.

In addition to flexibility of use and the diagnostic spectrum offered by the various methods, the principal advantage of point-of-care diagnostic testing resides in the rapid availability of the results. The time-consuming transport of the blood sample to the laboratory and the preparatory steps

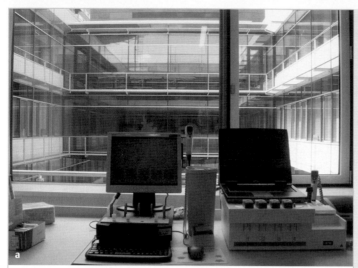

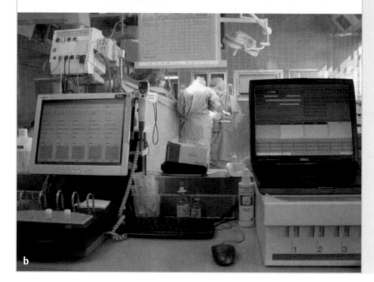

Fig. 4.3 Examples of locations where point-of-care coagulation testing is carried out in the perioperative setting. **(a)** Multiplate and ROTEM devices for point-of-care coagulation analysis at a central location in the anesthesiologic/surgical intensive care unit. **(b)** Bedside location in the main operating theater at Goethe University Hospital in Frankfurt, Germany.

needed in conventional laboratory analysis (including sample centrifugation, reagent preparation) are dispensed with. Most results are available within 10 minutes of starting measurement, even with more complex viscoelastic methods such as thromboelastometry, thus enabling quick decision-making on the course of treatment (Haas et al 2012).

General Limitations of Point-of-care Testing

None of the point-of-care methods currently available for coagulation analysis covers the body's entire hemostasis system. Often, several methods have to be combined and used in a complementary fashion in order to diagnose perioperative blood coagulation disorders, which are frequently of multifactorial etiology. However, even when combining several methods, certain potential causes of perioperative coagulopathy cannot not be diagnosed. For example, it is not possible to evaluate

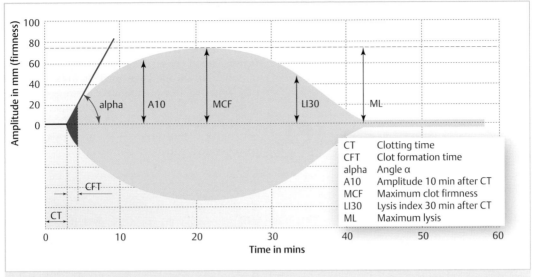

Fig. 4.4 Display of thromboelastometry results on a ROTEM device. CT, clotting time (comparable with R on the TEG), surrogate for plasma coagulation; MCF, maximum clot firmness (comparable with MA on the TEG), mainly determined on the basis of platelet count and fibrinogen concentration; LI30, lysis index (comparable with LY30 on the TEG); ML, maximum lysis, for the analysis of (hyper)fibrinolysis; ROTEM, rotational thromboelastometry; TEG, thromboelastogram. (Reproduced with kind permission of Tem International GmbH, Munich.)

the influence of low-molecular weight heparins, factor Xa inhibitors, direct or indirect platelet inhibitors, antithrombin, or protein C or S. The standard temperature of 37 °C used in viscoelastic and aggregometry testing precludes an analysis of hypo- or hyperthermia-induced coagulation disorders; other pathophysiological conditions influencing hemostasis (acidosis, hypocalcemia, anemia) cannot be reliably evaluated either by conventional testing.

Occasionally, when treating critically ill patients who have major blood loss and require a massive transfusion, there will not be enough time to analyze and record the results of point-of-care diagnostic tests. It is therefore recommended that all health care workers (physicians and nurses) involved in the treatment of bleeding patients are familiar with the use of point-of-care diagnostic tests. The cumulative costs for the performance of point-of-care tests (e.g., equipment costs, reagents, test cuvettes, control solutions, servicing) are higher than those for conventional coagulation analysis. However, the extra expenditure can be recovered through more restrictive transfusion regimens and more efficient use of other hemotherapeutic agents.

Quality Control

In Germany, the guideline on quality assurance in medical laboratories from the German Medical Association (BAEK 2015) sets out binding requirements for quality control that also apply to point-of-care methods. This guideline may serve as a good model for best practice. Based on these provisions, regular internal checks must be carried out, usually with control samples from the manufacturer. Besides, participation in multicenter studies is recommended for external quality control purposes. Since there is a time limit on the stability of whole blood, it is not suitable for use in multicenter studies; therefore, lyophilized plasma should be used for viscoelastic point-of-care testing in multicenter studies. For point-of-care methods where corresponding laboratory tests are available, a comparison of the point-of-care and laboratory results can serve as an external control mechanism.

Note

Point-of-care diagnostic testing can help to reduce the rate of allogeneic blood transfusions. Often, several point-of-care methods have to be combined for comprehensive coagulation testing.

Conclusion

The use of point-of-care methods as diagnostic tests and in treatment algorithms enables the efficient treatment and management of patients with coagulation disorders and can have a positive influence on their clinical outcome.

4.3 Use of Allogeneic Blood Conservation Strategies

C. von Heymann, L. Kaufner

4.3.1 Introduction

▶ **Shortage of blood products.** Transfusion of allogeneic RBC concentrates is currently the most commonly used treatment not only for acute but also for chronic anemia. Based on present scenarios and prognoses, the number of potential blood donors in the population is declining, while there is a rising need for RBC concentrates, in particular to treat elderly patients (Greinacher et al 2010). There are therefore concerns that there will be a critical shortage of allogeneic RBC concentrates in the future.

▶ **Transfusion safety.** In addition to concerns over the availability of allogeneic RBC concentrates, a growing number of scientific publications have raised doubts over the safety of treatment with allogeneic RBC transfusions. Studies have shown that the perioperative transfusion of RBC concentrates is associated with a significantly higher incidence of infectious, pulmonary, and thromboembolic complications (Glance et al 2011, Pedersen et al 2009). Apart from a significantly higher morbidity rate, most studies also identified a higher mortality rate among transfused patients (Bernard et al 2009, Karkouti et al 2004). The conclusion drawn from these studies is that the indication for RBC transfusion should be based on a strict

individualized risk–benefit assessment (ASATF 2015).

▶ **Alternatives to allogeneic red blood cell transfusion.** Blood conservation strategies play an important role in operative medicine because they may improve the preoperative condition of the patient (e.g., correction of preoperative anemia) and reduce the exposure to allogeneic blood products, and can thus improve the prognosis and the postoperative outcome.

Note

Allogeneic blood conservation strategies will be of paramount importance in the future, because perioperative RBC transfusion is associated with an increased rate of complications and there is a growing shortage of allogeneic blood products.

The exact perioperative allogeneic blood conservation techniques used depend on the transfusion probability and on structural aspects of the hospital or the responsible transfusion medicine institution.

This chapter describes the pre- and intraoperative (less commonly postoperative) allogeneic blood conservation techniques predominantly performed by anesthesiologists:
- Preoperative autologous blood donation (PAD).
- Acute normovolemic hemodilution (ANH).
- Intra- and postoperative cell salvage.

4.3.2 Preoperative Autologous Blood Donation

For PAD, blood is repeatedly drawn from the patient in the weeks preceding surgery and, depending on the method, stored either as whole blood or separated into autologous RBC concentrate and autologous FFP. Autologous RBC concentrates can be stored for 35 to 49 days. Retransfusion during or after the operation has to be carried out within this time period if the transfusion of blood products is indicated. Unused autologous RBCs have to be discarded because it is not permitted to transfuse autologous blood products to other patients.

▶ **Requirements.** PAD requires specialized personnel (e.g., personnel licensed to prepare blood products), technical equipment, and premises, as well as a medical indication.

For the donor, the requirements are the same as for allogeneic blood donors (Biscoping et al 2013). For example, according to guidelines governing the collection of blood and blood components in Germany, the absolute contraindications to PAD include suspected gastrointestinal infection, unstable angina pectoris, main trunk stenosis > 50%, symptomatic aortic valve stenosis, and acute infection with suspected hematogenous dissemination (BAEK 2010).

The hemoglobin concentration before PAD in Germany must be at least 11.5 ± 0.5 g/dL (BAEK 2011a). This threshold is relatively low compared with other countries; for example, in France (Rosencher et al 2008) and Canada (Freedman et al 2008), PAD may only be performed if the hemoglobin value is more than 13 g/dL. Each autologous blood donor must also be tested for HIV-1/2 antibodies, anti-HCV antibodies, and hepatitis B surface (HBs) antigen. Furthermore, PAD is governed by the same safety standards as allogeneic blood donation. Therefore, in addition to determination of the blood group (ABO/Rhesus system), autologous blood must be tested for alloantibodies that might cause incompatibility reactions, and for infections such as HIV (AIDS), hepatitis B and C, and lues (syphilis).

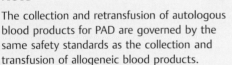

Note

The collection and retransfusion of autologous blood products for PAD are governed by the same safety standards as the collection and transfusion of allogeneic blood products.

▸ **Administration and effectiveness.** In most countries, PAD is primarily used in orthopaedic surgery. The effectiveness of PAD benefits from an "intense" blood donation schedule, with two or more autologous donations within a short period of time (1 week) as long as the patient's clinical condition allows it. Although this approach results in a larger drop in the hematocrit, in fact making the patient anemic, it also leaves a longer time period for RBC regeneration before surgery. The gain in RBC mass depends on the RBC count prior to donation and on the extent of erythropoiesis stimulation, which is stronger if the patient's hemoglobin value has dropped to around 10 g/dL or less (Eckhardt et al 1993). However, despite this favorable effect, the yield in autologous RBCs is smaller in anemic than in nonanemic patients. At the time of surgery, nonanemic patients also have a higher hemoglobin value after PAD and, as a consequence, a relatively lower transfusion risk. In addition, nonanemic patients often have more units of autologous blood—with a higher hematocrit—available, which often results in a waste of autologous blood units. Therefore, and because of the availability of less invasive, blood-sparing surgical techniques, the indication for PAD needs to be revised (Singbartl 2007, Singbartl et al 2009).

Note

In the context of PBM, the use of PAD is controversial, because most patients become anemic after the donation, which thwarts the first pillar of PBM.

▸ **Safety of autologous blood donation.** The responsible physician should bear in mind that autologous blood carries the same risks of blood product mix-up and bacterial contamination as allogeneic blood—especially in cases of inappropriate venipuncture technique or uncritical patient selection (BGSS 2005). Several studies have also demonstrated a higher infection rate in association with the transfusion of autologous RBC units (Bierbaum et al 1999, Freedman et al 2008). In addition, storage damage (e.g., reduced ATP and 2,3-bisphosphoglyceric acid content, reduced deformability of the RBC membrane) reported for allogeneic RBCs is also present in autologous units and increases in line with the storage duration (Lion et al 2010). These negative storage effects might have clinical implications, because the transfusion of allogeneic RBC concentrates older than 14 days was associated with higher rates of sepsis and mortality among patients who had cardiac surgery (Koch et al 2008, Rogers et al 2009). Whether storage damage in autologous RBC concentrates is also associated with higher rates of clinical complications and mortality is unknown at present, and must be investigated in clinical studies (Lacroix et al 2015).

Note

An increased infection rate has also been reported for autologous RBC transfusion.

▸ **Individual indication.** A Cochrane meta-analysis found that the risk of receiving an allogeneic

RBC transfusion was reduced by around 64% through PAD (Henry et al 2002). Therefore, PAD is an effective allogeneic-blood conservation strategy. However, the authors point out that the risk of being transfused in the first place (whether with autologous or with allogeneic blood) is increased by a factor of 1.33 after PAD. This finding underlines the need for the presence of an appropriate, individual indication for the donation and transfusion of autologous blood. This is also of paramount importance in terms of cost-effectiveness, because this is assured only if there is an actual reduction in allogeneic blood consumption. The implications for everyday clinical practice are that autologous blood products should not be transfused simply because they are available. Overtransfusion must be avoided at all costs (Lion et al 2010).

> **Note**
>
> PAD reduces the risk of allogeneic RBC transfusion, but increases the risk of receiving a transfusion in the first place.

4.3.3 Acute Normovolemic Hemodilution

In the operating theater, ANH can be used preoperatively in patients with an adequate hematocrit to obtain autologous whole blood with a high hematocrit. The withdrawn blood is then retransfused during the operation. Through concurrent replacement of the withdrawn blood, the patient's hematocrit is reduced so that the blood lost during surgery has a lower hematocrit. To maintain normovolemia, the withdrawn volume is replaced by electrolyte or colloid infusion. Depending on the baseline hematocrit, two to three 500-mL units of whole blood (each unit containing around 100 mL of a standard stabilizer solution) can be prepared and—after labelling with the patient data, date, and time—stored close to the patient at room temperature for up to 6 hours. Apart from reducing the hematocrit, hemodilution reduces the blood viscosity, increases the cardiac output, and improves the rheological properties of the blood (Messmer et al 1972). To avoid a negative impact on oxygen transport because of the removal of RBCs and the ensuing anemia, the minimum hematocrit has to be adapted to the patient's cardiac performance before and during surgery. For pa-

tients with normal cardiovascular function, early studies recommend that the hematocrit should not be reduced to values below 30% before starting the operation (Klövekorn et al 1981).

> **Note**
>
> The reduction of the hematocrit through withdrawal of whole blood and the concurrent replacement of the withdrawn volume through electrolyte or colloid infusion have to be tailored perioperatively to match the patient's cardiac performance.

▶ **Effectiveness and use.** The effectiveness of this method would certainly benefit from a further reduction in the hematocrit, provided the patient's cardiopulmonary status allows this. It is possible that lower hematocrit values will be tolerated during ANH if the patient's cardiovascular function is continuously monitored with advanced hemodynamic monitoring (Oriani et al 2011). No consensus has been reached in the scientific literature as to whether ANH helps to reduce the use of allogeneic RBC concentrates. The maximum saving has been estimated at 1 to 1.5 units (BAEK 2011a). These contradictory findings and the limitations of the technique (in particular in the case of patients with reduced cardiopulmonary tolerance and those undergoing tumor surgery) may explain why this simple, relatively inexpensive procedure, which is not subject to any technical requirements, has failed to prevail in operative medicine. The Federal Statistical Office of Germany reports that ANH was used only 1580 times during 2010.

▶ **Contraindications.** Contraindications to ANH comprise refusal by the patient, limited cardiopulmonary reserve, tumor surgery, and septic surgery with probable bacteremia. In the two latter cases, retransfusion of the whole blood obtained by ANH might lead to tumor cell dissemination or bacterial spread.

4.3.4 Cell Salvage

Cell salvage involves the recovery of the patient's blood from the surgical site during and/or after an operation with major blood loss, and the subsequent processing of the recovered wound blood for retransfusion. A separate suction device draws blood from the wound; in a second lumen, the device adds an anticoagulant solution to the salvaged blood to prevent coagulation of the activated wound blood (the anticoagulant used is generally unfractionated heparin in 0.9% saline, but citrate can also be used in cases of type II heparin-induced thrombocytopenia [HIT II]). The blood from the wound is first collected in a reservoir pending processing of the salvaged blood until retransfusion is indicated. Only then is the centrifugation system set up. The blood is processed by washing and separating the RBCs through centrifugation. The processed suspension corresponds to an RBC concentrate with a hematocrit of 50–70% depending on the device, since the plasma and all cellular components apart from the RBCs are removed through the centrifugation. This method can be tailored to the anticipated magnitude of the blood loss, making it cost-effective.

▶ **Cell salvage systems.** Various cell savage systems are on the market. While their technical principles may differ, their end product is essentially an RBC concentrate that should be retransfused immediately at room temperature; only in exceptional cases can it be stored for up to 6 hours until retransfusion. For clinical use, certain suppliers offer pediatric and adult systems; hence, smaller volumes of surgical blood can also be processed and retransfused. There are also different washing methods, washing speeds, and levels of washing quality to meet the respective clinical situation (e.g., more rapid and greater volume loss in aortic surgery or polytrauma). Further details on this topic are provided in a review article by Hansen and Seyfried (2011).

Note

Cell savage is cost-effective if the intraoperative blood loss is large enough and cell salvage can be continued postoperatively.

▶ **Indications.** Based on the recommendations of the Association of Anaesthetists of Great Britain and Ireland, cell savage is indicated for blood loss of > 1,000 mL or > 20% of the circulating blood volume, rare blood groups, irregular antibodies, preoperative anemia, or if allogeneic RBC transfusion is refused by the patient (AAGBI 2009). The German Medical Association and other societies recommend the use of cell salvage in operations where major blood loss is expected (e.g., ortho-

paedic or vascular surgery) or for acute emergency operations (BAEK 2011a, Ferraris 2011a, ASATF 2015). The indication of a volumetric blood loss (> 1,000 mL) is not appropriate in all cases (pediatric surgery, including pediatric spinal column surgery), because salvage of even small blood volumes can help to avoid an allogeneic RBC transfusion in subgroups of patients. Apart from operations with major blood loss, cell salvage can also be used in patients with preexisting anemia to avoid allogeneic RBC transfusions. However, it must be borne in mind that the (cost-) effectiveness of cell salvage, in terms of the RBC mass needed to produce a surgical RBC concentrate, depends on the intraoperative hemoglobin value. Although to date there are no prospective studies on the use of cell salvage for anemic patients, cell salvage appears to be a valuable, potentially cost-effective process when employed as part of a multimodal strategy to avoid allogeneic RBC transfusions in patients with preoperative anemia.

Note

Salvage even of small blood volumes can help to avoid allogeneic RBC transfusions, in particular in children and small-sized adults.

▶ **Areas of application.** Retransfusion of salvaged RBC concentrates in line with the current transfusion indications reduces the need for allogeneic RBC transfusion. Cell salvage is used on a regular basis primarily in orthopaedic, cardiac, and trauma surgery. Its use is not restricted to the intraoperative phase; it can also be applied postoperatively, for example in the ICU, if there is persistent blood loss.

▶ **Effectiveness.** In orthopaedic surgery, cell salvage reduces the relative risk of requiring an allogeneic RBC transfusion by 54% (Carless et al 2010b). Hence, cell salvage is an effective allogeneic blood conservation technique that should also prove to be cost-effective if used for the correct indications. No side effects or complications have been reported. However, the authors acknowledge that the inadequate methodological quality of the studies to date (e.g., lack of blinding) may have biased the findings in favor of cell salvage. The data from international studies and meta-analyses, in particular, also point toward a reduction in the rate of allogeneic RBC transfusions in other surgical disciplines such as obstetrics (Fong et al 2007), vascular surgery (Takagi et al 2007), pediatric cardiac surgery (Golab et al 2008), adult cardiac surgery (Wang et al 2009), and neurosurgery (Cataldi et al 1997). These data confirm that cell salvage has a place in the arsenal of measures to avoid perioperative blood loss and allogeneic RBC transfusion, especially in elective operations associated with a high bleeding risk—provided the undisputed contraindications are observed.

> **Note**
>
> In elective operations with a high bleeding risk, cell salvage is a cost-effective measure to avoid allogeneic RBC transfusions, and this does not just apply to orthopaedic surgery. However, specific contraindications, e.g., sepsis, must be taken into account.

▶ **Contraindications.** Systemic infection (sepsis) of the patient and bacterial contamination of the wound blood are indisputably the main contraindication for the use of cell salvage. Even in supposedly "sterile" operations, up to 33% of salvaged blood was found to be contaminated (mainly with skin bacteria) (Sugai et al 2001). The use of a leukocyte filter is not always effective in preventing bacterial contamination of the wound blood. Therefore, depending on the national recommendations, the use of cell salvage is contraindicated if there is any likelihood that the wound blood is contaminated (in particular with intestinal bacteria) (BAEK 2011a). However, this issue is still a focus of debate in the international literature (Ashworth and Klein 2010). The use of cell salvage in obstetrics is controversial because of the risks of fetal cell transfusion and amniotic fluid embolism. By contrast, the German Medical Association recommends the use of cell salvage in tumor surgery provided the wound blood concentrate is irradiated with 50 Gy before retransfusion (Hansen et al 2002, BAEK 2011a).

4.3.5 Comparison of the Effectiveness of Different Allogeneic Blood Conservation Strategies

The use of allogeneic blood conservation strategies is determined, on the one hand, by the suitability of the patients receiving treatment, the type of surgical procedure, and the availability of the technical devices. On the other hand, the cost-effectiveness of these therapies is crucial. Because of cost pressures in the health care sector, economic factors play an increasing role in decisions about the use of allogeneic blood conservation methods. Therefore, the proposed techniques themselves have to be cost-effective when used under the given circumstances, and/or be embedded in an overall PBM strategy that involves the treatment of preoperative anemia, the minimization of perioperative blood loss, and consequently the reduction of allogeneic RBC transfusions.

▶ **Evidence-based assessment.** Data on the aforementioned intraoperative modalities have been compared with other allogeneic blood conservation strategies in the field of orthopaedic surgery and subjected to evidence-based assessment (Muñoz et al 2009). The strength of the evidence was based on the methodological quality of the respective studies, and served as the basis for the recommendation level for each allogeneic blood conservation strategy (**Table 4.1**). **Table 4.2** shows the results of an analysis of the effectiveness of PAD, ANH, and cell salvage. Based on this analysis, PAD and cell salvage are deemed to be effective methods for the avoidance of anemia and allogeneic RBC transfusions (Muñoz et al 2009). By contrast, it was not possible to issue a general recommendation for ANH, because a meta-analysis covering various surgical disciplines did not identify a clinical benefit for ANH (Carless et al 2004a).

> **Note**
>
> For ANH, no benefit in terms of a reduction in allogeneic RBC transfusions has been demonstrated to date, despite its low costs and few technical demands.

Table 4.1 Definitions of evidence and recommendation levels

Evidence level		Recommendation level	
I	RCT with large number of cases, meta-analysis, systematic review	A	Supported by at least two level I studies
II	RCT with small number of cases	B	Supported by one level I study
III	Observational study with concurrent controls	C	Supported by level II studies
IV	Observational study with historical controls	D	Supported by level III studies
V	Case study, expert opinion	E	Supported by level IV and V studies

Abbreviation: RCT, randomized controlled trial.

Table 4.2 Evidence and recommendation levels for allogeneic blood conservation strategies in orthopaedic surgery

Strategy, use of autologous blood	Evidence level	Recommendation level
Preoperative autologous blood donation	I–III	B*
Cell salvage (intra- and postoperative)	I–III	B
Acute normovolemic hemodilution	I	Not recommended

* For scoliosis surgery.

Conclusion

Allogeneic blood conservation strategies will play an increasing role as part of PBM, because of the rising costs, diminishing donor blood supplies, and growing evidence of complications associated with allogeneic blood products. The few contraindications that apply to the techniques described must be observed to assure patient safety. By embracing a concept aimed at the treatment of preoperative anemia and the avoidance of perioperative allogeneic RBC transfusion, using a combination of strategies (e.g., PAD and cell salvage), the complication rate can be reduced and the patient outcome improved.

4.4 Surgical Technique and Minimally Invasive Surgery—Limitations and Prospects

J. W. Erhard

4.4.1 Perioperative Blood Loss

The second of the three pillars of PBM is aimed at preserving the patient's blood volume as far as possible under the given interventional or surgical conditions. Any form of bleeding during surgery can ultimately result in clinically relevant blood loss. Bleeding and blood loss represent a danger to the patient for three reasons:
• Need for allogeneic RBC transfusion.
• Risk of hemorrhagic shock/ischemia.
• Increase in morbidity and mortality.

The term *blood loss* already suggests that a patient "loses" blood because of an illness or injury, or for treatment-related reasons (surgery). In general, blood loss in the surgical setting is something that tends to be accepted rather than critically appraised. For certain elective procedures, it is legally required to document the perioperative blood loss. After all, the indication for RBC transfusion may be based on this blood loss. To date, there has not been sufficient debate about the reasons for such blood loss, the implications for the patient, and the consequences of minor or major blood loss.

In a chapter entitled "Hemorrhagic complications in surgery," F.S. Morrison noted in 1981 that the individual surgeon's technique ranked first among the causes of perioperative bleeding, followed by impaired platelet function and coagulation disorders as well as other causes that are rarer. He considered the surgeon and the surgical technique to be the key factors determining perioperative blood loss (Hardy 1981).

Note

Surgical technique is a key determinant of perioperative blood loss.

▶ **Interdisciplinary treatment.** PBM is an interdisciplinary treatment approach for patients who are at risk for anemia because of anticipated blood loss during elective surgery and/or patients who are already anemic at the time of treatment. Both anemia and blood loss (with or without the need for transfusion) are associated with increased morbidity and mortality in the perioperative phase (Gombotz 2012, Musallam et al 2011).

Note

Anemia during the perioperative phase is a key risk factor for increased morbidity and mortality, and this risk is further aggravated by the transfusion of allogeneic blood.

4.4.2 Indication for Surgery

▶ **Elective procedures.** For elective procedures, all medical specialists involved in the treatment of the patient should formulate an interdisciplinary strategy for individualized hemotherapy and its implementation (**Table 4.3**). The various specialists must be familiar with the standards (algorithms) for the given elective procedure, including the evidence-based probability of RBC transfusion (Erhard et al 2003, Shander et al 2012a; Ferraris 2011a; Carson et al 2012b; ASATF 2015). At the same time, the surgeon, anesthetist, internist, and intensivist must have reached an agreement on a hemotherapy strategy for the individual patient.

▶ **Emergency procedures.** In an emergency situation where an urgent or lifesaving operation is needed, the implementation of an individualized hemotherapy approach may be vital for the disease course and the survival of the patient. In any case, the number of transfused blood units should be decided by mutual agreement. In an emergency situation, it is particularly important to reach a consensus on the patient's surgical risk and on the impact of the patient's circulating RBC volume.

If the patient is already experiencing severe hemorrhagic shock or ischemia before the operation and this can only be treated with oxygen carriers, an acute allogeneic RBC transfusion may be needed (emergency).

In an emergency situation, it must also be promptly established whether there is a bleeding source that can be treated immediately (e.g., acutely bleeding vessel), whether there is diffuse bleeding (bleeding in the presence of a coagulopathy), or whether a critically ill patient has a combination of both problems (disastrous coagulation disorder, active bleeding). In the event of polytrauma or another form of severe bleeding, a differential coagulation analysis must be carried out in parallel with immediate treatment, preferably using a point-of-care method. Today, thanks to systems such as rotational thromboelastometry

Table 4.3 Algorithm for perioperative PBM

Preoperative	Intraoperative	Postoperative
Indication/risk: • Medical history (medications) • Disease • Anemia (diagnosis, treatment)	Elective/emergency: • Time-out, hemotherapy? Surgical strategy: • Positioning, approach, MIS • Technical equipment, cell salvage • Normovolemia/normothermia • Normal acid–base balance • Blood pressure, blood loss, hemostasis	ICU/normal ward: • Information/documentation • Normovolemia/normothermia • Secondary bleeding? Reoperation?
Conclusion: Individualized hemotherapy	**Conclusion: Is the strategy effective? Change?**	**Conclusion: Communication**

Abbreviations: ICU, intensive care unit; MIS, minimally invasive surgery.

(ROTEM) by Tem Innovations and Multiplate by Hoffmann-La Roche, it is possible to monitor the coagulation status and treatment process on site before and after the transfusion of blood and blood products (Theusinger et al 2009, Spahn and Ganter 2010, Meißner and Schlenke 2012).

> **Note**
>
> An individualized preoperative hemotherapy strategy must be formulated and implemented for patients at risk for RBC transfusion or for those with a perioperative anemia that might aggravate the course of disease.

4.4.3 PBM and Surgery

The second pillar of PBM entails organization of the surgical procedure in such a way that the patient's own RBC volume will be preserved as far as possible, i.e., the patient will not experience any relevant blood loss during surgery.

Individualized Surgical Technique

▶ **Blood loss.** "Individual surgical technique is highly variable and probably remains the most relevant factor." This statement by John Taylor on the topic of surgical methods to minimize blood loss places a great responsibility on the surgeon to avoid blood loss (Thomas et al 2005). Today, most surgical procedures are performed in accordance with a standardized technique that must be transmittable and reproducible. Such surgical techniques are the cornerstone of any young surgeon's continuing education program. It is precisely for that reason that continuing training courses should highlight the paramount importance of avoiding perioperative blood loss.

▶ **Tissue destruction.** A surgical procedure is always associated with tissue destruction. Apart from local trauma, the ensuing inflammatory process can trigger other reactions affecting the entire body, which in turn impacts hemostasis (e.g., generalized inflammation following major operations, septic reaction, or shock) (Thomas et al 2005).

> **Note**
>
> The surgeon is an important risk factor for perioperative blood loss. Through an optimal surgical technique, surgical blood loss can be reduced by up to 80%.

Anesthesia and Patient Positioning

The importance of teamwork in achieving a successful surgical outcome is borne out by the close cooperation with anesthesiologists: optimal patient positioning in itself is sufficient to significantly reduce venous pressure in a surgical area. Lateral, head-up, or head-down positioning, a change of the position, and monitoring of the central venous pressure can considerably help to reduce blood loss. Likewise, the type of anesthesia (e.g., regional anesthesia), anesthesia depth, and relaxation have a major impact (Erhard et al 2003).

For example, it is current standard practice to perform liver resection with the upper part of the body slightly raised, with a low venous pressure, and with no positive end-expiratory pressure. The different operative steps must be carefully coordinated within the team (Erhard et al 2003).

Apart from these measures based on patient positioning, anesthesia depth, and active reduction of the venous pressure, it may be advisable in certain operations to perform vascular occlusion of a region/organ system; for example: performance of the Pringle maneuver during liver surgery; application of a tourniquet in orthopaedic surgery of the extremities; embolization of highly vascularized tumors; cross-clamping of the aorta in deep pelvic surgery, a type of operation that used to be associated with major blood loss.

▶ **Maintenance of the coagulation cascade.** The measures described are supported by a functional coagulation cascade, with maintenance of the acid–base balance and normothermia playing a pivotal role. The biochemical reactions and corresponding enzymatic activities are directly dependent on the ambient temperature. For example, if there is a 5 °C drop in the local tissue temperature, the potential for coagulation will be decreased by 50% (Rohrer and Natale 1992). Apart from maintaining an optimal room temperature, there are now modern warming systems for infusions and warming mats that can be tailored to the patient's body and that should preferably already be used in the preoperative room.

> ### Note
>
> Optimized positioning, maintenance of normothermia and normovolemia, avoidance of acidosis, antihypertensive treatment, and lowering of the venous pressure help to considerably reduce the perioperative blood loss.

Surgical Anatomy

Surgical technique is aimed at minimizing tissue trauma. To that effect, anatomical avascular zones should be observed during the dissection. Apart from markedly reducing blood loss, an approach based on anatomical landmarks that takes account of natural boundaries can also improve the surgical outcome. An example is the technique of total mesorectal excision in rectal carcinoma surgery. Thanks to the improved oncologic results obtained with this technique, it is now possible to perform such a procedure without allogeneic blood transfusion. However, this only applies for tumors confined within anatomical organ boundaries. If the tumor has spread beyond a given organ, multivisceral resection may be needed. Here, too, the anatomical boundaries should be noted (Kim et al 2012b).

> ### Note
>
> Basic surgical rule: regardless of its nature, bleeding should always be staunched as quickly and effectively as possible.

Cell Salvage

The techniques used to collect and process wound blood intraoperatively continue to play a key role in allogeneic-blood conservation (Hansen and Seyfried 2011). The method is well established, especially for trauma surgery and elective orthopaedic surgery, but also for elective cardiac surgery. The algorithm used for blood conservation measures should be able to indicate for both elective and emergency procedures when and how cell salvage should be used. Apart from logistic considerations, such as assigning responsibilities and upgrading equipment, financial aspects should also be taken into account. For example, there is no

point in making preparations for cell salvage if there is a high probability that blood loss will be negligible for a specific operation (personal experience, evidence). Modern cell salvage systems can collect wound blood without first having to start elaborate processing. If the wound blood volume is at least around 1,000 mL, the use of cell salvage can be deemed beneficial in medical and financial terms. However, there continues to be uncertainty about its use in obstetrics (leukocyte depletion) or in the surgical resection of malignancies (Ashworth and Klein 2010). Wound blood containing tumor cells can be safely retransfused after irradiation with 50 Gy. The use of a leukocyte depletion filter to process wound blood merely reduces the tumor cell content and cannot be recommended without reservations. Likewise, preference should be given to automated processing as opposed to the retransfusion of unwashed wound blood.

> ### Note
>
> In the hands of an experienced user, cell salvage is eminently suited to minimizing perioperative blood loss. Its use is cost-effective if the wound blood volume is at least around 1,000 mL.

4.4.4 Specific Surgical Techniques

Preparations for Blood-sparing Surgery

Any surgical indication decisions must take the need for individualized hemotherapy into account.

▶ **Medical history.** When taking a medical history, exact details must be obtained on any medications that can cause a considerable increase of the patient's bleeding risk (coumarin, platelet aggregation inhibitors, new-generation anticoagulants [Spahn and Korte 2012], combination products [often containing nonsteroidal anti-inflammatory drugs]). Taking a bleeding history is mandatory. It may also be necessary to consider the medical history data obtained by colleagues (Erhard et al 2003).

▶ **Indication.** The surgical indication should also be reviewed to assess whether the diagnostic findings point to a particular risk for bleeding (e.g., tumor, blood supply). If this is the case, it should be considered whether the bleeding risk can be reduced in advance, for example through interventional embolization of the supplying blood vessels (de Jong and Wertenbroek 2011, Gombotz 2012).

▶ **Briefing.** The widespread practice of holding a documented "time-out" for briefing at the start of an operation should also include a review of the individualized hemotherapy measures (Haynes et al 2009).

▶ **Technical equipment.** High-frequency ultrasonic dissectors or similar technical equipment must be available for use in elective surgical procedures where there is a risk of bleeding. It is important that such tools are available from the beginning of the operation so that they can be employed without delay. Thanks to the fact that there are now reusable versions of these devices, their use on a large scale is also economically feasible (Soper et al 2009).

It is advisable to have a range of different facilities (e.g., mono- and bipolar current; ultrasound equipment; Cavitron ultrasonic surgical aspirator; water-jet technology) available to be able to respond to the specific demands of an operation.

> **Note**
>
> Medical history taking and surgical indication decisions should take the need for individualized hemotherapy into account.

Minimal Access Surgery—Surgical and Technical Requirements

▶ **Minimally invasive procedures.** Perioperative blood loss can be reduced through the extensive use of minimal access surgery/minimally invasive surgery (MIS). No randomized studies have been carried out to investigate this matter, but reliable data attest to the superiority of MIS over conventional surgery with regard to blood loss (Soper et al 2009, Kim et al 2012b). Besides, the choice of surgical approach is a prime determinant of blood loss, regardless of the use of MIS or conventional surgery—for example, blood loss can be further minimized if there is a good view of the surgical site, the approach can be extended without causing much injury, or appropriate retraction systems and positioning aids are being used. (Erhard et al 2003).

▶ **Technical systems.** Three-dimensional optical systems, optimized instruments for open and laparoscopic surgery, and robotic systems can enhance the dissection technique and help to reduce blood loss even further. Robotic surgical procedures are already well established in orthopaedic surgery, cardiac valve surgery, and prostate and kidney surgery (Binhas et al 2012, Nepple et al 2012).

To what extent the use of such systems can actually reduce blood loss has not been systematically investigated so far. However, it can be assumed that the detailed planning of each operative step, as is required for such methods, will help to further minimize blood loss. Similar meticulous planning is needed for conventional operations.

▶ **Feedback.** Even for experienced surgeons and their teams, it is not always possible to estimate the amount of blood lost during an operation. This calls for good feedback communication between the surgical and anesthesia personnel (tip: include this in the operating-room rules and regulations). This will enable the surgeon, for example, to pack the wound, stabilize the patient, and resume surgery the following day under noncritical circumstances (**Fig. 4.5**) (Erhard et al 2003, Gombotz 2012).

> **Note**
>
> MIS can help to reduce blood loss. However, this requires detailed planning, use of the optimal surgical approach, and availability of the relevant technical equipment.

4.4.5 Postoperative Period and Surgical Intensive Care Medicine

▶ **Communication.** The algorithm used in perioperative blood management must also take account of the postoperative phase (**Table 4.3**). Any information relating to an operation must be forwarded without fail to the persons responsible for the follow-up treatment of the patient; whenever possible, this information should be passed on in person and documented, especially for complex or uncommon surgical procedures. Details must include the surgical technique, any occurrence of bleeding, the exact location of the drains, the cardiovascular status, transfusions, hemostasis, and patient positioning. The more elaborate and

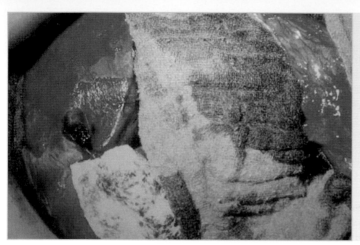

Fig. 4.5 Perihepatic packing as a stabilization and blood conservation measure in the context of perioperative PBM.

uncommon an operation, the more detailed the information that needs to be passed on. It is advisable to include a sketch depicting the operation that also shows the location of the drains.

▶ **Reintervention.** Early reoperation is not equivalent to personal failure by the surgeon or the intensive care physician, even if bleeding is suspected. If the patient is normothermic, normovolemic, and hemodynamically unstable despite catecholamine therapy, and if there is continuous blood loss from the drain(s) (even if minute), the indication for reoperation must be evaluated in a timely fashion. RBC transfusion is not a substitute for reintervention!

Note

Information on the surgical procedure must be passed on, in particular because this information is crucial in managing any secondary bleeding.

4.4.6 Quality of the Results

Since the Transfusion Requirements in Critical Care (TRICC) trial, published in 1999, other studies have been initiated in the surgical and conservative treatment setting to further investigate the benefits of a more restrictive versus a liberal indication for RBC transfusion. The clear trend is toward a paradigm shift in favor of restricting RBC transfusion. Carson et al (2011) demonstrated in a U.S. study of high-risk patients undergoing ortho-

paedic surgery that transfusion did not bestow any benefit if the hemoglobin value was above 8 g/dL. Similar findings were reported for Europe (Muñoz et al 2009). For cardiac surgery, Moskowitz and coauthors (2010) demonstrated impressively that the consistent implementation of a PBM strategy reduced the morbidity and mortality. By contrast, the Austrian Benchmark Study, which focused on blood consumption in standard operations, revealed a striking variability in the transfusion rates of elective surgical procedures even in leading hospitals (Gombotz et al 2007).

4.4.7 Implications for Routine Practice

In addition to aptitude and skill, surgeons possess a multifaceted armamentarium to minimize blood loss and achieve effective perioperative hemostasis. However, surgeons should be in no doubt that they themselves can represent a major risk factor for perioperative blood loss. They should improve the surgical and hemotherapeutic outcome for their patients by formulating a well-thought-out indication, engaging in interdisciplinary risk assessment (hypervascularized tumor, anticoagulants, patient-specific risk factors), and pursuing an optimal surgical strategy. With operative experience, access to the technical and pharmacological facilities described, and the absolute will to minimize blood loss, blood as a resource can be sustainably conserved and the patient morbidity and mortality reduced in the short, medium, and long terms (Erhard and Hofmann 2005, Gombotz 2012).

In routine clinical practice to date, too little account is taken of reaching pre, peri-, and postoperative interdisciplinary agreement on an individualized hemotherapy strategy. The operating-room rules and regulations, transfusion committee meetings, interdisciplinary conferences held when setting up new centers provide enough platforms to discuss and establish standards in hemotherapy. The critical situation of a patient who during surgery slips into a desolate coagulation and bleeding state (exception: emergencies) can have its origin in a suboptimal preparation (patient, anesthetist, surgeon), missing or inadequate standards, and poor communication. This should be avoided at all costs.

> **Conclusion**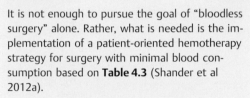
>
> It is not enough to pursue the goal of "bloodless surgery" alone. Rather, what is needed is the implementation of a patient-oriented hemotherapy strategy for surgery with minimal blood consumption based on **Table 4.3** (Shander et al 2012a).

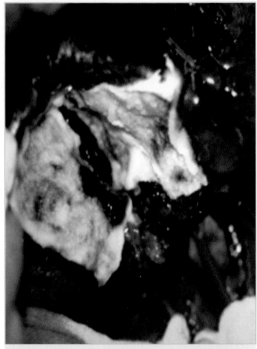

Fig. 4.6 Example of an "active compress" liver resection surface following right hemihepatectomy, with a collagen fleece that has been applied with slight pressure.

4.5 Local and Systemic Promotion of Perioperative Hemostasis

J. W. Erhard

4.5.1 Introduction

The control of intraoperative bleeding is vital for the success of an operation and possibly for the survival of the patient, especially in operations on parenchymatous organs and in cardiac and neurosurgery (Cox et al 2009). Hemostasis can be improved through topical measures, possibly in conjunction with systemic treatment, in particular if there is extensive bleeding (Inaba et al 2013). Topical applications range from powders through active compresses to sealants (**Fig. 4.6**).

Hemostatic agents are medicinal products used to stop bleeding. Nonspecific topical agents include cellulose, gelatin, and collagen; specific agents (with potential or proven procoagulant properties) include chitins and chitosans, zeolites, aluminum magnesium silicates, kaolins, glucosamines, and fibrin products (Arnaud et al 2009,

Inaba et al 2013). In some cases, combinations of different substance classes are used, to which thrombin or fibrinogen may be added. The main systemic hemostatic agents used are antifibrinolytics such as tranexamic acid. In critical situations with unexpectedly heavy blood loss (e.g., severe trauma), fibrinogen and—in exceptional cases—recombinant factor VIIa are used.

> **Note**
>
> Surgical hemostasis needs a subtle approach. Topical or systemic hemostatic agents should only be used to supplement anesthesiology and surgical measures.

4.5.2 Topical Hemostatic Agents

The main topical products are listed in **Table 4.4**.

▶ **Cellulose.** Cellulose, e.g., in the form of oxidized cellulose (Tabotamp; Ethicon, Johnson & Johnson), has been used successfully as a local agent for several years. There are no recent studies available.

Table 4.4 Selected topical hemostatic agents and their properties

Active substance	Application	Comments
Cellulose	Small-area bleeding	Has been in use for a long time, absorbable, moderate efficacy
Chitin/chitosan (polysaccharides)	Large-area bleeding of moderate severity	Biopolymers, MOA based on local vasoconstriction, nonallergenic
Magnesium aluminum silicate	Large-area bleeding of moderate severity	MOA based on local fluid removal, exothermic, has procoagulant activity, associated with thrombotic complications
Zeolite (aluminum silicate)	Large-area bleeding of moderate severity	Difficult to use (granules), highly exothermic with risk of tissue damage
Kaolin (aluminum silicate)	Large-area bleeding of moderate severity	Good effect, associated with endothelial swelling
Fibrin sealants, fibrin compresses	Parenchymal oozing, large-area bleeding	Absorbable, has been in use for a long time, expensive
Collagen with thrombin and fibrinogen	Large-area bleeding of moderate severity	Absorbable, has tissue-sealing properties
Collagen with PEG and thrombin	Parenchymal oozing, large-area bleeding	Absorbable, strongly adherent, no large studies so far
Tranexamic acid, topical	To date only in orthopaedic surgery	Very promising, indication spectrum still narrow, no large studies so far

Abbreviations: MOA, mechanism of action; PEG, polyethylene glycol.

The products are absorbable, inexpensive, and useful for small-area bleeding.

▶ **Chitin and chitosan.** Chitin and chitosan are polysaccharides and belong to the group of biopolymers. Their hemostatic action appears to be based on local vasoconstriction. Enhanced platelet adhesion in damaged tissue is observed in the case of chitosan (Arnaud et al 2009). Efficacy in terms of local bleeding control is deemed to be good provided there is no heavy bleeding (Cox et al 2009). Chitosan is also marketed as Celox (Med-Trade Products). It is available as a powder. A successor product is currently being tested.

▶ **Magnesium aluminum silicates.** The magnesium aluminum silicates, e.g., WoundStat (Trauma-Cure), have a mechanism of action that is similar to that of the zeolites (aluminum silicate, Quick-Clot, Z-Medica); it is based on local fluid removal from tissues and an increased local concentration of substances with procoagulant activity (Kozen et al 2008). These products form a gelatinous mass with a potential sealing effect. It remains unclear to what extent these products can also activate the coagulation cascade (Kheirabadi et al 2010). Thrombotic complications have so far proved to be an obstacle to their use on a broad scale (Kozen et al 2008).

▶ **Kaolin.** Kaolin is assigned to a similar group (aluminum silicate). It has a proven ability to activate the coagulation cascade (Combat Gauze, Z-Medica) (Kheirabadi et al 2010, Sena et al 2013).

Aluminum silicates have the drawback that they are not absorbable and they generally give rise to an exothermic chemical reaction at the application site. It is therefore possible that they might cause injuries.

▶ **Fibrin products.** In addition to sealants, fibrin products include Fibrin Pad and Fibrinkompresse (Ethicon, Johnson & Johnson). In fibrin products, human fibrinogen is combined with thrombin. The resulting hemostasis is deemed to be good (de Boer et al 2012, Fischer et al 2013). Tissue-sealing is an additional beneficial effect. However, the products are very expensive.

A similar approach is used for combination products consisting of collagen with fibrinogen and thrombin. Tachosil (Nycomed) is available as an adhesive, thin-walled sponge. Apart from providing hemostasis, which is judged to be good, the product is also claimed to have tissue-sealing properties (Vida et al 2014).

A collagen matrix with polyethylene glycol and thrombin is available under the name of Hemopatch (Baxter). Attention is drawn in particular to its rapid adhesion effect. So far, no large studies on its use have been conducted (Lewis et al 2014).

The topical use of tranexamic acid in total hip replacement has been reported in a randomized trial with orthopaedic patients. Total hip joint replacement was carried out after intra-articular injection of tranexamic acid. In total, 161 patients were randomized to receive tranexamic acid or no injection. Blood loss and the transfusion rate were significantly lower in the group treated with tranexamic acid (Alshryda et al 2013). These results were corroborated by another study group in a further, albeit retrospective, controlled trial with 211 patients (Chang et al 2014a).

4.5.3 Systemic Hemostatic Agents

Massive bleeding or the need for massive transfusion inevitably results in coagulopathy. To assure adequate hemostasis in such a situation despite these obstacles, any missing or consumed coagulation substrates must be replaced (Moskowitz et al 2009). At present, fibrinogen (factor I) is the first substrate to be replaced—with concurrent monitoring of the clot firmness (e.g., ROTEM)—in patients with such a severe coagulopathy (Weber et al 2012, Weber et al 2014).

The dosage recommendations are not standardized. The timely administration of high doses is recommended for dilutional coagulopathy (Fenger-Eriksen et al 2008). A multicenter publication has confirmed that the prophylactic use of fibrinogen in cardiosurgery reduces blood consumption and the need for transfusions (Sadeghi et al 2014).

▶ **Antifibrinolytics.** Antifibrinolytics are currently being used on a much broader scale in the intra- and perioperative time window. Any severe coagulopathy inevitably results in fibrinolysis. Systemic administration of antifibrinolytics is therefore advisable in cases where elevated local fibrinolysis is to be expected. In elective surgery, this includes major surgical procedures on parenchymatous organs and major orthopaedic operations. There are sufficient data available on tranexamic acid to justify its prophylactic use when planning such procedures (Karkouti et al 2010, Lin et al 2012, Zhou et al 2013). Tranexamic acid blocks plasminogen by irreversibly binding to the binding site with lysine, thus preventing the activation of plasminogen. However, caution is advised when using tranexamic acid in patients who have a history of thrombotic or thromboembolic complications (Zufferey et al 2010).

▶ **Desmopressin.** Desmopressin is a synthetic analogue of antidiuretic hormone. It is licensed as an antihemorrhagic agent for the treatment of moderate hemophilia A and von Willebrand disease. Within a very short time of its administration, it leads to a three- to fourfold rise in von Willebrand factor and factor VIII.

However, a Cochrane analysis did not detect any significant reduction in the perioperative transfusion rate (Carless et al 2004b). The product is often administered perioperatively to increase the active platelet count in patients who have been treated with platelet aggregation inhibitors (e.g., acetylsalicylic acid) before surgery.

▶ **Recombinant activated factor VII.** Recombinant factor VIIa (NovoSeven, Novo Nordisk) was originally developed and licensed for the treatment of congenital or acquired hemophilia A or B. In 1999, the first report on its off-label use for traumatic bleeding was published (Boffard et al 2005). A number of studies carried out in the field of traumatology and among patients with massive bleeding identified reductions in bleeding and blood consumption (Theusinger et al 2009, Wade et al 2010). No significant improvement has been achieved to date with regard to mortality.

Note

Apart from antifibrinolytics such as tranexamic acid, the use of hemostatic agents should at present be limited to a few exceptions. However, their well-targeted use can save lives.

Conclusion

Local and systemic hemostatic agents are adjuvants in the scenario of surgical hemostasis. Systemically, tranexamic acid should be used for limited indications such as huge parenchymal resections or extensive orthopaedic surgery. Locally, there is a tendency to use combined products, with thrombin being the most commonly added agent. If the decision arises to apply such products, they should be used immediately as appropriate and not as a last resort.

Chapter 5

**Third Pillar of PBM—
Harnessing and Optimization
of the Patient's Physiological
Tolerance to Anemia**

5.1 Perioperative Optimization of the Anemia Tolerance

J. Meier, K. Zacharowski

5.1.1 Tolerance to Low Hemoglobin Values

Throughout the evolutionary history of *Homo sapiens*, the primary effect of acute bleeding was hypovolemia with no decline in the hemoglobin concentration, because blood loss could only be compensated secondarily through the influx of intracellular and interstitial fluid into the vascular system. However, in 1866 the physiologist Hugo Kronecker observed that patients with hypovolemia, hitherto fatal, were able to survive on infusion of a saline solution; with this discovery, artificial volume expanders such as crystalloids and colloids gained their present-day significance in medicine (Kronecker 1886). Although the use of such solutions to compensate for blood loss is a very modern phenomenon in terms of the evolutionary history, the human body is in most cases capable of compensating dilutional anemia resulting from intravenous volume expansion. There are case reports of patients who survived surgery with almost no circulating oxygen carriers (Dai et al 2010). The fact that nonphysiological low hemoglobin concentrations can be compensated if normovolemia is maintained makes it possible to dispense with the immediate transfusion of red blood cell (RBC) concentrates in cases of bleeding.

There are widespread inter- and intraindividual variations in the ability to tolerate low hemoglobin values. Depending on a patient's underlying diseases and cardiac reserve and on the specific clinical situation, very different hemoglobin concentrations can still be compensated or will lead to tissue hypoxia with subsequent injury to the patient. In the following section, we shall elaborate on various influencing factors and on ways to optimize a patient's tolerance to anemia.

5.1.2 Individual Tolerance to Anemia

▶ **Oxygen demand and oxygen supply.** All organs of the human body have their own specific oxygen demand. However, the oxygen demand does not only vary from one organ to another, but it can also vary greatly for the same organ depending

on the given situation and its related metabolic effects. If one adds the oxygen demand of all organs, one obtains the body's total oxygen demand. The oxygen supply, on the other hand, can be calculated as the product of arterial oxygen content and cardiac output. Under resting conditions, the oxygen supply outstrips the oxygen demand by a factor of 4–5. Among other things, this "luxury" supply can balance out transient peaks in the oxygen demand of individual organs. The key determinant of adequate oxygen delivery to the body tissues (DO_2) is the regional oxygen supply, which is in turn determined by the oxygen content of the arterial blood and the regional blood flow in the respective organ. The latter differs greatly depending on the underlying disease, which might mean that individual organs are more affected by a limited oxygen supply than others. In the worst case, tissue hypoxia can develop in some organs despite an adequate oxygen supply in the body overall.

>
> **Note**
>
> Even if the oxygen supply is theoretically sufficient to assure adequate tissue oxygenation, individual organs might be affected by tissue hypoxia.

▶ **Compensatory mechanisms in anemia.** If the blood volume lost in an acute bleeding situation is replaced with crystalloids or colloids, this results in hemodilution, i.e., the dilution of all blood components, leading to anemia. The subsequent drop in the arterial oxygen content is compensated by a rise in cardiac output and enhanced arteriovenous oxygen extraction. This means that young, healthy patients can tolerate dilutional anemia even if it is extreme. Only at very low hemoglobin concentrations can the loss of circulating oxygen carriers no longer be compensated by a rise in cardiac output. In such a situation, the safety margin of tissue oxygenation is completely exhausted, with the ensuing onset of tissue hypoxia. It is impossible to predict which organs will be affected by tissue hypoxia, as this depends on the perfusion and the resulting oxygen demand of each organ during anemia.

These compensatory mechanisms form the basis for optimization of the perioperative anemia tolerance and thus for the measures of the third pillar of PBM, which should be employed in everyday clinical practice (Goodnough and Shander 2012):

1. Preoperative preparation of the patient.
2. Intraoperative optimization of oxygen transport and tissue oxygenation, and application of evidence-based transfusion thresholds.
3. Postoperative balancing of DO_2 and oxygen consumption (VO_2).

5.1.3 Preoperative Quantification of the Anemia Tolerance

The body's ability to compensate for acute anemia can vary greatly from one patient to another. Surprisingly, to date there is no routine clinical test to predict the level of acute dilutional anemia that would critically restrict the DO_2 to individual organs, or the entire body, in a given patient. This is because parameters such as regional perfusion and VO_2 vary widely between patients in different clinical situations. Therefore, it is currently not possible prior to an operation to determine the hemoglobin concentration that can be deemed "safe" for a patient in terms of compensation for acute anemia. However, this does not mean that it is generally impossible to estimate the potential risk through taking a detailed preoperative medical history and evaluating the patient.

▶ **Evaluation of the cardiac reserve.** Since the compensatory rise in cardiac output during acute anemia is mainly compensated by a rise in stroke volume, the cardiac reserve is a key determinant of the amount of acute anemia that can be compensated. For this reason, it is recommended that the compensatory ability of the patient's heart is evaluated prior to surgery with anticipated major blood loss (Habler et al 2006). However, it is not known what kinds of preoperative assessment would be best suited to predict and avoid the development of intraoperative tissue hypoxia. Potential options include the use of standardized evaluation forms, preoperative electrocardiography (ECG), and more complex procedures such as exercise ECG. However, to date there are no clinical studies to demonstrate the superiority of these investigations to a standardized medical history in this context. It is therefore no surprise that preoperative tests aimed at determining the anemia tolerance of individual patients are only rarely performed in routine clinical practice (van Gelder et al 2012).

▶ **Other organ systems.** If the evaluation is confined to the cardiovascular system alone, there is a risk of overly focusing on a single organ system without taking other organs into account whose tissue oxygenation is equally at risk. Growing evidence indicates that there are major differences in the ability of various organs to compensate for acute anemia (Torres et al 2005). For example, a hemoglobin concentration of less than 7 g/dL in cardiopulmonary bypass patients led to a marked deterioration in the postoperative renal function, whereas other organs, such as the brain, were not affected by the restricted oxygen supply (Habib et al 2003, Habib et al 2005, Karkouti et al 2005a). Therefore, the preoperative evaluation should include all organ systems that are susceptible to anemia-induced injury, so as to determine the hazard potential for each individual organ.

> **Note**
>
> In routine clinical practice, there are many obstacles to estimating a patient's ability to compensate for anemia. This makes it much more difficult to set physiological transfusion thresholds.

▶ **Transfusion threshold based on hemoglobin.** For the reasons outlined above, a different approach tends to be taken in clinical practice. Typically, the decision to administer intra- and postoperative transfusions is based on a hemoglobin threshold value. This value is often determined on the basis of the preoperative tests that have been carried out, but in the vast majority of cases it is well above what the body can actually compensate for.

The range given in the literature is generally between 6 g/dL and 10 g/dL. Whereas a transfusion will generally be required to prevent long-term tissue hypoxia if the hemoglobin concentration is less than 6 g/dL, there is virtually no patient with a hemoglobin concentration of more than 10 g/dL who must receive a transfusion to improve the tissue oxygenation. With hemoglobin values between 6 g/dL and 10 g/dL, the decision depends on comorbidities, local circumstances, and other needs, but in most patients without cardiac impairment a hemoglobin concentration of 8 g/dL is more than sufficient. This approach has been repeatedly verified in clinical studies, both intraoperatively and in intensive care patients (Marik and Corwin 2008, Hajjar et al 2010, Carson et al 2011, Vuille-Lessard et al 2012). Based on these data, it can be postulated that an intraoperative hemoglobin concentration of over 8 g/dL is not needed in the majority of patients with good cardiac health.

The transfusion of RBC concentrates once this generally accepted transfusion threshold has been reached guarantees a safety margin to ensure the maintenance of tissue oxygenation in all organs; however, it has the drawback that many patients receive an RBC transfusion—with all its associated risks—before this is actually warranted by their tissue oxygenation status.

Even though the literature agrees on a transfusion threshold of 8 g/dL for restrictive transfusion regimens, impressive data from the SOAP (Sepsis Occurrence in Acutely Ill Patients) and ABC (Australian Breakthrough Cancer) studies demonstrate that the average hemoglobin concentration in asymptotic patients approaches a value of 10 g/dL, both from previously lower and previously higher values, after a 14-day stay on the intensive care unit (ICU) (Vincent et al 2002, Sakr et al 2010). This phenomenon, which was observed in both studies, suggests that in routine clinical practice a hemoglobin concentration of 10 g/dL has been knowingly or unknowingly adopted as the "transfusion threshold" for all patients, regardless of the published evidence. However, it is beyond doubt that there is no justification to take measures aimed at achieving a hemoglobin concentration of 10 g/dL in ICU patients regardless of their clinical situation and concomitant diseases.

> **Note**
>
> The typical hemoglobin-based transfusion thresholds are 6 g/dL for patients with good cardiac health, and 8 g/dL for those with cardiac impairments. Only in individual cases can a hemoglobin concentration of 10 g/dL be justified.

5.1.4 Preoperative Estimation of the Anticipated Blood Loss

Preoperatively, it is easier to estimate the anticipated blood loss than to predict a patient's tolerance to anemia. Estimation of the anticipated blood loss does not only help to identify how many RBC units the blood bank should issue preoperatively, but it also helps to determine the

scope of the measures that need to be in place to reduce the need for perioperative allogeneic transfusions (see also Chapter 2.3).

5.1.5 Intraoperative Optimization of the Oxygen Demand to Oxygen Supply Ratio

Within the framework of the third pillar of modern PBM, optimization of the ratio of oxygen demand to oxygen supply represents the most important measure to optimize a patient's tolerance to anemia. By reducing the intraoperative oxygen demand and increasing the oxygen supply, it will be possible for the patient to tolerate lower hemoglobin values than would otherwise be the case.

Intraoperative Reduction of the Oxygen Demand

Therapeutic Hypothermia

There are various methods to achieve an intraoperative reduction of the body's oxygen demand. One of the best known is, no doubt, lowering of the core temperature, thus inducing therapeutic hypothermia (Azmoon et al 2011). Therapeutic hypothermia also reduces the oxygen demand of individual organs by around 7% per degree Celsius, thus increasing the tolerance to hypoxia (Polderman 2009). For example, hypothermia significantly improves the likelihood of survival during cardiopulmonary resuscitation (Bernard et al 2002).

However, data from an animal model did not demonstrate unequivocally that therapeutic hypothermia could significantly improve the physiological tolerance to anemia (Perez-de-Sá et al 2002). Besides, this modality has another drawback that militates against its use on a broad scale in clinical practice: therapeutic hypothermia leads to a marked deterioration in the coagulation activity of plasma (Watts et al 1998) and platelets (Kermode et al 1999), and can therefore aggravate intraoperative bleeding. For this reason, all guidelines on the treatment of intraoperative bleeding published to date recommend maintenance of a normal body temperature. Hence, therapeutic hypothermia has a very low priority as a measure to increase the tolerance to anemia in cases of acute bleeding.

Choice of Volume Expander

Depending on the clinical situation, local circumstances, and the treating physician, blood loss is initially replaced using either crystalloids or colloids, or a combination of both. The choice of intravenous fluid to be used for volume expansion is determined by numerous considerations, such as its impact on the microcirculation, kidney function, blood coagulation, and development of interstitial edema. Until recently, it was not known whether the choice of intravenous fluid also had implications for the tolerance to anemia. Whereas the choice did not appear to have any effect in earlier studies with animal models (Van der Linden et al 1993), a study of trauma patients carried out in 2010 revealed that the administration of a hetastarch solution significantly reduced the mortality compared with administration of a purely crystalloid intravenous fluid (Ogilvie et al 2010). This finding was confirmed in an animal study that investigated the effects of lactated Ringer, gelatin, hydroxyethyl starch (HES) 130, and HES 450 solutions on an individual's tolerance to anemia. The results showed that it is possible to increase the tolerance to anemia through the use of HES 130 compared with all the other solutions, in particular in comparison with lactated Ringer solution (Pape et al 2012b). These more recent findings suggest that modern colloidal solutions are indeed able to increase the perioperative tolerance to anemia. However, since the use of colloids is associated with other problems and no large clinical trials have been conducted in this context, their use cannot be generally recommended for the purpose of increasing the perioperative tolerance to anemia, even if the initial results are promising.

Effects of Anesthesia on the Tolerance to Anemia

The induction of general anesthesia leads to a considerable drop in a patient's VO_2. This phenomenon seems to hold out interesting prospects in terms of increasing the perioperative tolerance to anemia.

However, the link between anesthesia depth and tolerance to anemia has proved to be much more complex in clinical practice. In experiments with dogs, Van der Linden et al demonstrated that the deepening of general anesthesia with halothane did not result in a significant reduction in the so-called *critical hemoglobin concentration* and therefore in the maximum tolerable amount of acute anemia (Van der Linden et al 2000, Van der Linden et al 2003). Surprisingly, the drop in VO_2 induced by this measure was accompanied by a marked decline in the compensatory mechanisms at play in acute anemia. Compared with less deeply anesthetized animals, a reduction in the hemoglobin concentration in the deeply anesthetized dogs did not result in a substantial increase in cardiac output. In the case of halothane, this can be easily explained by the cardiodepressive effects of this inhalational anesthetic. However, Van der Linden et al demonstrated the same effect for Ketanest, which has far weaker cardiodepressive effects (White 1982). Thus, the physiological mechanisms responsible for tolerance to anemia can certainly be influenced by changing the depth of anesthesia; however, the relationship between tolerance to anemia and depth of anesthesia is not linear but probably has an inverted U-shape. In a clinical situation, the optimum anesthesia depth with respect to a patient's individual tolerance to anemia is difficult to predict. In particular, it is not known whether there are significant differences in the anemia tolerance of sedated versus awake patients.

More recent studies suggest that it is possible to increase the tolerance to anemia through sufficient muscle relaxation. Pape et al (2012a) showed in an animal model that the critical hemoglobin concentration could be significantly reduced by muscle relaxation. Whether these findings can be extrapolated to the clinical situation is currently unclear.

> **!**
>
> **Note**
>
> A patient's tolerance to anemia can be increased by maintaining an optimal intravascular volume during surgery and by adapting anesthesia.

Intraoperative Optimization of the Oxygen Supply

The supply of oxygen to the body tissues (the DO_2) is calculated as the product of cardiac output and arterial oxygen content. From a physiological point of view, it seems beneficial to increase the DO_2 in acute anemia using several different methods. In theory, this can be achieved either by increasing the cardiac output (optimization of cardiovascular function) or by augmenting the arterial oxygen content.

Optimization of the Cardiovascular Function

In acute anemia, the drop in blood viscosity and the ensuing reduction in endothelial shear forces give rise to an increased release of endothelial nitric oxide, resulting in peripheral arteriolar vasodilatation. This leads to a drop in the mean arterial pressure, regardless of the rise in cardiac output. If the limits of dilutional anemia are reached, this results not only in a critical impairment of all DO_2 parameters, but also in a dangerous drop in the coronary perfusion pressure. In animal experiments, the concurrent use of acute normovolemic hemodilution with vasodilator administration did not lead to a disproportionate impairment in cardiac output, but the perfusion pressure of individual organs dropped below the minimum pressure needed (Crystal et al 1991).

▶ **Vasopressors and inotropes.** One way to counter the phenomenon described would be to administer vasopressors to maintain the organ-specific perfusion pressure. Animal experiments have shown that the tolerance to anemia can be improved through stabilization of the coronary perfusion pressure with noradrenaline (Meier et al 2007). The use of inotropes can also increase the tolerance to anemia (Pawlik et al 1975, Pawlik et al 1976). In both cases, the positive effects of the respective therapeutic approach outweighed the side effects. By contrast, increasing the cardiac output only through raising the heart rate does not appear to improve the tolerance to anemia (Kertscho et al 2012). However, it must be pointed out that almost all data published to date on this topic are based on animal models. Whether the various effects also occur in humans to the same extent, and whether it is indeed possible in the clinic to increase the tolerance to anemia by combining the measures described, has not yet been confirmed by evidence-based research.

Increasing the Arterial Oxygen Content

The oxygen content of arterial blood is determined by the oxygen bound to hemoglobin and the oxygen physically dissolved in plasma. Since there is a decline in the oxygen bound to hemoglobin in acute anemia, the arterial oxygen content can be expanded only by increasing the amount of oxygen physically dissolved in plasma. However, for many years now physiology textbooks have unanimously upheld the view that the amount of oxygen that is physically dissolved in plasma is very small compared with that bound to hemoglobin, and is thus negligible. However, this view fails to properly explain the physiological processes at play in acute anemia.

▶ **Increasing the inspired oxygen concentration.** An increase in the concentration of inspired oxygen translates into a direct proportionate increase in the partial pressure of oxygen (PO_2) in arterial blood. With an inspired oxygen concentration of 100%, the PO_2 of arterial blood can assume values of more than 500 mmHg. Because of the large difference to the PO_2 in tissues (< 20 mmHg), the oxygen that is physically dissolved in plasma is ideally suited to be utilized for tissue oxygenation. As the amount of oxygen bound to hemoglobin continues to decline in the presence of anemia, the dissolved plasma oxygen plays an increasing role in tissue oxygenation through hyperoxia. Thus, the dissolved oxygen is an important contributor to tissue oxygenation.

In animal experiments, the use of hyperoxic ventilation once the critical hemoglobin concentration had been reached resulted in improved survival rates (Meier et al 2004), an increased tolerance to anemia (Kemming et al 2003), and maintenance of tissue oxygenation even in the presence of extremely low hemoglobin concentrations (Habler et al 1998, Kleen et al 1998, Kemming et al 2003).

It is therefore no surprise that in most case reports of patients with an extremely low hemoglobin value and no possibility of acute RBC transfusion, the shortage of circulating oxygen carriers was addressed through ventilation with pure oxygen (Zollinger et al 1997, Dai et al 2010). The combination of data from animal experiments and patient case reports justifies the recommendation to administer oxygen in patients with an extremely low hemoglobin concentration to assure tissue oxygenation. However, to date there are no large clinical studies to prove that the use of hyperoxia in acute anemia does indeed improve tissue oxygenation in the clinic. It is also not known whether ventilation with high oxygen concentrations has a positive impact on long-term survival in patients with moderate anemia. In the worst-case scenario, it is conceivable that the side effects of hyperoxia (e.g., hyperoxic arteriolar vasoconstriction, formation of radicals, neurologic toxicity, atelectasis) outweigh the positive effects on oxygen transport and tissue oxygenation.

Note

A patient's tolerance to anemia can be improved through intraoperative optimization of the cardiovascular function with inotropes and vasopressors and by raising the arterial oxygen content.

5.1.6 Postoperative Optimization of the Oxygen Demand to Oxygen Supply Ratio

In general, the therapeutic principles described above also apply to the postoperative phase, even though the opportunities to influence oxygen supply and demand are more limited than during the intraoperative phase because of less extensive monitoring.

Besides, it was a longstanding belief that an increase in the postoperative hemoglobin concentration, with its accompanying increase in oxygen supply, has a positive impact on the patient's functional recovery. Therefore, the transfusion thresholds recommended for the postoperative phase were generally higher than those recommended for the intraoperative phase. Only recently has it become clear that this is not the case. Two independent groups demonstrated in patients undergoing orthopaedic surgery that a restrictive transfusion regimen is just as safe as a liberal regimen in terms of postoperative functional recovery, regardless of the patients' cardiac health (Carson et al 2011, Vuille-Lessard et al 2012).

▶ **Infections with a septic course.** During the postoperative phase, special attention should be paid to the development of infections with sepsis. For physiological reasons, it can be assumed that the onset of sepsis is accompanied by an increased oxygen demand (Regueira et al 2012) and severely impaired oxygen utilization, resulting in a reduced perioperative tolerance to anemia. It could be shown that the critical DO_2 in septic animals was significantly higher than that in healthy animals

(Morita et al 2003); however, the critical hemoglobin concentration did not differ significantly between septic and nonseptic animals (Lauscher et al 2011). Even though sepsis is associated with generalized impairments in the microcirculation, oxygen extraction, and oxygen utilization, the septic body retains some tolerance to anemia. In intensive care patients with sepsis, the 30-day mortality was independent of whether a restrictive or a liberal transfusion strategy was applied (McIntyre et al 2004).

Note

Because of the limited possibilities for monitoring, it is much more difficult to manage the oxygen supply and demand during the postoperative phase than during the intraoperative phase.

Conclusion

The third pillar of modern PBM (optimization of the anemia tolerance) is a very effective instrument in the hands of anesthesiologists to influence the perioperative consumption of allogeneic blood. Of paramount importance in this regard are the preoperative preparation of the patient, the intraoperative optimization of oxygen transport and tissue oxygenation, the application of evidence-based transfusion thresholds, and the postoperative balancing of DO_2 and VO_2. To achieve the maximum benefit, it is important to use a combination of these strategies in line with the needs of the patient rather than using a single measure.

5.2 Determinants of the Decision to Transfuse Red Blood Cells

D. Meininger, K. Zacharowski

5.2.1 General Considerations

Allogeneic RBC transfusion, which enables a myriad of surgical procedures involving major blood loss, is considered to be one of the most important medical achievements of the 20th century. Meticulous care must be taken with such blood products because of the transmission risk for certain diseases and the raised perioperative morbidity and mortality of transfused patients. Notwithstanding these risks, blood conserves also save lives, and some patients with postpartum bleeding or severe trauma are unlikely to survive without the transfusion of allogeneic blood. It is only thanks to the supply of allogeneic blood that certain complex operative procedures are possible, and blood products prolong the lives of patients with a hematopoietic disorder caused by, e.g., bone marrow disease. The costs incurred for the transfusion of blood products account for approximately 1.5% of the budget of an average-sized hospital (Shander et al 2010). Whereas the infection risk posed by transfusion used to be the prime consideration, today there is a growing awareness of other complications of blood products unrelated to infections. These are particularly important for patients who are ill or seriously ill. Therefore, the use of blood products must be targeted and based on strict indication criteria.

> **Note**
>
> The general framework for transfusion is set out in the guidelines from various medical societies and associations (Napolitano et al 2009, BAEK 2011a, Ferraris et al 2011a, Carson et al 2012b, American Society of Anesthesiologists Task Force on Perioperative Blood Management 2015).

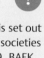

▶ **Demand for blood products.** In the past, homologous blood products were mainly used in perioperative medicine; however, in recent years this trend has changed with RBC concentrates now being increasingly transfused for nonsurgical indications such as gastrointestinal bleeding and impaired erythropoiesis. This change is driven by novel surgical techniques and, of course, by the availability of perioperative blood conservation methods. Since the worldwide implementation of blood conservation strategies, the overall incidence of RBC transfusion in medical and surgical patients has decreased, along with a decrease in the pretransfusion hemoglobin level (Roubinian et al 2014b). At the same time, in line with the trend toward aging societies in high-income countries, there is a rise in the number of hematologic and oncologic diseases requiring transfusion. A prospective study of the indications for RBC transfu-

sion published in 2006 revealed that only 33% of the transfusions were administered in the perioperative setting, and only 5% were for gynecologic/obstetric procedures. Nonsurgical indications were predominantly related to blood diseases (18.2%), gastrointestinal bleeding (13.8%), and nonhematologic tumors (8.8%) (Wallis et al 2006). Transfused patients were on average 66 years old; only 25% of the transfused RBC concentrates were administered to persons younger than 55 years. Patients aged 40 to 50 years received only 20 units of RBC concentrates per year per 1,000 patients, whereas patients aged 80 years and over received 10 times this amount (200 units per year per 1,000 patients).

▶ **Indications.** The main indications for transfusion are:
• Acute anemia (e.g., because of traumatic blood loss).
• Chronic intractable anemia (e.g., bone marrow disease).
• Treatment-resistant chronic anemia.

▶ **Transfusion criteria.** RBC concentrates are transfused to prevent overt anemic hypoxia. However, since the clinical symptoms of anemia are nonspecific, a rational indication must be based on the hemoglobin concentration or the hematocrit and on consideration of the following criteria:
• Cause, duration, and severity of anemia.
• Extent and progression of blood loss.
• Individual ability to compensate for reduced oxygen supply.
• Comorbidities that may restrict the compensatory ability in acute anemia.
• The patient's current clinical condition.
• Presence or absence of physiological transfusion triggers (**Table 5.1**).
• The patient's intravascular volume status (RBC deficiencies cannot be reliably identified in hypovolemia).

In addition to these criteria, the latest findings from clinical studies on the relationship between anemia, RBC transfusion, and outcome must be taken into account. The etiology of any form of anemia must be investigated and causal treatment must be initiated whenever possible. The timely transfusion of RBC concentrates is vital in the presence of active bleeding, signs of hypoxia, or hemorrhagic shock. In such situations, the deci-

Table 5.1 Physiological transfusion triggers

Symptoms/examination results	
Cardiopulmonary symptoms	• Tachycardia • Hypotension • Hypotension of unknown origin • Dyspnea
Typical ischemia-related changes on ECG	• New-onset ST depression or elevation • New-onset arrhythmias
Changes on ECG	• New-onset regional myocardial contraction disorders
Global indices of inadequate oxygen supply	• Rise in global O_2 extraction > 50% • Drop in O_2 extraction > 10% of baseline • Drop in mixed venous O_2 saturation < 50% • Drop in mixed venous PO_2 < 32 mmHg • Drop in central venous O_2 saturation < 60% • Lactic acidosis (lactate > 2 mmol/L)

Abbreviations: ECG, electrocardiography; PO_2, partial pressure of oxygen.

sion to administer a transfusion is based on the hemodynamic parameters and the symptoms of anemia with consideration of the incurred and anticipated blood loss.

> **Note**
>
> Causal therapy of anemia should be initiated whenever possible.

5.2.2 Transfusion in Otherwise Healthy Patients

A normovolemic decrease in the hemoglobin concentration to around 5 g/dL (hematocrit 15%) is generally well tolerated by patients with normal cardiovascular function (Weiskopf et al 1998). If the hemoglobin value is less than 6 g/dL, there is a risk that individual organ systems will not receive the critical minimum supply of oxygen. At these values, even young, otherwise healthy persons can have ECG changes, impaired cognitive function, or a subjective feeling of tiredness. These changes can be reversed by increasing the hemoglobin value to above 7 g/dL or administering additional oxygen (Weiskopf et al 2002). For this reason, the administration of oxygen is viewed as an emergency measure for the treatment of acute anemia. Based on clinical observations, a hemoglobin value of 4.5 to 5 g/dL (hematocrit ~ 15%) is considered to represent a critical threshold, in particular in the presence of risk factors; if this

threshold is exceeded, a transfusion may be needed. However, the patient's current intravascular volume status must also be taken into account when making a decision about the indication for transfusion. Laboratory values alone do not represent reliable transfusion triggers in patients with intravascular hypovolemia (**Table 5.2**).

A Cochrane analysis published in 2012 containing data on 6,264 patients demonstrated that the use of a restrictive transfusion threshold (hemoglobin < 7–9 g/dL) reduced the risk of an individual patient receiving an RBC transfusion. The study authors concluded that patients without acute coronary heart disease and no active bleeding should only receive a transfusion if the hemoglobin value is below 7 to 8 g/dL. The benefits of avoiding transfusion are all the greater against a background of doubtful blood product safety (Carson et al 2012a).

> **Note**
>
> A transfusion trigger should serve as a discussion point and not as a strict indication to transfuse (Koch 2014).

5.2.3 Transfusion in Critically Ill Patients

Critically ill patients who are monitored and treated in an ICU can benefit in terms of their morbidity and mortality if a restrictive transfusion

Table 5.2 Recommendations for the transfusion of red blood cell concentrates in acute anemia, taking account of the current hemoglobin value, the patient's compensatory ability, risk factors, and physiological transfusion triggers (Carson et al 2012b)

Hemoglobin	Ability to compensate for anemia, risk factors	Transfusion	Level of evidence
≤ 6 g/dL	—	Yes [a]	1C+
>6–8 g/dL	Adequate compensation, no risk factors	No	1C+
	Limited compensation, risk factors (e.g., coronary heart disease)	Yes	1C+
	Presence of physiological transfusion triggers	Yes	1C+
8–10 g/dL	Presence of physiological transfusion triggers	Yes	2C
>10 g/dL	—	No [b]	1A

Level of evidence
1C+: no randomized controlled trials, but unequivocal data ("should")
2C: observational studies, case reports ("may")
1A: randomized controlled trials, no major methodological limitations, clear-cut results ("should")

[a] Individual patients with risk factors may be able to tolerate a lower hemoglobin value without transfusion if their compensatory response is adequate.
[b] In individual patients, a transfusion may be indicated despite a hemoglobin value of more than 10 g/dL.

strategy with hemoglobin values between 7 and 9 g/dL is used (Hébert et al 1999a) (**Table 5.2**).

5.2.4 Transfusion in Patients with Cardiovascular Disease

Unfortunately, because of the paucity of data available it is currently not possible to establish a transfusion threshold for patients with coronary heart disease, heart failure, or cerebrovascular disease. However, despite the limited data it can be inferred that hemodynamically stable patients with cardiovascular risks and no physiological transfusion triggers have no morbidity or mortality benefits from RBC transfusion at hemoglobin values between 8 and 10 g/dL (Carson et al 1996). In stable patients with cardiovascular risks, hemoglobin values of 7 to 8 g/dL are tolerated without any long-term hypoxic injury; however, hemoglobin concentrations below 7 g/dL are associated with elevated morbidity and mortality (Carson et al 2002a).

Murphy et al (2015b) compared the postoperative use of a restrictive transfusion threshold (hemoglobin <7.5 g/dL) with that of a liberal transfusion threshold (hemoglobin <9.0 g/dL) in 2,003 cardiac-surgery patients. No benefit for a liberal transfusion threshold was found in terms of the primary outcome. The authors' suggestion of a possible benefit for liberal transfusion in terms of 90-day mortality in this trial needs to be viewed with caution because this was not a primary endpoint and there was no difference between the groups in terms of periprocedural complications (Spertus 2015).

In a study of 2,016 patients with suspected or diagnosed coronary heart disease who underwent hip surgery, a liberal transfusion strategy (transfusion if hemoglobin <10 g/dL) was compared with a restrictive strategy (transfusion in the presence of anemia symptoms or at the discretion of the physician if hemoglobin <8 g/dL). The authors of this study concluded that a liberal transfusion strategy did not improve the mortality, the ability to walk independently within 60 days, or the morbidity during hospitalization (Carson et al 2011).

Cardiovascular risk patients with chronic anemia, in particular those with severe heart failure, appear to benefit from higher hemoglobin concentrations in terms of their mortality, resilience, and quality of life (Ezekowitz et al 2003) (**Table 5.2**). However, hemoglobin as an independent predictor of performance failed to differentiate between patients who had received transfusions and those who had not (Ranucci et al 2011b).

5.2.5 Transfusion in Patients with Acute Blood Loss

During the acute phase of massive or uncontrolled bleeding (e.g., polytrauma), it may be advisable to transfuse not only RBC concentrates, but also plasma, coagulation products, and platelets. A hemoglobin value of 10 g/dL should be targeted in patients with massive, uncontrolled bleeding because higher hemoglobin values have beneficial effects on primary hemostasis (Hardy 2004).

Note

The combination of signs of tissue hypoxia and laboratory-diagnosed anemia in the presence of normovolemia constitutes a physiological transfusion trigger, indicating that the transfusion of RBC concentrates should be initiated immediately, regardless of the hemoglobin value.

5.2.6 Patients with Chronic Anemia

In chronic anemia (e.g., renal or tumor-associated anemia), long-term adaptation processes take place that—under normal circumstances—assure tissue oxygenation. Chronic anemia can adversely affect the clinical course of disease. Therefore, an increase in the hemoglobin value can improve the objective resilience and the subjective wellbeing of patients with chronic anemia, and reduce the inpatient treatment rate. The indication for transfusion is based on assessment of the overall clinical picture, rather than on laboratory values alone. If patients with chronic anemia experience acute blood loss, the same compensatory mechanisms seen in patients without chronic anemia come into play. The presence of chronic anemia as such does not imply an enhanced tolerance to low hemoglobin concentrations. If there is a further drop in the hemoglobin concentration, patients with chronic anemia must therefore be treated based on the same criteria as patients without chronic anemia (**Table 5.2**).

In patients with chronic anemia and no concomitant cardiovascular disease, a transfusion is not indicated even with hemoglobin values of 7.0–8.0 g/dL, unless typical anemia symptoms are exhibited. Based on observational studies, which produced compelling results despite absence of a control group, a moderate recommendation was issued to administer RBC concentrates in patients with chronic anemia if the hemoglobin concentration is below 7.0 to 8.0 g/dL (Foley et al 2008, Buser et al 2010, Koch 2014).

In patients with chronic anemia because of primary or secondary bone marrow insufficiency, transfusions should generally be used sparingly, in particular if there is the possibility of bone marrow or stem cell transplantation at a later stage.

Conclusion

The general framework for transfusion is set out in clinical practice guidelines from various medical societies and associations (Napolitano et al 2009, BAEK 2011a, Ferraris et al 2011a, Carson et al 2012b, American Society of Anesthesiologists Task Force on Perioperative Blood Management 2015). Transfusion triggers should serve as discussion points rather than as strict indications to transfuse.

5.3 Functions of Circulating Blood Other Than Oxygen Transport

B. Friesenecker

5.3.1 Functions of Red Blood Cells

One of the most important functions of blood is the transport of oxygen bound to the hemoglobin molecule. However, hemoglobin must be enclosed inside a sheath, the RBC, since free hemoglobin is a potent nitric oxide scavenger that would adversely affect microvascular perfusion (Vermeulen et al 2012). Moreover, the oxygen uptake in the lungs and the DO_2 are strongly dependent on RBCs. In addition to their role in oxygen transport, RBCs—being the most abundant cellular component of blood—are the main determinant of the hematocrit and therefore of the viscosity of the circulating blood.

▶ **Oxygen carrying capacity.** The perioperative setting, trauma, and diverse underlying diseases and critical illnesses are associated with blood loss of varying severity and therefore with dilutional anemia. The common therapeutic response is RBC transfusion, which is generally initiated to improve the oxygen carrying capacity of the circulating blood, which will have been compromised by the anemia, and thus to avert the danger of hypoxia. In recent years, the transfusion threshold has gradually been lowered because it has emerged that the number (Corwin et al 2004) and age ("storage lesions") (Frenzel et al 2009) of transfused RBC concentrates are both independently associated with an increased morbidity and mortality (Reeves and Murphy 2008). This means that anemia should be tolerated without transfusion as long as there are no clinical signs of anemic hypoxia (arrhythmia, tachycardia, hypotension, dyspnea, typical ECG signs, regional myocardial contraction disorder on ECG, or changes in global oxygen transport parameters [DO_2, oxygen extraction, central or mixed venous oxygen saturation]). Patients at cardiac risk (Hébert et al 1999a) generally need a higher hemoglobin target, but this should never exceed a hemoglobin level of 10 g/dL.

▶ **Viscosity.** However, their effect on the blood's oxygen carrying capacity is only one of the reasons why RBCs are very important and indispensable components of the circulating blood. In addition to their function as oxygen carrier and their role in oxygen delivery to the tissues, RBCs (hematocrit) are also responsible for the viscosity of the circulating blood and act as a mechanical component, which is crucial for the regulation of microvascular perfusion. RBCs therefore also play a key role in the maintenance of capillary perfusion (Tsai et al 2010). Even though the oxygen carrying capacity of stored and retransfused RBCs is poor during the first hours after transfusion (Marik and Sibbald 1993, Fitzgerald et al 1997, Fernandes et al 2001), it is nevertheless the clinical impression that hemodynamically unstable patients with anemia stabilize rapidly after the transfusion of RBC concentrates—an immediate effect that cannot be attributed to improvements in the oxygen carrying capacity of the circulating blood, but must be ascribed to an increase in its viscosity. The underlying mechanisms will be discussed in detail in the following sections.

>
>
> **Note**
>
> Transfused RBCs only play an active role in oxygen transport after a latency period of up to 24 hours. However, RBCs are responsible for the viscosity of the circulating blood, and are therefore an important determinant of the maintenance of microvascular perfusion.

5.3.2 Determinants of Capillary Perfusion

▶ **Microvascular blood flow and functional capillary density.** The most important determinants of microvascular perfusion are the microvascular blood flow, which is the mathematical product of vessel diameter and blood flow velocity, and the functional capillary density, which is defined as the number of capillaries perfused with RBCs per microscopic field of view. Maintenance of the microvascular perfusion, and in particular of the capillary flow, is vital: Kerger et al (1996) demonstrated in a hamster model that capillary perfusion was the only microvascular parameter that significantly determined survival during hemorrhagic shock. In addition, data on children with septic shock show an association between the mortality and alterations in the capillary blood flow (Top et al 2011). The functional capillary density also serves as a measure of the homogeneity of tissue perfusion (Tsai et al 1995). Based on studies of the human sublingual microcirculation, Edul et al (2012) reported that sepsis results in microvascular hypoperfusion and in an increased heterogeneity of the capillary perfusion (heterogeneity index). This phenomenon was much more pronounced among nonsurvivors. Using the same technique, Trzeciak et al (2007) reported that abnormalities in markers of early microcirculatory perfusion (flow velocity score, flow heterogeneity index, and capillary density) during severe sepsis and septic shock were more pronounced among nonsurvivors and with increasing severity of systemic cardiovascular dysfunction.

▶ **Mean arterial pressure and interstitial pressure.** What are the factors that affect capillary perfusion? The mean arterial pressure (Lindbom and Arfors 1985) and the interstitial pressure (Mazzoni et al 1990) are important and counteracting determinants of capillary perfusion. The administration of vasoactive drugs and fluids therefore has a direct influence on the regulation of the microcirculation. The microvascular system is a metabolically active and oxygen-consuming system that is composed of blood vessels of varying sizes. These vessels are not rigid tubes; because of the muscular activity of the myocytes in the vascular wall, blood vessels can change their diameter and accordingly their flow rate—a phenomenon called *vasoactivity*. Vasoconstriction significantly reduces the number of perfused capillaries (Friesenecker et al 2004, Friesenecker et al 2006a, Friesenecker et al 2006b), whereas vasodilatation increases the functional capillary density (Friesenecker et al 2007). Using a mathematical model, Tsai and Intaglietta (1993) demonstrated that vasomotion—the rhythmic changes between vasoconstriction and vasodilatation—facilitates oxygen diffusion in the capillary bed, promoting a more homogeneous distribution of oxygen in the tissues. In critically perfused tissues, this has the positive effect that fewer cells are exposed to a low PO_2.

Of note, in contrast to widespread belief, oxygen delivery to the microcirculation does not take place at the level of the capillaries: it was demonstrated in the hamster window chamber model that the biggest drop in intra- and perivascular PO_2 occurs between the large feeding arterioles (A0) and the A3/A4 arterioles, whereas the intravascular PO_2 in the small arterioles and capillaries is identical with the surrounding tissue PO_2. This means that there is basically no PO_2 diffusion gradient from the small arterioles and capillaries to the tissues (Friesenecker et al 2004, Tsai et al 2006).

> **Note** ❗
>
> The maintenance of capillary perfusion is of vital importance. Clinically, alterations in the capillary flow are associated with mortality. Important determinants of capillary perfusion are the mean arterial pressure and the interstitial pressure (tissue pressure). Vasomotion is a natural mechanism aimed at improving the capillary perfusion under pathophysiological conditions.

Last but not least, there is another important mechanical parameter that affects capillary perfusion: the viscosity of the circulating blood.

5.3.3 Relevance of the Blood Viscosity for Capillary Perfusion

Blood is a viscous fluid (viscosity of blood = 4.47 cP [centipoise]; viscosity of plasma = 1.7 cP; viscosity of water = 1.0 cP); its viscosity is mainly determined by the number of RBCs. Depending on the extent of anemia, the viscosity of the circulating blood may be greatly reduced.

▶ **Role of shear stress.** Maintenance of the viscosity of the circulating blood is important because viscous fluids induce shear stress on the surface of endothelial cells. This shear stress acts as a mechanical stimulus leading to the release of nitric oxide and vasoactive substances such as prostacyclin, which in turn causes vasodilatation in the downstream microvascular bed and improves capillary perfusion (McIntire et al 1987). Martini et al (2006) demonstrated in the hamster model that a moderate rise in hematocrit by around 10% from baseline leads to significant reductions in blood pressure and systemic resistance, an effect attributed to higher shear stress and consecutive nitric oxide release.

▶ **Effects of high-viscosity plasma expanders.** In the hamster model, it was also demonstrated that the decrease in viscosity of the circulating blood after hemodilution with a low-viscosity plasma expander (6% dextran-70; viscosity = 2.8 cP) led to a reduction in the arteriolar/venular microvascular blood flow and a significant drop in the number of perfused capillaries. Conversely, hemodilution with a high-viscosity plasma expander (6% dextran-500; viscosity = 6.4 cP) increased the arteriolar/venular blood flow in the last and critical hemodilution step (hematocrit = 11 g/dL, hemoglobin = 2–3 g/dL) to a value that was higher than the baseline value, while capillary perfusion was maintained (Tsai et al 1998). In the same animal model, it was demonstrated that high-viscosity solutions were even better at preserving capillary perfusion during hemorrhagic shock than was the retransfusion of RBC concentrates (Kerger et al 1996).

Cabrales et al (2004) showed that during extreme hemodilution, the functional capillary density is directly proportional to, and a linear function of, the capillary pressure. Administration of a low-viscosity plasma expander during extreme hemodilution (hematocrit ~ 11%) led to a significant drop in the capillary pressure, whereas the capillary pressure was maintained within the normal range when a high-viscosity plasma expander was used. Here, too, the maintenance of capillary function—specifically the functional capillary density—is the only critical microvascular parameter that makes a difference in the mortality of patients with severe hemorrhagic shock. It can be concluded that restoration of the blood pressure by raising the blood viscosity creates a state that facilitates transmission of the central blood pressure in the large vessels to the capillary level, thus increasing the capillary pressure throughout the entire capillary compartment and improving tissue perfusion. Hence, the functional capillary density is highly dependent on the central blood pressure, the plasma viscosity, the microvascular tone (microvascular resistance), and the shear stress exerted on vascular endothelial cells. This study showed that by using high-viscosity plasma expanders during extreme hemodilution, it is possible to generate pressure in the macro- and microcirculation (capillary pressure), thus maintaining a functional microcirculation through the restoration of capillary perfusion. Under extreme hemodilution, this effect is independent of the local tissue PO_2 (Cabrales et al 2004).

During moderate hemodilution (40% blood exchange), the changes in cardiovascular geometry arising from the increased viscosity of the circulating blood have positive effects on cardiovascular function, such as maintenance of cardiac power and reduction of the systemic vascular resistance (Chatpun and Cabrales 2010).

▶ **Improvement of the microcirculation.** The viscosity of the circulating blood is therefore one of the key factors in the maintenance of capillary perfusion. Our microcirculation is adapted to a certain level of shear stress, which declines in anemia because the viscosity is reduced. This leads to a reduction in the release of nitric oxide and can therefore considerably impair capillary perfusion. Poor capillary perfusion in various organ systems thus explains the clinical symptoms especially of severe anemia. It also explains why the clinical symptoms of anemia rapidly improve after the transfusion of RBC concentrates: the reason is bound to be the instantaneous rise in viscosity of the circulating blood, which translates into rapid improvement of the microvascular perfusion and therefore of the clinical picture. The improvement in the oxygen carrying capacity after administration of RBC concentrates, which is seen only after a delay of up to 24 hours, is a secondary mechanism to avert danger to organs at risk for hypoxia (Fitzgerald et al 1997).

Given the efforts to reduce the RBC transfusion rate in the future, there are currently attempts to produce plasma expanders with higher viscosity by means of chemical modification. This could help to further reduce the transfusion threshold

and—because of the higher viscosity of the circulating blood—good microcirculatory perfusion would be assured even under conditions of severe anemia. Thus, the tolerance to anemia could be markedly increased and RBC transfusions averted.

> **Note**
>
> In addition to the mean arterial pressure and the interstitial pressure, the viscosity of the circulating blood has a major effect on capillary perfusion. Viscous solutions induce shear stress on the surface of endothelial cells, and this acts as a mechanical stimulus for the release of nitric oxide and vasoactive mediators such as prostacyclin. The resulting vasodilatation in the downstream microvascular bed improves capillary perfusion.

5.3.4 Modern Plasma Expanders with High Viscosity—a Vision for the Future

The viscosity of currently available volume expanders is very different from that of blood—crystalloids have a viscosity that is similar to that of water. Even the viscosity of the colloid volume expanders normally used in the clinical setting (gelatins and starches) is, at body temperature, closer to that of water than it is to that of blood (e.g., Gelofusine and HES 130 have a viscosity of around 1.8 cP).

▶ **Polyethylene glycosylation.** One of the methods used to chemically modify low-viscosity solutions so that they will have a higher viscosity is polyethylene glycosylation. Studies with polyethylene glycol-conjugated albumin (PEG-albumin) and hemoglobin (PEG-hemoglobin; viscosity ~ 2.2 cP) revealed that the use of pegylated solutions during extreme isovolemic (normovolemic) hemodilution (hemoglobin ~ 2–3 g/dL, hematocrit ~ 11%) led to a significant increase not only in the functional capillary density but also in the cardiac index and the ratio of DO_2 to oxygen extraction; however, hemoglobin-containing solutions did not improve the tissue oxygenation (Cabrales et al 2005b). Martini et al (2008) demonstrated in a combined hemodilution/shock model that PEG-albumin in the hamster was better at maintaining microvascular function (functional capillary density, microvascular blood flow) than chemically unmodified HES.

A study by Sriram et al (2012) explains why PEG-albumin exerts such a positive effect on microvascular perfusion, producing a state of "supraperfusion." Blood in high-shear-rate zones of the circulation (heart, major vessels) is highly diluted when PEG-albumin is administered and now has a lower viscosity, whereas the microcirculation has an increased viscosity and shear stress, leading to the release of nitric oxide from the endothelium and vasodilatation in the downstream microvascular bed. The positive effect is caused by conversion of the fluid in the blood vessel core into a solid mass, with the result that the difference in viscosity between the macro- and microcirculation acts like a piston motor, driving the microvascular blood flow. The same phenomenon probably occurs in the microcirculation of the cardiac muscle and explains why, under the extreme conditions of hemodilution, the blood pressure is maintained and cardiac output is increased.

▶ **Other high-viscosity substances.** Another high-viscosity substance, polymerized human serum albumin, was compared with a hypertonic saline solution (7.5% NaCl) for use in intravenous infusion during hypovolemic hemorrhagic shock. Because of its greater molecular size and higher viscosity, it had positive effects on central hemodynamic parameters, microvascular blood flow, volume expansion, and persistence in the circulation (Messmer et al 2012).

Infusion of a lactated Ringer solution mixed with alginate—another substance with high viscosity—in the same hemorrhagic shock model resulted in significant improvements both in microvascular hemodynamic parameters and in oxygen transport parameters. Compared with infusion of a conventional lactated Ringer solution, there were significant increases in arteriolar/venular blood flow, functional capillary density, arteriolar PO_2, DO_2, and tissue PO_2 (Villela et al 2011).

A vision for the future would be the design of a chemically modified, inert high-viscosity volume expander that could be used instead of RBC concentrates for the treatment of anemia. This would avoid collapse of the microvascular circulation, observed after dilution with low-viscosity plasma expanders, and the microvascular rheology would be preserved. Thus, one could cut back on the use of blood products in general and of RBC concentrates in particular. In the long run, this is likely to substantially reduce mortality.

Note

Artificial plasma expanders that have a higher viscosity than currently available colloids (e.g., because of polyethylene glycosylation) and that have no effect on the coagulation system would be ideal volume expanders. Preservation of the viscosity of the circulating blood during anemia would make it possible to considerably lower the transfusion threshold without adversely affecting capillary perfusion.

5.3.5 Oxygen Transport or Blood Viscosity—Which Will Win the Race?

In a study of hemorrhagic shock (50% blood volume), Cabrales et al (2005a) demonstrated the complex and integrative link between blood, tissue PO_2, and pH. The tissue hypoxia seen in shock leads to the production of lactate, and the ensuing lactic acidosis results in a lower tissue pH (tissue acidosis). Infusion of PEG-albumin increased the functional capillary density, improved the microvascular blood flow, normalized the pH value, enhanced DO_2 and oxygen extraction, and increased the tissue PO_2. PEG-albumin was significantly better than HES across all parameters. With PEG-albumin, it was possible to eliminate acidosis and normalize the tissue pH through restoration of the DO_2, with improved oxygen supply to the microcirculation. Hence, improvement of the microvascular oxygen transport was only possible by first restoring the microvascular perfusion; this led to a normalization of the tissue metabolism with increasing lactate clearance.

Another study by Cabrales et al (2006) was specifically designed to answer the question of "oxygen transport or blood viscosity—which will win the race?" In an animal model of hypovolemic shock, three different infusion solutions were compared (plasma, oxygen carrying RBCs, and non-oxygen carrying RBCs). The blood viscosity was significantly lower in the group that received the plasma infusion. There were no differences between the groups infused with oxygen carrying versus non-oxygen carrying RBCs in terms of blood pressure, functional capillary density, DO_2, or oxygen extraction. However, a significant difference for all the aforementioned parameters was seen in comparison with the plasma infusion group, which can be attributed to the lower viscosity in the latter group (Cabrales et al 2007). This means that the maintenance of blood viscosity is the key factor in maintaining microvascular perfusion, regardless of the maintenance of the blood's oxygen carrying capacity. Thus, blood viscosity "wins the race," as pointed out in the paper published by Cabrales et al (2006).

> **Note**
>
> Under pathophysiological conditions (e.g., shock, anemia), microvascular oxygen transport will only function if it is possible to maintain microvascular perfusion. This means that the maintenance of blood viscosity takes priority over the administration of potential oxygen carriers!

5.3.6 Viscosity and Coagulation

Apart from the very positive effect on microvascular rheology described above, high blood viscosity also has undesirable effects, in particular on the blood coagulation system. It is well established that high-viscosity solutions increase the coagulation ability of blood and accordingly the tendency toward thrombosis (Schmid-Schönbein et al 1976, Smith and La Celle 1982). In particular, the use of starch products for volume expansion in bleeding situations makes it more difficult to counterbalance the lack of fibrinogen after hemodilution through administration of fibrinogen concentrates (Fries et al 2006). It is therefore possible that the positive effect of high-viscosity volume expanders on the microvascular rheology might be negated by an increased tendency toward bleeding or thrombosis. This is the focus of current investigations.

> **Note**
>
> Colloids and solutions with altered viscosity can have a negative effect on blood coagulation (both clotting and bleeding).

5.3.7 Anemia Threshold/Critical Hematocrit—Clinical Implications

Under healthy conditions, our body is a "luxury system." This applies equally to the hematocrit ("luxury hematocrit") and to oxygen carrying parameters ("luxury DO_2"), and means that the DO_2 in an unstressed state is three to four times greater than the VO_2. A decrease in the DO_2 with a constant VO_2 has initially no impact on the oxygen supply of the tissues. As such, in a healthy, unstressed state, the oxygen supply is independent of the oxygen demand (Aly Hassan et al 1997).

▶ **"Critical" hematocrit.** The hematocrit is defined as the proportion of all cellular components of blood and is largely determined by the concentration of RBCs, since they account for around 99% of all blood cells. Normal values range from 42% to 50% in men, and from 37% to 45% in women. "Luxury hematocrit" means that the microvascular (i.e., the capillary) hematocrit is kept constant over a wide range. Only after a 30–50% drop in the macrovascular hematocrit does the capillary hematocrit also begin to decline (Pries et al 1992). The "critical hematocrit" is reached if the physiological limits of tolerance to anemia are reached and the body develops tissue hypoxia, which ultimately leads to increasing lactic acidosis and death (Habler et al 2006).

▶ **"Safe" hematocrit.** The first reports on hemodilution in the literature date back to the 1970s and originate from the laboratory of Professor Konrad Messmer, one of the pioneers in the field of microcirculation. The values cited in the literature for a "safe hematocrit" in "healthy" patients are relatively uniform between 20% and 25%, which corresponds to a hemoglobin value of 6.5–7.5 g/dL (Klövekorn et al 1974, Kreimeier and Messmer 1996). At an arterial hematocrit of 25%, the capillary hematocrit in the microcirculation will decline by 30%, but the capillary RBC flow velocity will rise by 60%, thus leading to a homogenization and redistribution of the microvascular blood flow of the skin (Mirhashemi et al 1988). Several studies have demonstrated that hemodilution to a hematocrit of 20% does in fact increase the tissue PO_2 in the liver, pancreas, kidneys, small intestine, skeletal muscle, myocardium, and the brain (Messmer et al 1973, Chan and Leniger-Follert 1983, Forst et al 1987). Hutter et al (1999) showed that normovolemic hemodilution—a decrease in the hematocrit from 36% to 20% with 6% HES 200—led to significant rises in the cardiac index (a mechanism of natural tolerance to anemia) and muscle perfusion. The DO_2 in skeletal muscle and the tissue pO_2 were preserved.

> **Note**
>
> Clinically, this means that a hematocrit of around 20% (hemoglobin ~ 6.5–7.0 g/dL) is generally safe for patients who have the capacity to activate their mechanisms of natural tolerance to anemia, meaning that they can sufficiently raise their cardiac output under anemic conditions.

5.3.8 Outlook

If it were possible to produce high-viscosity solutions for volume expansion that can prevent microvascular collapse during anemia owing to their high viscosity (Salazar et al 2008), if these solutions were chemically inert, and if they had few disruptive effects on the coagulation system, it would probably be possible to lower the transfusion threshold even beyond a hematocrit of around 20%. This would help to cut back on the necessity to transfuse RBC concentrates and reduce transfusion-induced mortality. Other advantages of modern hemoglobin-free, high-viscosity volume expanders include easy transport, uncomplicated production in large quantities, simplified storage, and improved availability (emergency situations where no blood bank is available). Such solutions would make a valuable contribution to the safer and better care of patients with anemia.

5.3.9 Recommendations for the Use of Red Blood Cell Transfusions

▶ **Recommendations from the American Association of Blood Banks** (AABB 2014). As explained in detail in Chapter 5.3.7, hemodilution to a hematocrit of around 20% (hemoglobin ~ 6.5–7.0 g/dL) is safe with regard to preservation of the microvascular flow, which explains why young and healthy patients tolerate a decrease in hemoglobin to around 6 g/dL very well. If patients develop symptoms from anemia (e.g., arrhythmia, hypotension, typical ischemia-related changes on ECG) or if they have an underlying cardiovascular disease, the hematocrit should be raised to 25% to 30% (hemoglobin > 8 g/dL). This low transfusion threshold for healthy people in clinical practice, which is safe and beneficial in terms of the microcirculation, is in accordance with current recommendations from the American Association of Blood Banks (Carson et al 2012b) and with the most recent Cochrane analysis to date (Carson et al 2012a), as presented in **Table 5.3**.

▶ **Cochrane analysis.** The most recent Cochrane analysis to date endorses the general recommendation by the American Association of Blood Banks, suggesting that restrictive transfusion thresholds are good for most patients—including those with underlying cardiovascular disease (Carson et al 2012a). Restrictive transfusion strategies reduced the risk of receiving RBC transfusions by almost 40%, and the number of transfused RBC concentrates was reduced by an average of 1.19 units. Restrictive transfusion regimens led to a significant reduction in hospital mortality, but not in 30-day mortality. There was also no effect

Table 5.3 Recommendations for transfusion by the American Association of Blood Banks (Carson et al 2012b)

	Recommendation 1	Recommendation 2	Recommendation 3	Recommendation 4
Patient group	Hospitalized, stable	Hospitalized, underlying CVD, symptoms	Hospitalized, with ACS, hemodynamically stable	General recommendation
Transfusion strategy	Restrictive; target 7–8 g/dL	Restrictive; target > 8 g/dL	None	Symptoms and Hb as reasons for transfusion
Recommendation level	Strong	Weak	Uncertain	Weak
Evidence level	High quality	Moderate quality	Very low quality	Low quality

Abbreviations: ACS, acute coronary syndrome; CVD, cardiovascular disease; Hb, hemoglobin.

on functional recovery or on the length of hospital/ICU stay.

Conclusion

The maintenance of capillary perfusion is vital for survival. In addition to the two counteracting factors of mean arterial pressure (vasoconstrictors) and interstitial pressure (fluid administration), the blood viscosity—the physical/mechanical component in the regulation of microvascular perfusion—is a key factor responsible for the perfusion of the capillary bed. This is of particular clinical relevance during severe anemia, since a low viscosity of the circulating blood reduces shear stress on the surface of endothelial cells. This, in turn, means that fewer vasoactive substances (nitric oxide, prostacyclin) are released, leading to collapse of the capillary bed for purely mechanical reasons. Until chemically inert plasma expanders with a higher viscosity and no negative effect on the coagulation system become available in the clinical setting, the individual transfusion threshold may need to be raised, especially in patients with hemodynamic instability. For the time being, it is therefore not possible to avoid the transfusion of RBC concentrates.

5.4 Management of Profound Anemia in Patients Refusing Red Blood Cell Transfusion

P. Van der Linden

5.4.1 Refusal of Red Blood Cell Transfusion

The therapeutic efficacy of allogeneic RBC transfusion remains a matter of intense debate. Although it may save lives in some acute situations, it is also associated with increased morbidity and reduced survival after major surgery. Adult surgical patients may refuse allogeneic RBC transfusion, mainly for religious reasons, and their management represents a particular challenge for surgeons, anesthesiologists, and intensivists. However, such a management approach, based on a severe blood conservation strategy, does not seem to alter the patients' outcome after major surgery unless their hemoglobin level drops below 5–6 g/dL (Shander et al 2014c). A study using propensity methods reported that Jehovah's Witnesses do not appear to be at increased risk for surgical complications or long-term mortality after cardiac surgery when compared with patients who are not Jehovah's Witnesses (Pattakos et al 2012). It is beyond the scope of this chapter to discuss the ethical issues that arise when caring for this particular population of patients. However, it is important that a "therapeutic contract" is negotiated on an individual basis, specifying the mutual commitments and undertakings of all parties (Chassot et al 2006). The patient's autonomy must be respected at all times; this also requires the availability of colleagues who agree with the patient's position. The management of these patients implies that all members of the medical team demonstrate expertise in minimizing the risk of blood loss and in ensuring adequate oxygen transport to the tissues in the event of acute severe anemia. The present review will first describe the physiological mechanisms elicited during "isovolemic" anemia. Based on these mechanisms, several therapeutic approaches to improve the tolerance to anemia will be discussed.

5.4.2 Physiological Mechanisms to Compensate for Acute Isovolemic Anemia

Maintenance of the DO_2 at the level of oxygen demand during acute isovolemic hemodilution depends on both an increase in the cardiac output and an increase in the extraction of oxygen from blood (Van der Linden 2002, Hébert et al 2004). These two phenomena are directly linked to the decrease in blood viscosity that is associated with the acute reduction in RBC concentration (Kreimeier and Messmer 2002). Both experimental and clinical data have demonstrated that these phenomena also require the intervention of the sympathetic nervous system (Tsui et al 2010).

Cardiac Output Response

The cardiac output rises in response to isovolemic anemia, mainly through an increase in the stroke volume and, to some extent, through an increase in the heart rate. The increase in stroke volume essentially results from an improvement in the myocardial performance, which is in turn attributable to the decrease in blood viscosity during acute anemia: as a result of the decreased blood viscosity, the venous return increases and the peripheral vascular resistance is reduced. In addition, isovolemic anemia enhances arteriolar vasomotion, which contributes to peripheral vasodilatation and stimulates aortic chemoreceptors; this in turn increases the sympathetic-mediated myocardial contractility (Chapler and Cain 1986).

Tissue Oxygen Extraction

Tissue oxygen extraction also increases in response to isovolemic anemia, and this phenomenon entails mechanisms that occur at both the systemic and the microcirculatory level. At the systemic level, there is a redistribution of the blood flow to tissues with a high oxygen demand, such as the brain and the myocardium, at the expense of organs with a lower oxygen demand, such as the splanchnic area, the kidneys, and the skin (Fan et al 1980). An important mediator of this redistribution of the regional blood flow is α-adrenergic stimulation; however, it does not seem to be influenced by β-adrenergic blockade. At the microcirculatory level, the principal hemodynamic effect of isovolemic anemia is an increase in the velocity of RBCs, which stimulates arterial vasomotion (Messmer 1991). Increased flow velocity at the microcirculatory level favors the redistribution of RBCs to small-diameter capillaries, thereby reducing the heterogeneity of RBC distribution and improving the capacity of tissues to extract oxygen from their environment (Van der Linden et al 1993). However, these adaptive mechanisms have limitations, and with further progres-

sion of anemia the reduced viscosity of blood at very low hematocrit values could negatively affect its rheological characteristics in the microcirculation, resulting in a decreased DO_2 to the tissues (Cabrales and Tsai 2006).

Another adaptive mechanism involves an increase in the 2,3-bisphosphoglycerate level in RBCs, which is associated with a reduced affinity of hemoglobin for oxygen and therefore improves oxygen availability at the tissue level. However, this mechanism takes hours to develop and has been demonstrated only in chronic anemia (Rodman et al 1960).

Limits of Hemodilution

Thanks to the compensatory mechanisms described above, humans are highly tolerant to acute hemodilution. Although increases in both cardiac output and blood oxygen extraction have been observed in the early stages of isovolemic anemia (Spahn et al 1994), their relative contribution to the maintenance of adequate tissue oxygenation depends on the body's ability to recruit these mechanisms. In heathy individuals, these two mechanisms allow maintenance of the cellular oxygen balance until a hemoglobin concentration of about 3–4 g/dL (hematocrit 10–12%) has been reached. When the hemoglobin concentration falls below this "critical" value, oxygen delivery to the cells becomes insufficient and cellular hypoxia develops. Experimental studies have demonstrated this "critical" hemoglobin value to be around 3–4 g/dL in different animal species (Räsänen

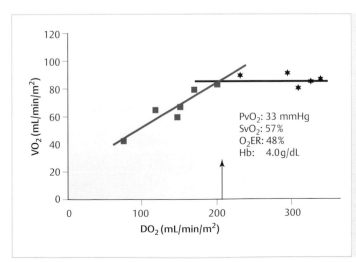

Fig. 5.1 Relationship between VO_2 and DO_2 in an 84-year-old Jehovah's Witness patient who eventually died from an untreatable hemorrhage after surgery for gastric cancer. The critical hemoglobin concentration (hemoglobin value below which the VO_2 becomes DO_2-dependent) was 4.0 g/dL. DO_2, oxygen delivery; Hb, hemoglobin; O_2ER, oxygen extraction ratio; PvO_2, mixed venous partial pressure of oxygen; SvO_2, mixed venous oxygen saturation; VO_2, oxygen consumption. The critical point was determined using the mathematical method proposed by Samsel and Schumacker (1988). Redrawn from data initially published by van Woerkens et al (1992).

In figure:
PvO_2: 33 mmHg
SvO_2: 57%
O_2ER: 48%
Hb: 4.0g/dL

1992, Van der Linden et al 1998, Van der Linden et al 2003). In healthy volunteers, Weiskopf et al (1998) reported that tissue oxygenation remains unaltered during isovolemic hemodilution up to a hemoglobin concentration of 5 g/dL. van Woerkens and colleagues (1992) reported a critical hemoglobin concentration of 4 g/dL in a Jehovah's Witness patient who eventually died from extreme anemia (**Fig. 5.1**).

> **Note**
>
> Adequate compensatory mechanisms enable the maintenance of adequate tissue oxygenation until the hemoglobin concentration falls to about 3 to 4 g/dL.

5.4.3 Therapeutic Approaches

Optimization of Tissue Oxygen Delivery

Optimization of the Circulating Blood Volume

The maintenance of adequate volume replacement is of paramount importance during acute anemia to achieve a better cardiac output response. Indeed, hypovolemia will markedly blunt the effects of the reduced blood viscosity on the venous return (Richardson and Guyton 1959).

▶ **Colloids versus crystalloids.** In this context, colloids appear superior to crystalloids as they maintain the colloid osmotic pressure and remain largely in the intravascular space. Studies in humans have demonstrated that the expanding effect of crystalloids during acute hemodilution is only 20% of the infused fluid, whereas it is 80–100% with albumin or hydroxyethyl starches (Jacob and Chappell 2013). As a consequence, a smaller volume of fluid is required when colloids are used, and the effects of these solutions on the cardiac output are greater than those obtained with crystalloids (Verheij et al 2006, van der Heijden et al 2009). Only a few studies have compared the effects of different plasma substitutes on the hemodynamic response to acute isovolemic anemia; these studies also showed that colloids appeared superior to crystalloids (Arya et al 2006, Otsuki et al 2007).

The choice of plasma substitute may also affect the ability of the tissues to extract oxygen. Tissue perfusion closely depends on the functional capillary density, which is determined by the perfusion pressure, the vascular resistance, and the blood viscosity (Villela et al 2009). Colloids maintain the functional capillary density to a better degree than crystalloids do, and they are associated with less fluid extravasation (Hoffmann et al 2002). An experimental study demonstrated that the tolerance to extreme anemia was higher when colloids were used as plasma substitutes (Pape et al 2012b).

▶ **Hydroxyethyl starch solutions.** Among colloids, tetrastarches—the latest generation of hydroxyethyl starch solutions—seem to be the best substitute in this context (Pape et al 2012b), whereas gelatins appear less efficacious, as do pentastarches or hetastarches (Van der Linden 1998, Pape et al 2012b).

Under physiological conditions, the viscosity of the blood, which has important effects on the functional capillary density, is mainly determined by the viscosity of its cellular components. However, during severe isovolemic anemia, the viscosity of the plasma may play a significant role as it appears to regulate systemic and microvascular perfusion (Cabrales and Tsai 2006). Therefore, an increase in plasma viscosity through the use of "viscogenic" plasma expanders might be associated with an improvement in the functional capillary density, improving the tolerance to severe isovolemic anemia (Villela et al 2009). These experimental observations (Villela et al 2011) need to be confirmed in clinical practice.

▶ **Hemoglobin-based oxygen carriers.** Hemoglobin-based oxygen carrier (HBOC) solutions might represent the plasma substitute of choice in patients with severe anemia who refuse RBC transfusion. On the one hand, these solutions possess oncotic properties that are interesting for the maintenance of the intravascular volume. On the other hand, they possess oxygen carrying capacities contributing to the delivery of oxygen to the tissues. In South Africa, HBOC-201 (bovine hemoglobin glutamer-250, marketed as Hemopure [Biopure Corporation]) has been approved for the treatment of adults with surgical anemia (Evaluate 2011). In Western countries, the development of HBOCs has stagnated because of safety issues.

Studies suggest that HBOCs have considerable side effects such as myocardial infarction, stroke, acute renal failure, deleterious increases in arterial blood pressure, methemoglobinemia, and death (Natanson et al 2008). However, when RBC transfusion is not an option in patients with severe anemia and signs of ischemia, the Food and Drug Administration has authorized the compassionate use of such solutions (Mozzarelli et al 2010).

Mackenzie et al (2010) reviewed 54 patients with anemia who were treated with HBOC-201. Overall, the mortality rate was 52%. No serious event was attributed to HBOC-201. Survival was more likely if the duration and magnitude of a low hemoglobin concentration was minimized before treatment with the HBOC. In a review article, Weiskopf and Silverman (2013) compared the risks associated with HBOC infusion in patients with severe anemia (hemoglobin <6 g/dL) with the risks associated with a further small decrease in the hemoglobin concentration (Weiskopf and Silverman 2013). They concluded that at such a low hemoglobin concentration, the risks of anemia greatly exceed the risks of HBOC infusion.

▶ **Monitoring.** Optimization of the circulating blood volume also requires adequate hemodynamic monitoring to avoid hypervolemia, which might be as deleterious as hypovolemia (Bellamy 2006). In mechanically ventilated and sedated patients, dynamic parameters such as stroke volume variation or pulse pressure variation appear more reliable than static parameters, such as the cardiac filling pressure (Marik et al 2009). Esophageal Doppler monitoring represents an interesting alternative (Bundgaard-Nielsen et al 2007), but requires skill and expertise.

Maintenance of Myocardial Function

▶ **Vasoactive agents.** Extreme anemia alters myocardial performance through decreases in the arterial oxygen content and the coronary artery perfusion pressure because of the vasodilatation associated with severe hemodilution. Maintenance of the coronary artery perfusion pressure through the use of vasoactive agents such as norepinephrine might therefore increase the tolerance of patients to extreme anemia. This hypothesis has been verified in a pig model of extreme hemodilution (Meier et al 2007). Although norepinephrine titrated to maintain a mean arterial pressure

of >60 mmHg was associated with a significant increase in 6-hour survival in the animals, lactic acidosis appeared, indicating the development of tissue hypoxia in association with vasoconstriction of the peripheral organs. Therefore, the use of norepinephrine during extreme anemia should be considered as a short-term intervention; its long-term use is not advised.

> **Note**
>
> Norepinephrine should only be used as a short-term intervention during extreme anemia.

▶ **Influence of anesthesia.** Patients undergoing severe isovolemic anemia are most often sedated and mechanically ventilated in an attempt to reduce the metabolic demand of the tissues. However, anesthesia can alter the physiological adjustments to isovolemic hemodilution at several levels. The most striking effect of anesthesia appears to be a decreased cardiac output response, mainly related to a complete blunting of the increase in heart rate (Ickx et al 2000, Kungys et al 2009). In an experimental study in anesthetized dogs, Crystal and Salem (2002) reported complete restoration of the cardiac output response after the administration of small isoproterenol doses. Although interesting from a theoretical point of view, this observation needs to be confirmed in humans.

Hyperoxic Ventilation

Ventilation with a high inspired oxygen fraction increases the physically dissolved part of the arterial oxygen content. Physically dissolved plasma oxygen is highly available and covers up to 75% of the body's total oxygen demand in conditions of extreme dilutional anemia (Habler 2011). Experimental studies have shown that hyperoxic ventilation improves tissue oxygenation and survival during extreme dilutional anemia (Meier et al 2004, Pape et al 2013). These beneficial effects have been attributed to the increased arterial oxygen content, but also to increases in the mean arterial pressure and the coronary artery perfusion pressure caused by hyperoxic arteriolar vasoconstriction (Kemming et al 2004). Although hyperoxia may result in microcirculatory dysregulation in normal physiological conditions, the effect is counterbalanced by the increase of organ blood flow induced by dilutional anemia, which leads in turn to an increase in shear stress and induces the release of nitric oxide (Meier et al 2011).

>
> **Note**
>
> Hyperoxic ventilation improved tissue oxygenation and survival during extreme dilutional anemia in experimental studies.

Only a few studies have investigated the effects of hyperoxic ventilation in humans. Weiskopf and colleagues (2002) reported that hyperoxic ventilation in healthy volunteers completely reversed the deficits in cognitive function and memory associated with the induction of profound isovolemic anemia (Weiskopf et al 2002). Spahn et al (1999) observed that hyperoxic ventilation reversed a preset transfusion trigger in patients undergoing major orthopaedic surgery. Although the long-term administration of hyperoxic gas mixtures might be associated with some toxicity (mainly pulmonary toxicity), their short-term administration appears safe and is even associated with a reduced incidence of postoperative wound infection (Belda et al 2005).

Control of the Tissue Oxygen Demand

The individual tolerance to acute dilutional anemia does not only depend on the integrity of the compensatory mechanisms responsible for maintenance of the DO_2, but also on the tissue oxygen demand. For a given cardiac output and oxygen extraction response, any increase in the tissue oxygen demand will require a corresponding increase in the hemoglobin concentration. Therefore, reducing the tissues' metabolic demand represents another therapeutic approach to increase the tolerance of patients to severe anemia.

Sedation

The use of sedative agents may be useful to reduce the tissues' metabolic demand in mechanically ventilated patients. This effect results more from the decrease in muscular work associated with spontaneous ventilation and the decrease in sympathetic activity associated with stress, pain, and anxiety than from a reduction in the basal cellular metabolism. Indeed, general anesthetics cannot be considered as general metabolic depressant agents (Mikat et al 1984).

In addition, as stated above, anesthetic agents interfere considerably with the cardiac output response elicited during acute isovolemic hemodilution, mainly through a complete blunting of the heart rate increase. On the one hand, this effect may be beneficial to the patient because it decreases the myocardial oxygen demand. On the other hand, this effect can be deleterious because it decreases the cardiac output and therefore the amount of oxygen delivered to the tissues (Ickx et al 2000). An experimental study assessed the effects of anesthetic depth on the tolerance to acute dilutional anemia in dogs (Van der Linden et al 2003). The authors observed that increasing the depth of anesthesia with either halothane or ketamine is associated with a decreased tolerance to anemia, mainly through a complete blunting of the cardiac output response. Several studies have demonstrated that almost all anesthetic agents decrease the cardiac output response to isovolemic anemia.

Therefore, although it appears judicious to maintain patients with severe anemia who refuse RBC transfusion under sedation, the level of sedation must be titrated carefully to avoid too light and too profound a level of anesthesia, either of which could be associated with a decreased tolerance to anemia.

>
> **Note**
>
> Although it appears judicious to maintain patients with severe anemia who refuse RBC transfusion under sedation, the level of sedation must be titrated carefully.

Muscular Relaxation

Neuromuscular blocking agents are often used during general anesthesia to facilitate not only endotracheal intubation and mechanical ventilation but also abdominal and thoracic surgical procedures. The effects of these agents on the body's total VO_2 and energy expenditure remain debated and probably depend on the depth of anesthesia or sedation (Pape et al 2012a). It might also depend on the type of agent used, as these drugs possess different effects on the cardiovascular system. An experimental study demonstrated that rocuronium increased the tolerance to extreme dilutional anemia in pigs anesthetized with propofol, midazolam, and fentanyl (Pape et al 2012a). The authors hypothesized that rocuronium might reduce the muscular oxygen consumption and the regional blood flow to the skeletal muscles, enabling a redistribution of oxygen delivery in favor of the vital organs. Extrapolation of these results in humans appears difficult, and complete muscular relaxation may hide a level of sedation that is too low in patients with severe anemia. Therefore, the use of neuromuscular blocking agents to increase a patient's tolerance to profound anemia is not recommended on a routine basis.

Hypothermia

Through its effect on the basal cellular metabolism, mild hypothermia (32–35 °C) may improve the balance between oxygen supply and demand when the DO_2 is acutely reduced. However, it is not known whether the reduction in the oxygen demand will counterbalance the cardiovascular depression induced by hypothermia or whether it will compensate for the decreased oxygen availability caused by the increased hemoglobin affinity for oxygen. An experimental study assessed the effects of mild hypothermia (32 °C) on the tolerance to acute normovolemic anemia in anesthetized and paralyzed pigs (Perez-de-Sá et al 2002). The authors were not able to demonstrate a clear-cut protective effect of mild hypothermia. These results, together with the potential deleterious effects of hypothermia on the cardiovascular and hemostatic systems, indicate that the induction of hypothermia is not recommended in patients with severe anemia.

> **!**
>
> **Note**
>
> The induction of hypothermia is not recommended in patients with severe anemia.

5.4.4 Stimulation of Erythropoiesis

▶ **Administration of erythropoiesis-stimulating substances.** Ideally, the stimulation of erythropoiesis in surgical patients should have begun before commencing the actual procedure. However, this is not always possible. With adequate supportive treatment, erythropoiesis can be increased to approximately four times the level of basal marrow RBC production (Goodnough 2011). Administration of recombinant human erythropoietin (rHuEPO) is required to achieve this response. However, the optimal dosage of rHuEPO is not known. Goodnough et al (2011) reported a good correlation between the rHuEPO dose (administered twice per week over 3 weeks) and the response in terms of RBC production. The currently recommended rHuEPO doses in patients scheduled for elective surgery range from 300 U/kg to 700 U/kg twice per week over 3 weeks. Data regarding the use of rHuEPO in the postoperative period are scarce. In a small study addressing the management of Jehovah's Witness patients undergoing cardiac surgery, McCartney et al (2014) reported the use of 20,000 units of rHuEPO administered daily subcutaneously up to the fourth postoperative day in patients with clinically significant anemia. In a case report, doses of 150 U/kg to 350 U/kg per day up to the 20th postoperative day were used in a Jehovah's Witness patient with extreme postoperative anemia (de Araújo Azi et al 2014). This aggressive erythropoietin therapy was associated with a rise in the patient's hemoglobin level of 240% in 10 days. The only side effect reported was an increase in the platelet count, which peaked on the eighth day. Erythropoietin administration does not only cause a rise in the platelet count, but it can also increase platelet reactivity (Wolf et al 1997).

▶ **Iron substitution.** To support such high rates of erythropoiesis, oral iron will not be sufficient and intravenous iron therapy should be considered.

The total iron deficit (TID) can be calculated using the Ganzoni formula (Del Vecchio and Locatelli 2011):

> **Formula**
>
> TID (mg) = [Weight (kg) × (Target hemoglobin – Actual hemoglobin) (g/dL) × 0.24] + Depot iron (500 mg)

Different products exist and their administration needs to take into account their specific pharmacokinetic and pharmacodynamic properties (Muñoz et al 2011). To minimize the risks of iron overload, the following iron targets have been recommended in patients undergoing hemodialysis: serum ferritin 200–500 ng/mL and transferrin saturation > 20% (Del Vecchio and Locatelli 2011).

These targets should probably also be used to monitor iron therapy in patients with severe anemia. A systematic review reported that although intravenous iron appears effective in increasing the hemoglobin concentration and reducing the need for allogeneic RBC transfusion, it could potentially increase the risk of infection (Litton et al 2013).

Vitamin B_{12} and folic acid deficiency should also be excluded; these are more frequent in patients older than 60 years (Muñoz et al 2011).

Conclusion

Humans are highly tolerant to acute anemia if the intravascular volume is adequately maintained. Fulfilment of the tissue oxygen demand during acute anemia depends on both an increase in the cardiac output and an increase in the peripheral oxygen extraction. Any factor that reduces these two compensatory mechanisms will decrease the tolerance to anemia.

Several therapeutic approaches exist that can considerably increase the tolerance of patients to severe anemia. However, most of these approaches can only be used for a relatively short period.

- Optimization of the cardiac output response with adequate fluid loading and hyperoxic ventilation represents the best therapeutic strategy to improve the tolerance of patients to acute anemia. In mechanically ventilated patients, the use of parameters such as pulse pressure variation or stroke volume variation is highly recommended to dynamically evaluate the response to fluid loading.
- From a theoretical point of view, decreasing the tissue oxygen demand through anesthesia and hypothermia could be helpful to increase a patient's tolerance to acute anemia. However, the depth of anesthesia should be carefully titrated to avoid the depressant effects of anesthetic agents on the cardiovascular system. Hypothermia is not recommended because of its deleterious effects on hemostasis.
- The management of profound anemia in patients who refuse RBC transfusion requires adequate erythropoiesis stimulation through the administration of subcutaneous erythropoietin and intravenous iron. Folic acid and vitamin B_{12} deficiencies should also be corrected if present.
- The use of HBOC solutions remains limited to compassionate cases.

Chapter 6

PBM in Surgical Settings

6.1 PBM in Cardiac Surgery

H. M. Mueller

6.1.1 Introduction

The transfusion rate in cardiac surgery is much higher than that in other surgical disciplines (Gombotz et al 2007, Maddox et al 2009, Bennett-Guerrero et al 2010, Likosky et al 2014, McQuilten et al 2014). For example, in the Austrian Benchmark Studies, on average more than 50% of patients received transfusions even for uncomplicated coronary bypass operations, despite a decline in perioperative blood loss over the years (Gombotz et al 2014). Besides, there continues to be widespread variability in the consumption of allogeneic blood and allogeneic blood derivatives between different centers (Gombotz et al 2007, Maddox et al 2009, Bennett-Guerrero et al 2010, Gombotz et al 2014, Likosky et al 2014). The disease severity and the presence of concomitant diseases (a factor that is increasing in prevalence) have, of course, a prominent impact on the indication for transfusion and affect the disease course (Dixon et al 2013, Roubinian et al 2014a). The avoidance of perioperative anemia through the reduction of perioperative surgical blood loss does not only help to decrease the frequency of unnecessary allogeneic blood transfusions, or preempt them altogether, but it also enhances patient safety and improves the disease course (Bracey et al 1999, Oliver et al 2009, Howard-Quijano et al 2013, Goodnough et al 2014a, Willems et al 2014). The cardiac surgeon is therefore confronted with the particular challenges associated with a perioperative multidisciplinary strategy, such as PBM, to improve outcome through the avoidance of surgical blood loss (Moskowitz et al 2010, Vivacqua et al 2011, Gombotz 2012, Dixon et al 2014, Frank et al 2014b).

This chapter presents a number of techniques and operative strategies based on the author's own experience.

6.1.2 Preoperative Measures

The prevalence of anemia among patients undergoing cardiac surgery is as high as 50% (Gombotz et al 2007, Van Mieghem et al 2011, David et al 2013, Gombotz et al 2014, Kim et al 2015a). In addition to preexisting conditions such as iron deficiency, possible causes include blood loss secondary to preoperative interventions such as coronary angiography, or simply frequent blood draws (Ereth et al 2000, Hung et al 2015). Despite the fact that even moderate preoperative anemia—when left untreated—leads to a two- to threefold rise in the transfusion rate and negatively affects the course of disease, it continues to go untreated in more than 90% of patients (Gombotz et al 2007, Kulier et al 2007, Dunkelgrun et al 2008, Karkouti et al 2008a, De Santo et al 2009, Patel and Carson 2009, Weber et al 2009, Carrascal et al 2010, Gombotz 2011, Musallam et al 2011, Ranucci et al 2012, Gupta et al 2013, Gombotz et al 2014, Miceli et al 2014).

The preoperative diagnosis and treatment of existing anemia is of paramount importance for the subsequent course of disease (Gombotz 2011). It reduces the probability of allogeneic red blood cell (RBC) transfusion and improves the outcome. Therefore, patients undergoing cardiac surgery should—whenever permitted by the urgency of the operation—be referred as soon as possible to a preanesthesia clinic or similar institution (Sowade et al 1997, Goodnough and Shander 2012, Gombotz and Hofmann 2013). Ideally, such clinics will investigate and treat not only the anemia but also any other relevant concomitant diseases, including coagulation disorders, while making the necessary preparations for anesthesia.

Since it is very hard to predict the bleeding risk (Vuylsteke et al 2011, Gombotz and Knotzer 2013), it is crucial to take a detailed bleeding and coagulation history and to discontinue anticoagulants and platelet inhibitors in a timely fashion (Harder et al 2004, Nuttall et al 2006, Levi et al 2011, Tafur et al 2012, Emeklibas et al 2013). In special cases, required antiplatelet therapy can be provided by short-acting platelet inhibitors (Savonitto et al 2010). If the patient responds to the treatment of anemia, a hemoglobin rise of around 1 g/dL per week can be expected (Doodeman et al 2013).

The treatment of preoperative anemia can result in greater logistical efforts because of changes to the surgical schedule. However, the short-term use, or even a single dose, of erythropoietin a few days before surgery can significantly reduce the transfusion requirement (Yazicioglu et al 2001, Weltert et al 2010, Yoo et al 2011). Since erythropoietin gives rise to a relative iron deficiency, iron deficiency must be ruled out or treated before and during the course of therapy (Sowade et al 1997). A hematologist should be consulted in complex cases.

Preoperative autologous blood donation increases the risk of anemia, and it is time-consuming and expensive. It is therefore no longer used as a global measure (Gombotz et al 2000, Singbartl 2007).

The use of proton pump inhibitors to avoid gastrointestinal bleeding complications and to administer antibiotic prophylaxis is standard.

> **Note**
>
> Patients undergoing elective surgery should be referred to the preanesthesia clinic as early as possible—ideally once the surgical indication has been established. Timely referral does not only enable the treatment of potential anemia but also the preoperative management of other risk factors.

6.1.3 Intraoperative Measures (Second Pillar of PBM)

The views presented here are subjective perceptions, based on the author's own experiences; the methods have stood the test of time over several years of using a restrictive transfusion approach, including approaches in patients who declined transfusion. Experience has shown that it is rarely an isolated measure but rather the combination of various measures that leads to the desired outcome. Of the many ways to minimize blood loss, I would like to present the most important methods actually implemented in our department, which were also used for the 19 cardiac operations in Jehovah's Witness patients described below.

▸ **The sternum.** The sternum plays a major role as a cause of continuous intraoperative bleeding because of its structure, with widely open red-bone-marrow sinusoids following sternotomy. In surgical terms, it should therefore be viewed as a parenchymatous organ. Although blood entering the surgical area can be collected, continuous aspiration with the cardiotomy suction device of the heart–lung machine causes hemolysis and leukocyte activation because the blood is exposed to air and the RBCs are mechanically destroyed by the roller pumps (Osborn et al 1962, El-Sabbagh et al 2013). During embryological development, the sternum forms from a paired ossification center, thus assuring the symmetrical perfusion of both

sides of the body. Hence, precise midline sternotomy can reduce blood loss.

▸ **Bone wax.** Bone wax is commonly used in cardiac surgery to minimize blood loss. It is composed of a nonabsorbable mixture of 75% white beeswax (cera alba), 15% paraffin wax, and 10% isopropyl palmitate as a softening agent. It does not have hemostatic activity; rather, its action derives from mechanical hemostasis. Once applied to the bone surface, bone wax is usually not resorbed (Sudmann et al 2006, Vestergaard et al 2010). Furthermore, bone wax acts as a physical barrier that inhibits osteoblasts from reaching the bone defect and thus impairs bone healing (Alberius et al 1987, Allison 1994, Vestergaard et al 2010). The use of bone wax is a major risk factor for the development of sternocutaneous fistulas (Steingrimsson et al 2009). Experimental studies have shown that when a bone defect is treated with bone wax, the number of bacteria needed to initiate an infection is reduced by a factor of 10,000 (Johnson and Fromm 1981, Nelson et al 1990, Gibbs et al 2004, Vestergaard et al 2010). Radiological bone healing assessed by a radiologist using computed tomography at 3 and 6 months postoperatively was significantly impaired in the bone wax group (Vestergaard et al 2014).

▸ **Alternatives to bone wax.** Given the drawbacks of conventional bone wax, we use a variety of commercially available local hemostatic products, including TachoSil (Takeda Austria) and SeraSeal (Wortham Laboratories). TachoSil is a sponge impregnated with a hemostatic agent based on equine collagen, human fibrinogen, and human thrombin. TachoSil has been used in cardiac surgery to seal graft anastomoses, bleeding from aortic sutures, bleeding from atrial sutures, etc. (Maisano et al 2009, Alizadeh Ghavidel et al 2014, Vida et al 2014). It is also suitable for immediate sealing of the sternum following sternotomy (**Fig. 6.1**).

Another way to minimize bleeding from the sternum is to use SeraSeal, which is a liquid hemostatic agent containing agar and activated factors II, VII, IX, and X. SeraSeal is sprayed directly onto the bony surface of the sternum, where it forms a clot. Once the clot has formed, the surface should not be touched (e.g., with swabs) for a few minutes, until its structure has stabilized.

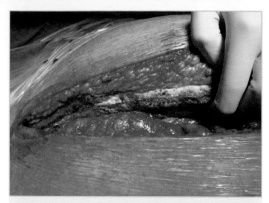

Fig. 6.1 Sealing the sternum with TachoSil.

Note

The traditional use of bone wax should be replaced by the use of modern local hemostatic products.

▶ **Crucial point: harvesting the vein.** The blood lost during vein harvesting for coronary artery bypass graft (CABG) surgery is taken up by the drapes and swabs and can normally not be retransfused (Markar et al 2010). A meticulous surgical technique is absolutely necessary to reduce this avoidable blood loss. We prefer the suturing of bleeding veins to the customary use of diathermy. The saphenous stumps are precisely ligated. Sternotomy and vein harvesting should be carried out as a collaborative effort. It is unfair to open the sternum as quickly as possible without allowing the assistant enough time to remove the leg vein. Enough time must be allowed especially under

difficult circumstances, e.g., varicose veins, anatomical variations, or obesity (**Fig. 6.2**).

Note

Sternotomy and vein harvesting should be carried out as a collaborative effort.

6.1.4 Cell Salvage, Cardiotomy Suction, Minimally Invasive Extracorporeal Circulation Technologies, Swabs

▶ **Cell salvage.** Extensive use of a cell salvage device is imperative in blood-sparing cardiac surgery (Vonk et al 2013). After all, it ensures that fully functional RBCs are retransfused. However, if the volume of salvaged blood is large, the coagulation potential can be reduced because of the loss of plasma coagulation factors (Rollins et al 2012).

▶ **Cardiotomy suction.** The action of the roller pumps and the aspiration process due to cardiotomy suction can cause hemolysis and leukocyte activation because of the mechanical destruction of RBCs and the exposure of blood to air (Osborn et al 1962, Lau et al 2007, El-Sabbagh et al 2013). Timely and meticulous surgical hemostasis is absolutely necessary to interrupt the vicious circle of continuous bleeding and continuous aspiration from the sternum and the cannulation sites. These drawbacks can be reduced by setting the flow rate on the cardiotomy suction device to "low" and avoiding "excessive suctioning" (Svitek et al 2010). Make sure that the assistant or the instrument nurse does not confuse the cell salvage

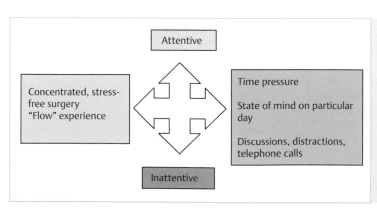

Fig. 6.2 Factors influencing the work of cardiac surgeons.

or cardiotomy suction device with the normal operating-room suction device (nonretransfusable). This could lead to the unintentional loss of large quantities of blood! Such mistakes are not uncommon when new members of the team are not thoroughly briefed at the start of the operation as regards the use of the three different suction systems. The best approach in our opinion is to use the handpiece of the operating-room (nonretransfusable) suction device only when required.

▶ **Minimally invasive extracorporeal circulation technology.** The use of minimally invasive extracorporeal circulation technology (MiECT) for CABG operations significantly reduces blood loss because of the centrifugal pumps (less hemolysis), smaller priming volumes, and autologous priming (less hemodilution), and decreases the risk of systemic inflammatory response syndrome thanks to the reduction of blood–polymer contact (Kofidis et al 2008, Anastasiadis et al 2013, Baikoussis et al 2014). The disadvantages resulting from MiECT as a closed system are the absence of a cardiotomy suction device and, in rare cases, restriction of the cardiopulmonary bypass (CPB) flow during heart luxation.

▶ **Swabs.** Frequent use of swabs results in extensive blood loss from the surgical area, especially if large numbers of blood-soaked swabs are discarded. We try to minimize the number of swabs used, an approach that has led to the "single-swab method." After its use, this single, blood-soaked swab is rinsed in saline, carefully squeezed out into a bowl by the instrumentation nurse, and reused by the surgeon. The recovered blood is later processed with the cell salvage device.

▶ **Disastrous bleeding.** We distinguish between expected bleeding (e.g., bleeding from the sternum or from cannulation sites) and disastrous bleeding (e.g., tearing of vital sutures and ligatures at the aortic and atrial cannulation sites as well as bleeding from major blood vessels) (Dyke et al 2014). Surgical redundancy is increased by repeat suturing of these vital sites because it minimizes the risk of failure of both sutures.

6.1.5 Postoperative Measures

Any increased bleeding tendency should be treated immediately at the end of the operation. Hypotensive circulatory situations can mask postoperative secondary bleeding and should be avoided. The body temperature should postoperatively be restored as soon as possible, and blood draws for laboratory diagnostic purposes should be limited to the absolute minimum. The use of point-of-care coagulation diagnostic tests has advantages over determination of the activated clotting time (Petricevic et al 2014). Their validity is on a par with that of conventional laboratory tests. However, they have only limited power to diagnose the underlying coagulation disorder (Pekelharing et al 2014, Welsh et al 2014). Nonetheless, point-of-care tests confer advantages such as rapid test results and therefore timely treatment intervention. Only weak evidence is available to support the repeated demand for a widespread use of fibrinogen—like all blood derivatives, this should only be administered when indicated (Warmuth et al 2012, Bilecen et al 2013, Wikkelso et al 2013, Lunde et al 2014). Conversely, the perioperative administration of tranexamic acid reduces blood loss, but—in rare cases—it is associated with the onset of generalized cramps (Dietrich et al 2008, Koster et al 2013).

If, despite all these measures, there is heavy postoperative bleeding, extensive rethoracotomy must be performed as soon as possible—definitely before the onset of coagulation disorders (Vivacqua et al 2011). Postoperative bleeding is not uncommon in cardiac surgery and is difficult to classify (Dyke et al 2014). Therefore, the indication for rethoracotomy must be tailored to the individual patient. Blood lost from the chest drains can be collected, for example, by the closed Drentech Emotrans system (Redax), and directly retransfused to the patient using a special connecting line to the cell salvage device. This does not only reduce the transfusion requirement, but it also helps to preserve the oxygen transport capacity, and ultimately improves the outcome (Axford et al 1994, Schmidt et al 1995, Dalrymple-Hay et al 1999).

> **Note**
>
> In case of postoperative bleeding, extensive rethoracotomy must be performed as soon as possible—definitely before the onset of coagulation disorders.

Based on the current data, the routine postoperative administration of iron and erythropoietin cannot be recommended and must be investigated in future studies (Madi-Jebara et al 2004).

6.1.6 Cardiac Operations in Jehovah's Witnesses

The religiously motivated refusal of blood transfusions by Jehovah's Witnesses constitutes an ethical challenge. However, surgical operations can be performed for Jehovah's Witnesses while utilizing all three pillars of PBM with comparable risk or even a better outcome (Gombotz et al 1985, Gombotz et al 1989, Stein et al 1991, Sparling et al 1996, Rosengart et al 1997, Gohel et al 2005, Stamou et al 2006, Casati et al 2007, Berend and Levi 2009, Emmert et al 2011).

Between 2008 and 2014, 46 operations—19 of which were cardiac surgery procedures—were carried out for Jehovah's Witness patients at the First Surgical Department for Cardiovascular and Thoracic Surgery at Linz General Hospital in Austria (**Table 6.1**). These operations were performed by two surgeons. No patient received a transfusion. Three patients would have accepted a transfusion if based on a vital indication, whereas the remainder categorically refused transfusions. Rethoracotomy was not needed in any of these patients and no patient died (**Table 6.2**).

As can be seen from **Fig. 6.3**, the hematocrit did not drop below 20% in any of the 19 patients.

Conclusion

The cardiac surgeon is confronted with the particular challenges associated with a perioperative multidisciplinary strategy, such as PBM, to improve outcome through the avoidance of surgical blood loss (second pillar of PBM). Of the various blood-sparing methods available, those acquired through many years of surgical experience have been presented here. Experience has shown that it is rarely an isolated measure but rather a combination of various measures that contributes to the desired outcome. Using this approach, we were able to successfully perform 19 cardiac surgery operations (between 2008 and 2014) for Jehovah's Witness patients without RBC transfusions. Clinical evidence shows that the use of appropriate blood conservation measures for patients who do not accept transfusions results in similar or better outcomes, compared with transfused patients (Pattakos et al 2012, Frank et al 2014b). We therefore believe that "every patient should be treated as a Jehovah's Witness."

Table 6.1 Cardiac procedures performed in 19 Jehovah's Witness patients at Linz General Hospital, Linz, Austria (2008–2014)

N	Type of procedure	Details
7	CABG	CABG ×4: n = 1; CABG ×3: n = 2; CABG ×2: n = 3; CABG ×1: n = 1 MiECT: n = 4
3	AVR	Mechanical valves Reoperation AVR: n=1
3	AVR + CABG	Biological valves CABG ×3: n = 1; CABG ×2: n = 2
1	AAR	
1	AAR + AVR	Biological valves
1	AAR + CABG (1x)	Biological valves
2	MV replacement	Mechanical valve: n = 1; biological valve: n = 1 SICTRA: n = 1
1	MV repair + TV repair	Annuloplasty + ring
19	Total	

Abbreviations: AAR, ascending aorta replacement; AVR, aortic valve replacement; CABG, coronary artery bypass graft; MiECT, minimally invasive extracorporeal circulation technology; MV, mitral valve; SICTRA, saline-irrigated cooled tip radiofrequency ablation; TV, tricuspid valve.

Table 6.2 Complications among 19 Jehovah's Witness patients who underwent cardiac surgery at Linz General Hospital, Linz, Austria (2008–2014)

Number of patients	Complication	Treatment
1	Paravalvular leak after AVR	Reoperation AVR (3 weeks postoperatively)
2	Postoperative third-degree AV block	Pacemaker implantation
2	Postoperative atrial fibrillation	Cardioversion

Abbreviations: AV, atrioventricular; AVR, aortic valve replacement.

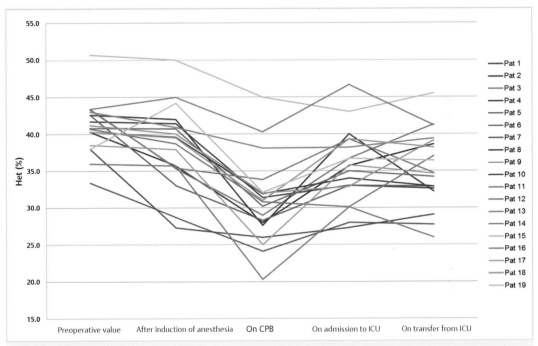

Fig. 6.3 Perioperative time course of the hematocrit in 19 Jehovah's Witness patients undergoing cardiac surgery at Linz General Hospital, Linz, Austria (2008–2014). CPB, cardiopulmonary bypass; Hct, hematocrit; ICU, intensive care unit; OR, operating room; Pat, patient.

6.2 PBM in Pediatric Cardiac Surgery

J. Meier, R. Mair

6.2.1 Introduction

Although many of the measures that are cornerstones of a modern PBM strategy in adults have to be modified to be applicable in children undergoing cardiac surgery, the underlying principles stay the same: optimization of the RBC mass, minimization of blood loss and bleeding, and utilization of the physiological tolerance to anemia. However, because of different time frames, measures especially focusing on the preoperative period are largely hampered. Many of the surgical procedures in pediatric cardiac surgery have to be performed in the first few days or weeks of life and, as a consequence, prolonged preparation of the patient is impossible. However, unnecessary transfusions can be avoided even in these patients if several arrangements are undertaken.

6.2.2 Risks of Anemia and Transfusion in Children with Congenital Heart Disease

In the last few years, it has been demonstrated convincingly in adult as well as in pediatric cardiac patients that anemia is associated with a higher risk of mortality (Kammache et al 2012). In both populations, anemia (not only extreme anemia but also moderate anemia) is an independent driver of undesirable outcomes (Musallam et al 2011). The most obvious solution for this problem seems to be transfusion, which is the only way to immediately increase the amount of RBCs. Although the application of blood products is safer than ever before, both transfusion-transmitted infections and noninfectious serious hazards of transfusion can occur, limiting the positive effects of the administration of allogeneic blood products. Taking recently published studies into account, it has to be stated that RBC transfusion does not only increase the morbidity but also the mortality because of a conflicting risk–benefit ratio (Pattakos et al 2012). Therefore, alternative approaches are also desirable in this patient group.

6.2.3 Optimization of the RBC Mass

In many cases, congenital heart disease has to be treated by surgery within the first days of life to reduce mortality (Donofrio et al 2014). This tight time frame reduces the options to optimize the RBC mass preoperatively. However, anemia is not rare in pediatric patients undergoing cardiac surgery. Depending on the population studied, a preoperative hemoglobin concentration as low as 11.8 g/dL is common in pediatric patients (Mulaj et al 2014). Unfortunately, preoperative anemia is also one of the most important drivers of intra- and postoperative RBC transfusion in these patients (Mulaj et al 2014). However, the measures that have been demonstrated to be effective in adults lack good evidence in this patient population.

> **Note**
>
> In children undergoing open heart surgery, preoperative anemia is one of the most important drivers for RBC transfusion and is associated with increased morbidity and mortality.

▶ **Iron supplementation and erythropoietin.** Furthermore, the Food and Drug Administration and the European Medicines Agency have placed severe restrictions on the use of many intravenous iron and erythropoietin preparations. This situation is not different to the use of other drugs in a pediatric patient population; however, only a limited number of studies exist that show the utility of these drugs in the environment of pediatric cardiac surgery. As a consequence, no general recommendation can be given to use these drugs in this situation.

However, the complete, general avoidance of iron and erythropoietin might exclude a potent strategy to adequately prepare pediatric patients. Anemia from iron deficiency is one of the most common alimentary deficits in children. Oral treatment with iron preparations may take months to correct the anemia. Modern intravenous iron preparations seem to be a safe alternative when a rapid reversal of iron deficiency anemia is necessary. The peak response following intravenous iron administration occurs in approximately 10 days. Modern iron preparations, such as ferrous gluconate and iron sucrose, are safer than the old ones, especially iron dextran, which may cause anaphylactic reactions in susceptible individuals. Low levels of iron and erythropoietin provide a rationale for the use of intravenous iron or erythropoietin in children. A recent randomized clinical trial (RCT) demonstrated that the combined treatment of high-dose erythropoietin (300 U/kg per day intravenously or 700 U/kg three times per week subcutaneously), iron (1.5 mg/kg per day intravenously or 9 mg/kg per day orally), folate (100 mg/kg per day orally), and vitamin E and B_{12} during the first weeks of life significantly reduced the transfusion need of infants with an extremely low birth weight (Haiden et al 2006).

To date, it is not known whether the short-term preparation of children with iron or erythropoietin in the cardiac surgery setting is effective in reducing the number of transfusions or in improving survival rates. Comparable studies in adults provide strong evidence that the application of iron or erythropoietin even some days before or after surgery might reduce the number of allogeneic RBC transfusions needed (Muñoz et al 2014b).

6.2.4 Minimization of Perioperative Blood Loss

Although most modern strategies to reduce perioperative blood loss have been developed in adult patients, some of the underlying ideas are also applicable to the pediatric patient population.

▶ **Cardiopulmonary bypass support.** Most patients who undergo surgery for congenital heart defects require CPB support. The CPB circuit is usually primed with a mixture of fluids to prevent abrupt intravascular volume depletion caused by the elongation of the circulatory pathway. In addition, it is often necessary to mix RBC components with the priming fluid to prevent excessive hemodilution. In adult cardiac surgery, a relatively small-volume RBC transfusion will suffice to maintain adequate levels of hematocrit during CPB. However, in neonates and infants, the volume of the total priming fluid may represent 200% to 300% of their total blood volume. Consequently, the RBC volume that is initially mixed with the priming fluid frequently exceeds 50% of the total blood volume. However, it is possible to reduce the priming volume considerably by so-called *mini-volume priming* methods. Among other things, oxygenators and hemofilters with small priming volumes, vertically aligned pump heads, vacuum-driven venous drainage, and small venous-circuit-tubing diameters might help to reduce the amount of allogeneic blood necessary to prepare the CPB circuit (Chang et al 2014b). In many centers, priming of the CPB circuit is additionally performed with fresh frozen plasma (FFP). However, the prophylactic use of FFP in the priming solution does not have obvious clinical benefits in pediatric patients undergoing cardiac surgery (Miao et al 2015).

> **Note**
>
> Minimizing the priming volume is one of the key measures in pediatric cardiac surgery.

▶ **Coagulation management.** As in adult cardiac surgery, intraoperative blood loss in pediatric surgery does not only depend on the surgical technique but also on the sophisticated management of coagulation. Timely correction of the coagulation potency during surgery is effective in avoiding unnecessary perioperative bleeding, and it is known for adult cardiac surgery that special emphasis on the perioperative management of coag-

ulation can reduce the number of necessary RBC transfusions. However, there is considerable variation in transfusion practice with respect to the threshold for FFP transfusion (Karam et al 2014), and it has to be stated that FFP transfusions are often prescribed for nonbleeding critically ill children.

▶ **Iatrogenic anemia.** Despite the fact that laboratory blood tests are essential for the monitoring and management of infants and children after heart surgery, excessive blood tests can lead to iatrogenic anemia and subsequent RBC transfusion. This is especially true in pediatric cardiac surgery patients, where the circulating blood volume is small and blood sampling is convenient because of indwelling catheters in most postoperative patients. Therefore, one very effective measure to reduce perioperative blood loss is to restrict postoperative laboratory tests as much as possible. Such an approach can effectively reduce the postoperative occurrence of anemia and thereby the transfusion of RBCs (Delgado-Corcoran et al 2014).

6.2.5 Utilization of the Physiological Tolerance to Anemia

It has been demonstrated convincingly in the last few years that survival does not depend on the physiological hemoglobin concentration. Depending on the individual situation, even very low hemoglobin concentrations can be endured. However, the situation is much more complex in patients with congenital heart disease. Two main reasons might be responsible for this situation. (1) Depending on the underlying pathophysiology (e.g., single ventricle, pulmonary volume overload), the ability of the patient to increase the cardiac output might be severely restricted. Since an increase of the cardiac output is one of the main compensatory mechanisms in acute anemia, it is very difficult to anticipate whether this restriction will critically limit the tolerance to anemia (see Chapters 5.1 and 5.4). (2) In some cardiac defects, general hypoxia is induced by significant right-to-left shunting. Only very little is known about the tolerance to anemia during hypoxia, and to date no trial exists that describes the tolerance to anemia in hypoxic pediatric patients. As a consequence, in daily clinical practice, cardiac patients receive more RBC transfusions than other critically ill children (Bateman et al 2008), despite the fact that it has been demonstrated convincingly in children with cardiac defects that the transfusion of RBCs is associated with a high morbidity and mortality (Karimi et al 2013, Iyengar et al 2013).

▶ **Necrotizing enterocolitis.** Besides the well-known hazards of RBC transfusion in children with hypoplastic left heart syndrome, necrotizing enterocolitis (NEC) might be of special interest. Although it is seen most frequently in infants with a very low birth weight, NEC is not unique to this population. Reports show that NEC occurs 10–100 times more frequently in the congenital heart disease population than in term infants without congenital heart disease. Depending on the severity of the lesion, the incidence of NEC may approach that seen among infants with a very low birth weight. In the case of hypoplastic left heart syndrome, the incidence is often considerably higher. Some investigations have indicated that the duration of RBC storage may increase the risk of NEC (Baxi et al 2014), and RBC transfusion therefore has the potential to induce catastrophic courses of pediatric cardiac surgery.

However, a restrictive RBC transfusion policy (hemoglobin threshold of 8.0 g/dL) during the entire perioperative period is safe, leads to a shorter hospital stay, and is less expensive, at least in patients with an acyanotic congenital heart defect undergoing elective cardiac surgery (de Gast-Bakker et al 2013). It can therefore be speculated that the compensatory ability of these patients is sufficient to tolerate moderate degrees of anemia.

Conclusion

In the pediatric population, the development of RBC storage lesions, and therefore the age of the RBCs (>21 days) used for transfusion, seems to influence the perioperative outcome (Gauvin et al 2010, Redlin et al 2014). Therefore, it seems advantageous to exclusively use fresh blood, especially in this population; however, nowadays this is not always possible.

An unresolved problem in pediatric cardiac surgery is the question of whether cyanotic cardiac defects can be treated in the same way as acyanotic cardiac defects. However, to date no clinical study exits that can answer this question. Therefore, a hemoglobin concentration of at least 10 g/dL is often targeted in this situation. This approach seems reasonable from a clinical point of view, but future studies will have to show whether this approach should be adapted.

6.3 PBM in Trauma Surgery

J. M. Hamdorf

6.3.1 Introduction

Trauma remains a common cause of death across all ages. Hemorrhage is responsible for up to half of all trauma deaths. Rapid hemorrhage control and the prevention and correction of trauma-related coagulopathy result in reductions in the mortality and morbidity. Although attention to the first-pillar activities of PBM is impossible for the trauma team, important elements of the second and third pillars certainly are. Measures to minimize blood loss and hemorrhage (second pillar) and efforts to harness and optimize physiological reserves (third pillar) may well be attended to.

▶ **Coagulopathy.** Trauma patients are at particular risk for the development of a coagulopathy (Gruen et al 2012, Davenport 2013), because of the combined effects of tissue injury and organ hypoperfusion. Activation of protein C is the initial driver for this development, which is exacerbated by hypothermia, acidosis, and hemodilution (Brohi et al 2007, Brohi et al 2008).

▶ **Hemodynamic shock: Classes I–IV.** One of the overriding principles of the traditional trauma care response is the prompt recognition and management of hemodynamic shock. The identification of the stage of shock and the class of hemorrhage then guides the treatment approach (Gombotz and Knotzer 2013).

Class I hemorrhagic shock is defined as loss of up to 15% of the circulating blood volume (roughly up to 750 mL in adults). The administration of intravenous crystalloids allows the restoration and maintenance of organ perfusion.

Class II hemorrhage is defined as loss of 15% to 30% of the circulating blood volume (between 750 and 1500 mL). Crystalloid fluid administration—generally 2,000 mL—is recommended; this will suffice to restore adequate organ perfusion in the majority of trauma patients; however, a proportion will not respond sufficiently or sustainably. Traditionally, RBC transfusion is then recommended.

Trauma patients with Class III hemorrhage, having lost 30–40% of the circulating blood volume, are confused and anxious, display tachycardia and tachypnea, may be hypotensive but will generally have a reduced pulse pressure, and will have a reduced urine output. Crystalloid fluid administration is initially recommended and instituted (2,000 mL in the first instance), but RBC transfusion is almost always considered necessary, too.

Class IV intravenous hemorrhage results from the loss of more than 40% of the circulating blood volume. This is considered to be a preterminal state featuring confusion and lethargy, marked tachycardia and tachypnea, hypotension, and a negligible urine output. In the resuscitation response, crystalloid fluid administration is rapidly followed by RBC transfusion (Mylankal and Wyatt 2013).

6.3.2 Potential Barriers to the Adoption of PBM Principles on the Trauma Ward

Without question, the team response to the severely injured is a most stressful and time-critical situation. The trauma management protocols employed are intended to be reliable, thorough, and suitable to be implemented successfully by a broad variety of trauma services. The modification of protocol-driven responses in the emergency and time-critical setting, which have global recognition and support, is challenging. Yet, clinicians have an obligation to consider the potential application of the principles of PBM. In particular, massive transfusion is accompanied by considerable morbidity and mortality, a substantial component of which may well be ascribed to transfusion. Efforts to reduce the reliance on blood products should be considered.

Given that trauma care is so heavily reliant on documented protocols, one might conjecture that the introduction of measures of proven therapeutic benefit would be entirely feasible employing a variety of modalities.

6.3.3 Early Administration of Tranexamic Acid

Tranexamic acid is a lysine derivative that, on intravenous administration, inhibits plasmin action. The use of tranexamic acid has enabled a significant blood-sparing benefit in elective surgery (Theusinger et al 2014a).

The rather extraordinary CRASH-2 study tested the use of tranexamic acid in trauma in an RCT of adult trauma patients presenting to more than 250 emergency departments in 40 countries, accruing over 10,000 patients in each of the treatment and control arms. The use of tranexamic acid resulted in a significant reduction in both all-cause mortality and risk of death from blood loss. Interestingly, the somewhat anticipated severe thrombotic side effects, particularly myocardial infarction and vascular occlusive events, were fewer in the treatment arm (Shakur et al 2010).

While the CRASH-2 study protocol employed a dose of 1 g intravenously over 10 minutes and then a further dose of 1 g over 8 hours, a subsequent systematic review suggested that a total dose of 1 g was probably adequate (Perel et al 2013). Hospital administration has been found to be both feasible and safe, and early administration (within 1 hour of presentation) is optimal. An estimate based on WHO data indicates that worldwide around 400,000 trauma patients die in hospital each year as a result of bleeding. Of these deaths, some 128,000 might be averted by the administration of tranexamic acid within 1 hour of injury; for administration within 3 hours, the corresponding number is 112,000 (Ker et al 2012b).

6.3.4 Modified Massive Transfusion Protocol

Massive transfusion is variably defined as the transfusion of more than 10 units of RBCs within 24 hours, replacement of the entire blood volume within 24 hours, or replacement of 50% of the blood volume within 3 hours. Perhaps 5% of trauma patients will fall into this category. The administration of massive transfusions has been associated with a high mortality rate of up to 70%. Massive hemorrhage results in acidosis, hypothermia, and coagulopathy. Transfusion-related coagulopathy in trauma may be particularly difficult to correct—attempts to prevent this should be promoted (Rossaint et al 2010).

> **Note**
> Approximately 5% of all trauma patients have massive bleeding.

The term *massive transfusion protocol* (MTP) refers to the management of a critical blood loss situation. Recently, consideration has been offered to replacing this terminology with one that is more focused on the problem, rather than on the solution (NBA 2011). Accordingly, the term *critical bleeding protocol* may well find its way into the critical care and trauma lexicon as a more appropriate description for a state in evolution.

Improved survival in patients whose life-threatening injuries result in the need to administer massive transfusions has been accomplished through damage control techniques, appreciation and correction of coagulopathy, patient rewarming, and improved overall resuscitation techniques.

MTPs are activated in situations where extraordinary transfusion requirements are anticipated. Although MTPs will vary from one site to the next, the key elements include: activation of the MTP by a designated senior clinician, agreed trigger for activation, communication to the relevant blood bank team, and the delivery of the MTP pack (combination of RBCs, FFP, and platelets) to the bedside.

The establishment of MTPs has resulted in a substantial reduction in mortality with various military and civilian centers documenting improvements of up to 50%.

> **Note**
>
> The implementation of MTPs has resulted in a substantial reduction in mortality.

The revision of MTPs has been the subject of some scrutiny especially in respect of the recommended proportions of the various components, the RBC:FFP:platelets ratio. Although various ratios have been proposed, the favored trauma protocol currently appears to be advocating a 1:1:1 target ratio over 6 hours. It needs to be noted that 1 unit of platelets provides the equivalent of 4 units of RBCs (Riskin et al 2009).

The administration of recombinant activated factor VII (rVIIa) may result in a reduction in the reliance on blood products. Multicenter RCTs have shown a promising reduction in transfusion requirements following rVIIa administration in blunt trauma (Boffard et al 2005, Lu et al 2014). However, a Cochrane review has concluded that its use in major trauma remains unproven and should be limited to clinical trials (Simpson et al 2012).

6.3.5 Point-of-care Testing

The early recognition and correction of coagulopathy will reduce blood loss, use of blood products,

and trauma patient morbidity and mortality. Thromboelastography and thromboelastometry measure the viscoelasticity of the developing and resolving clot, and the graphical display guides the administration of various products including FFP, cryoprecipitate, platelets, desmopressin, and tranexamic acid.

Point-of-care testing can provide meaningful results within 5 to 10 minutes versus the 30 minutes needed for standard laboratory results. The use of point-of-care testing is increasingly recommended and will attract further scrutiny (Theusinger et al 2014a).

6.3.6 Tolerance to Acute Anemia—Triggers for Transfusion in Trauma

Hemodynamic instability is the generally accepted trigger for resuscitation and blood product transfusion in trauma patients. Trauma guidelines will usually endorse a target hemoglobin value of 7 to 9 g/dL.

> **Note**
>
> The transfusion trigger should primarily be used as a discussion point and not as a strict indication for the transfusion of RBCs.

Of note, one group (Villanueva et al 2013a) randomized patients presenting with upper gastrointestinal hemorrhage to 7 g/dL versus 9 g/dL as a transfusion trigger. The group found significantly improved outcomes in the restrictive-strategy group compared with the liberal-strategy cohort. Notably, the protocol excluded massive exsanguinating bleeding, and also patients with occlusive vascular disease, recent transfusion, trauma, or surgery.

Although the ability of patients undergoing major elective surgery to tolerate very low hemoglobin levels has been well documented (Shander et al 2014c), this is an area that has not been tested in the trauma domain and, although feasible, large-scale RCTs may be challenging to initiate.

6.3.7 Permissive Hypotension

Vigorous resuscitative maneuvers in an attempt to restore a "normal" blood pressure in hemorrhaging trauma patients carries the risk of promoting further bleeding by raising the intravascular pressure, reducing the blood viscosity, and potentially allowing hemostatic clots to dislodge. The restriction of fluid resuscitation until satisfactory hemostasis has been achieved is referred to as *permissive hypotension*.

Such practice is not without risk because a systolic pressure of 70 to 90 mmHg is the target and there exists the potential for the compromised perfusion of vital organs. Where brain injury is present or suspected, allowing diminished cerebral perfusion can contribute to significant secondary injury (Mylankal and Wyatt 2013).

6.3.8 Damage Control Surgery

The principal aim of damage control surgery (DCS) is to limit the physiological stress imposed by surgery while controlling hemorrhage and contamination. For example, while the definitive management of a ruptured small bowel will include the formal resection of traumatized margins of the bowel and safe anastomosis with attention to the mesentery and its potential defects, in the DCS situation the traumatized ends may be sealed expeditiously to limit contamination using a surgical stapling device. Major abdominal hemorrhage may often be controlled by four-quadrant packing, and the use of perihepatic packing for major hepatic trauma is well documented. DCS will often enable a more rapid return of the patient to the intensive care unit for secondary resuscitation, with the definitive maneuvers being undertaken in a staged return to the operating room within 24 to 48 hours after various physiological deficits have been corrected (Finlay et al 2004, Lee and Peitzman 2006).

Note

DCS to stop bleeding and blood loss is key for the successful treatment of trauma patients.

Trauma patients who are likely to benefit from a DCS approach may be identified prior to the emergent surgery and include those involved in high-energy trauma; patients with multiple system involvement, especially abdominal and extra-abdominal involvement; and patients who are hypotensive, hypothermic, and/or coagulopathic on presentation. Perhaps special mention might be made of the growing number of patients receiving anticoagulants such as clopidogrel, dabigatran, apixaban, and rivaroxaban, whose reversal may be problematic and in whom DCS may play an increasing role in major trauma.

6.3.9 Topical Hemostatic Agents

A variety of topical agents are available for use in elective surgery and these are also increasingly considered in the emergency trauma setting. Ideally, a topical agent acts rapidly, is inert, is easily applied and able to be removed, and has few side effects. Factor concentrates and local hemostatics are effective in the management of arterial and venous bleeding. Fibrin sealants reduce blood loss and the need for RBC transfusion (Carless et al 2003). Surgical pads delivering procoagulant factors have shown substantial promise in elective surgery but their role in trauma surgery is yet to be demonstrated (Gruen et al 2012).

6.3.10 Fibrinogen Concentrate

Fibrinogen concentrate may have a role in helping to avoid the depletion of fibrinogen associated with trauma and has several advantages over other sources of fibrinogen (FFP and cryoprecipitate) in that it can be administered before hospital admission, may be administered as a relatively small volume, is not associated with transfusion-related acute lung injury or ABO incompatibility issues, and has a long shelf life (Aubron et al 2014). There may well be a role for fibrinogen concentrate in trauma resuscitation in the future.

6.3.11 Other Maneuvers

In situations where the surgeon is confronted by a large raw surface, for example following splenectomy or partial hepatectomy, the use of conventional suture ligation and electrosurgery (coagulation) to control surface ooze may not be effective. Modern energy sources such as laser (argon, carbon dioxide) or spray electrosurgery may provide useful adjuncts to other surgical techniques (Hohmuth et al 2014).

6.3.12 Endovascular Adjuncts

Temporary control of major vascular injuries may be provided by the introduction of proximally advanced balloon catheters via vascular cutdown. Radiological arterial embolization can be considered as an adjunct to surgery in certain situations in the trauma setting. In patients with isolated pelvic trauma, the radiological embolization of bleeding vessels (either of the internal iliac artery or more selectively) will often be effective in providing hemostasis. However, it is often the venous bleeding and fracture surface bleeding that is problematic, so radioembolization may play a secondary role to packing to effect pelvic tamponade and fracture fixation.

> **Note**
>
> Radiological arterial embolization can be considered as an adjunct to surgery in certain trauma situations.

Selective hepatic artery embolization may be effective in liver trauma, both primarily in the stable patient and as an adjunct in major trauma following perihepatic packing with incomplete hemorrhage control (Lee and Peitzman 2006, Gruen et al 2012).

6.3.13 Cell Salvage in Trauma Surgery

Experience with the use of cell salvage technology in the trauma setting, although promising, is limited. A small single-center RCT (Bowley et al 2006) reported a reduction in allogeneic RBC transfusion in patients with penetrating torso trauma undergoing laparotomy without impacting on the rates of mortality or sepsis. There are case reports and some considerable conjecture pertaining to the role of cell salvage in isolated massive hemothorax where local blood product supplies are threatened. Arguably, there is also an opportunity to limit transfusion in certain pelvic fractures (e.g., acetabular fracture) where blood loss may be considerable and surgical corrective procedures lengthy.

6.3.14 Additional Measures

Optimization of erythropoiesis should be considered in the recovering trauma patient, embracing the principles of the first pillar of PBM. There may well be an opportunity to optimize erythropoiesis in trauma patients with the use of intravenous iron. The Intravenous Iron or Placebo for Anaemia in Intensive Care (IRONMAN) RCT is examining the administration of intravenous ferric carboxymal-

tose in patients admitted to critical care units with a hemoglobin value of < 10 g/dL (Litton et al 2014); patient recruitment has been completed but the results are not yet available (A. Hofmann, personal communication, June 2015).

Desmopressin enhances platelet function, promoting adherence, and is used in patients with von Willebrand disease. It may have a role in patients receiving aspirin or clopidogrel, and the European trauma guidelines suggest that a single dose of desmopressin may be beneficial (Spahn et al 2013a). Otherwise, platelet transfusion may well be necessary in such patients.

Oral anticoagulants inhibiting thrombin (dabigatran) or activated factor X (apixaban, rivaroxaban) will increasingly present and trauma patient management is challenging because of the persistence of effective plasma levels. Hemodialysis may well need to be considered in patients requiring the elimination of such drugs (Meybohm et al 2013). The relatively high volume of distribution of these agents may demand repeated applications of hemodialysis.

> **Conclusion**
>
> Trauma patients are at risk of hemorrhage-related morbidity. Hemorrhage is responsible for up to half of all trauma deaths. Rapid control of hemorrhage and the prevention and correction of trauma-related coagulopathy result in reductions in both mortality and morbidity. Traumatic injury with organ hypoperfusion places patients at risk of coagulopathy. Traditional trauma management protocols hold that RBC transfusion is offered without delay in patients whose blood loss estimate exceeds 30% of the circulating blood volume. Accordingly, a time-critical trauma setting will challenge the introduction of PBM principles, whose success has for the most part been demonstrated in elective settings. Yet, the adoption of practical management strategies such as early administration of tranexamic acid and use of massive transfusion (or critical bleeding) protocols have been shown to reduce morbidity and mortality in the trauma domain. Surgical maneuvers such as permissive hypotension and DCS with various energy sources, topical hemostatic agents, endovascular agents, and the like are finding increasing application in the trauma surgeon's armamentarium.

6.4 PBM in Gynecology

J. J. Lee

6.4.1 Introduction

To date, no data are available in the literature that show the exact total number of gynecologic operations worldwide. **Table 6.3** provides hysterectomy numbers for representative countries.

6.4.2 First Pillar: Detection, Diagnosis, and Treatment of Anemia

▶ **Preoperative evaluation.** As with other surgical disciplines, during the preoperative health and risk assessment in gynecology it is essential to take a thorough medical and menstrual history and to perform a physical examination in order to identify any coexisting illness that might be a cause of anemia. If the hemoglobin level is lower than normal, additional laboratory tests such as serum transferrin saturation, ferritin, total iron-binding capacity, peripheral blood morphology, folic acid, vitamin B_{12}, and C-reactive protein should be conducted for the differential diagnosis of iron deficiency anemia. A proposed algorithm for the preoperative detection and treatment of preexisting anemia is provided in **Fig. 6.4**.

> **Note**
>
> Reversible anemia is generally a contraindication for elective surgery.

The most common cause of iron deficiency anemia in gynecology is acute or chronic uterine bleeding. In premenopausal women, the cause of iron deficiency anemia is often presumed to be hypermenorrhea, menorrhagia, increased menstrual blood loss due to uterine fibroids, or adenomyosis. Ultrasound is frequently used for the evaluation of a potential pathological condition underlying iron deficiency anemia.

In addition, careful management of anticoagulation is required. Agents that can adversely affect clotting (e.g., aspirin, nonsteroidal anti-inflammatory drugs, antiplatelet agents, or anticoagulants) must be discontinued throughout the perioperative period.

▶ **Oral iron therapy.** Oral iron has proved effective in the treatment of mild iron deficiency anemia (hemoglobin > 10 g/dL) and should always be considered as an initial treatment approach. The most common adverse effects of oral iron therapy are gastrointestinal side effects. One of the main indications for parenteral iron therapy is a poor tolerance of oral iron. Intravenous iron is an effective treatment for preoperative anemia because it is associated with the rapid recovery of hemoglobin levels. According to Muñoz et al (2014a), 3 to 4 weeks of intravenous iron therapy are necessary prior to a scheduled operation to adequately restore iron levels. In selected patients with anemia who are undergoing gynecologic oncology surgery after chemotherapy, preoperative intravenous iron therapy seems to be safe and effective in substantially reducing the need for transfusion (Dangsuwan and Manchana 2010, Athibovonsuk et al 2013).

Table 6.3 Approximate number of hysterectomies per year in various countries

Country	Number of hysterectomies	Source
Germany	153,000	Stang et al 2011
Sweden	9,000	Consultant et al 2000
United Kingdom	23,000[a]	Lundholm et al 2009
United States	600,000	Whiteman et al 2008
South Korea	50,000	Department of Health and Welfare, Republic of South Korea

[a] Hysterectomies for the treatment of menorrhagia only

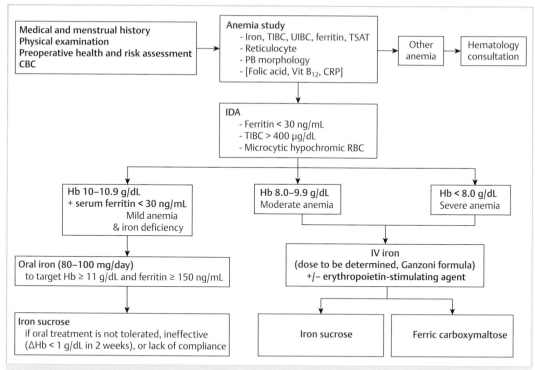

Fig. 6.4 Patient-specific management plan using appropriate blood conservation modalities to minimize blood loss, optimize RBC mass, and manage anemia. ΔHb, change in hemoglobin; CBC, complete blood count; CRP, C-reactive protein; Hb, hemoglobin; IDA, iron deficiency anemia; IV, intravenous; PB, peripheral blood; RBC, red blood cell; TIBC, total iron-binding capacity; TSAT, transferrin saturation; UIBC, unsaturated iron-binding capacity; Vit B₁₂, vitamin B₁₂.

▶ **Erythropoietin-stimulating agents.** The use of erythropoietin-stimulating agents (ESAs) to stimulate the production of RBCs has not yet received universal clinical acceptance. Iron therapy alone seems to be as effective in correcting preoperative anemia as a regimen of iron with ESAs (Krafft and Breymann 2011). Treatment with vitamin B₁₂ and/or folic acid also has a positive effect on erythropoiesis (Burns et al 1995). The use of ESAs should be closely monitored and adjusted to ensure that the potential benefits outweigh the risks. In patients of reproductive age without hematopoietic dysfunction (e.g., patients without chronic inflammation), ESAs are not recommended because the risk of side effects exceeds any potential benefit.

6.4.3 Second Pillar: Minimization of Blood Loss

▶ **Preventive measures.** In some cases, prophylactic interventional radiology and embolization are essential for preoperative assessment and planning (see also **Fig. 6.5**) (Laios et al 2014, Kröncke and David 2015). During surgery, a cell salvage machine can be used to collect, filter, and wash blood that has been removed by suction; the processed RBCs can then be reinfused. However, there are scant opportunities for using cell salvage in gynecologic surgery because the average blood loss volume is mostly less than 1,500 mL.

▶ **Less invasive surgery.** The development of less invasive approaches such as laparoscopic and vaginal procedures for gynecologic surgery may contribute to a reduction in the need for RBC transfusion (Ottosen et al 2000). The average blood loss volume during abdominal hysterectomy is approximately 500–700 mL (Rock and Meeks 2001); vaginal hysterectomy and laparoscopic approaches are associated with smaller blood loss volumes (Wood et al 1997).

▶ **Robotic surgery.** Robotic surgery is currently the most innovative minimally invasive approach in the field of gynecology, and is employed with increasing frequency. The da Vinci Surgical System (Intuitive Surgical) offers a number of advantages, including a lower blood loss volume compared with conventional laparoscopy (El Hachem et al 2015, Sinha et al 2015).

▶ **Advanced energy-based devices.** Further technological advances that help to minimize blood loss include the development of energy-based devices. Many forms of energy are used, including electrocautery, electrothermal bipolar energy, high-frequency ultrasonic energy, argon-beam energy, and radiofrequency energy. The Harmonic Scalpel (Ethicon) uses ultrasonic energy to simultaneously dissect and seal vessels using a rapidly vibrating tip. This instrument acts at a lower temperature (80 °C) than electrocautery devices, resulting in less thermal damage to the surrounding tissues and less smoke (Spitzer et al 2008).

The Thunderbeat (Olympus) platform delivers two different types of energy—ultrasonic and advanced bipolar energy—in a single multifunctional instrument. This platform allows the surgeon to simultaneously seal and cut vessels of up to and including 7 mm in size with minimal thermal spread. Moreover, it provides a faster dissection speed and more acceptable thermal spread than other commercially available devices (Milsom et al 2012, Fagotti et al 2014).

Note

The development of less invasive approaches contributes to the minimization of blood loss and hence to a reduction in RBC transfusions.

▶ **Normovolemic and hypervolemic hemodilution.** See Chapters 4.3.3 and 4.3.4.

▶ **Gauze pressure.** Pressure with gauze has historically been the primary way to control hemorrhage. Gauze pressure is not only used in laparotomy—it is also the main method of local hemostasis used in minimally invasive surgery.

▶ **Local hemostatic agents.** See also Chapters 4.4 and 6.1.3.

Since 1945, gelatin derived from porcine skin has been used as a topical hemostatic agent in many operations. The most recently developed gelatin preparations are available in powder form or as pliable film material (Nandi et al 2012, Watrowski 2014, Wysham et al 2014).

Collagen hemostatic agents are available from various manufacturers. Collagen is extracted from bovine material. Platelets accumulate around the helical collagen molecules, leading to platelet activation and, finally, stimulation of the clotting cascade. Collagen is absorbed within 3 months. Recent collagen preparations include FloSeal Matrix (Baxter) and SurgiFlo Hemostatic Matrix (Johnson & Johnson) (Nandi et al 2012, Watrowski 2014).

Absorbable hemostats (Surgicel; Johnson & Johnson) are preparations containing oxidized regenerated cellulose at a low pH in the form of knitted fibrous mesh. Diverse mechanisms are thought to promote hemostasis. These products are also available in a microfibrillar form (Surgicel Fibrillar; Johnson & Johnson).

Fibrin sealant products all share the common feature of combining fibrinogen and thrombin (Carless et al 2003). Tisseel (Baxter) is the first commercial fibrin sealant approved by the Food and Drug Administration and is used in hemostasis, tissue sealing, and suture support (Kim et al 2012a, Kim et al 2015b, Kaidarova et al 2015).

Note

The use of local hemostatics optimizes hemostasis and reduces intra- and perioperative blood loss.

▶ **Physiological monitoring.** Careful attention to vital signs and frequent measurement of hemoglobin/hematocrit, serum lactate, and base deficit to monitor tissue perfusion and tissue oxygenation are important to prevent and treat perioperative blood loss. The respiratory function should be optimized, and the intravascular volume and the cardiac function should be monitored in critical cases.

The body temperature should be continuously monitored to prevent coagulopathy induced by hypothermia (body temperature < 35 °C). Warming systems such as Bair Hugger (Arizant) and Buddy (Belmont Instrument Corporation) may be used for this purpose (Bräuer et al 2007).

▶ **Pharmacological measures.** Intraoperative pharmacological measures to prevent blood loss include the temporary use of vasoconstrictors. Lysine analogues (tranexamic acid and ε-aminocaproic acid) also reduce intraoperative bleeding and the frequency of RBC transfusion.

6.4.4 Third Pillar: Harnessing and Optimization of the Physiological Tolerance to Anemia

Understanding an individual patient's tolerance to anemia is an important part of determining the need for RBC transfusion. When making a decision about transfusion, the patient's individual ability to endure, and recover from, a severe decrease in the hemoglobin concentration must be considered. A "general" hemoglobin threshold that can be used as a reliable transfusion trigger does not exist.

Note

A "general" hemoglobin threshold that can be used as a reliable transfusion trigger does not exist in gynecology.

The signs and symptoms of inadequate tissue oxygenation can be considered as relevant transfusion triggers; they can occur at diverse hemoglobin concentrations depending on the patient's underlying conditions and include relative hypotension, new ST-segment change, new wall motion abnormality, and decreased central venous oxygen saturation (Madjdpour and Spahn 2005). These physiological transfusion triggers are gradually replacing hemoglobin-based transfusion triggers (Ferraris et al 2011, Carson et al 2012b).

There is no RCT to determine whether restrictive and liberal RBC transfusion strategies produce equivalent results in the field of gynecology.

Frequent blood sampling may contribute to anemia. Therefore, it is critically important to prevent blood loss related to phlebotomy for diagnostic laboratory tests in patients with severe anemia.

6.4.5 Evidence Base for Transfusion Thresholds

Despite advances in medical knowledge, there is no clear evidence for an optimal trigger for allogeneic RBC transfusion. The extent of a hemoglobin decrease that can be safely tolerated is highly debated. The decision to administer an RBC transfusion should be based on clinical and hematologic evidence. A transfusion is rarely indicated in stable patients with a hemoglobin value of more than 10 g/dL, and it is almost always indicated when the hemoglobin concentration is less than 6 g/dL (Murphy et al 2001, Carson et al 2012b).

The factors that determine the decision to transfuse should include individual patient characteristics and the patient's symptoms, rather than simply the hemoglobin level. Clinical judgment is an important component of the decision-making process.

▶ **Transfusion thresholds in obstetrics.** Up to one-quarter of all pregnancies are complicated by unpredictable uterine bleeding complications, especially after delivery. At term, the uteroplacental circulation receives an estimated 700 mL of blood per minute. It is therefore not surprising that uncontrollable postpartum bleeding can result in life-threatening hemorrhage. Despite medical advances, postpartum hemorrhage is still a leading cause of maternal mortality and morbidity worldwide. Therefore, the implementation of a multidisciplinary PBM concept for the early detection and treatment of substantial bleeding is essential. For a discussion of PBM in obstetrics and maternity, see also Module 5 of the Australian PBM guidelines (NBA 2015).

Several studies in the field of obstetrics have been published that have used a specific hemoglobin concentration as the transfusion threshold. So-Osman et al (2010) used a hemoglobin value of 6.4 g/dL in postpartum patients with limited blood loss, and a hemoglobin value of 8.1 g/dL in postpartum patients with massive blood loss. In a study by Butwick and colleagues (2009), a hemoglobin value of 7.6 g/dL was used as the transfusion threshold in patients with obstetric hemorrhage or postpartum anemia.

Conclusion

Gynecology patients who have no underlying conditions can overcome severe perioperative anemia relatively easily. The necessity of RBC transfusion should be determined after an individualized assessment. A reduction of the need for transfusion is not only favorable in terms of the patient's welfare, but it is also beneficial in terms of cost-effectiveness (Prick et al 2014). Whether a restrictive RBC transfusion strategy is safe in the setting of obstetrics and gynecology is currently uncertain. An RCT would provide the appropriate level of evidence with regard to the critical timing and the amount of transfusion.

6.5 PBM in Orthopaedic Surgery

A. Kotze

6.5.1 Introduction

Orthopaedic surgery makes substantial demands on blood donors and blood transfusion systems. In the United Kingdom, elective hip and knee replacement surgery consistently accounts for 8% to 10% of all RBC administrations (Wells et al 2002, Boralessa et al 2009). Moreover, the number of major elective orthopaedic procedures performed per annum is increasing across Europe (Pedersen et al 2009, SAP 2009) and North America (Belatti and Phisitkul 2013). Audits in the United Kingdom (Boralessa et al 2009) and across Europe (Rosencher et al 2003, Gombotz et al 2007) show that transfusion practice for similar procedures varies greatly between institutions. Unwarranted variation is often seen as an indication that practice may be improved (Brunskill et al 2015).

Preoperative anemia, postoperative anemia, and allogeneic transfusion are all strongly associated with the occurrence of complications and with poorer functional recovery after elective and emergency orthopaedic surgery (Lawrence et al 2003, Spahn 2010). Although evidence from RCTs shows that the reliance on allogeneic transfusion is reduced by the implementation of PBM (Wong et al 2007), evidence for an improvement in patient outcomes with PBM is largely observational (Kotze et al 2012). There are, however, strong public health reasons why a reduced reliance on transfusion is in itself a good thing, even if there were no patient benefits. The blood supply is by definition a finite and vulnerable resource, and the implementation of PBM in high-volume fields such as orthopaedic surgery potentially conserves this resource for patients who truly have no viable alternative to allogeneic blood, for example those with exsanguination and marrow failure.

There is also a good economic argument for PBM in orthopaedic surgery. These are high-volume operations that place a significant and increasing economic burden on society, whether via taxation, insurance, or direct funding. PBM programs in the United Kingdom (Kotze et al 2012) and Europe (Spahn et al 2012, Theusinger et al 2014b) have shown financial benefits related to reduced spending on RBCs, reduced nursing

time related to administration, shorter hospital stay, and fewer complications.

The three pillars of PBM have been well described and this author does not propose to deal exhaustively with each pillar in turn. The reader is instead referred to the other chapters in this book and to the growing literature on the topic. Instead, the importance of an *organized* institutional PBM program will be emphasized, while making specific reference to the relevance of each pillar to orthopaedic surgery.

6.5.2 Elective Orthopaedic Surgery: The Importance of an Organized Response

In many ways, elective major orthopaedic surgery represents the ideal scenario for the implementation of PBM. As discussed above, the total burden of transfusion is high. The procedures are furthermore scheduled rather than emergent, and a relatively small range of procedures accounts for the majority of transfusions. These are hip and knee replacement, revision arthroplasty, and major spinal surgery, e.g., intervertebral fixation for degenerative disease or scoliosis repair.

> **Note**
>
> Elective major orthopaedic surgery represents the ideal scenario for the implementation of PBM.

Preoperative patient education regarding the possibility of transfusion, and the alternatives thereto, is best practice. It may not be reasonable to expect patients to give fully informed consent to transfusion in an urgent perioperative situation when opportunities for discussion before surgery were missed. Patients may also require investigation and treatment of anemia. It is therefore imperative that surgical pathways are structured so as to allow the implementation of PBM without delay to surgery. If first contact with the PBM program is left until near the date of surgery, it is unlikely that all necessary interventions will consistently be achieved without postponement of surgery. A PBM program therefore requires collaboration between interested surgeons, anesthesiologists, nurses, and hospital managers.

Strategies

It is this author's experience that a number of different strategies to organize PBM for orthopaedic surgery may deliver good results. These include:
- Involving the patient's general practitioner (or family physician) in the evaluation of possible anemia.
- Conducting initial screening for anemia in the surgical outpatients department as soon as the surgeon advises an operation, with anesthesiologists then coordinating the management of anemic patients.
- If the hematology service has capacity, they may provide expert management and investigation of anemia.

Note

A PBM program requires collaboration between interested surgeons, anesthesiologists, nurses, and hospital managers.

What is important is therefore *local discussion and agreement* regarding the timing of tests, referral patterns, etc. It is legitimate for each institution to develop its own pathways and operating procedures. The following questions should be considered explicitly when developing such a program:
- Preoperative patient education regarding the risk of anemia and transfusion.
  - Where is this to take place, at what stage, and using what methods (e.g., leaflets)?
- Anemia screening.
  - Is this to take place at referral, in the surgical outpatients clinic, or at a later date (e.g., in a pre-assessment clinic)?
  - How are the results communicated, and who has responsibility for action?
  - In the event of serious unexpected anemia (indicating, e.g., the possibility of an unexpected cancer diagnosis), what referral is to be made for investigation?
  - What treatment modalities are to be used? For example, is surgery to be postponed for oral iron therapy to be given time to work, or should intravenous iron be used to expedite surgery?
- Minimization of intraoperative blood loss.
  - For which procedures performed locally is cell salvage indicated?

- How is the use of antifibrinolytic therapy to be integrated into care, bearing in mind local thromboprophylaxis protocols?
  - Are wound drains to be used? If they are, the evidence suggests that using reinfusion drains reduces RBC transfusion.
- Institutional transfusion triggers should be evidence-based, agreed, and regularly audited.

It is important that hospitals audit their own practice in advance of setting up a PBM program. This will allow them to target their efforts appropriately. It would, for example, likely be wasted effort to concentrate only on preoperative anemia management if overtransfusion is common postoperatively. The use of algorithms (Goodnough et al 2011, NBA 2012) to guide treatment decisions is beneficial, but such algorithms must be adapted for local circumstances.

6.5.3 Selected PBM Techniques Applicable in Orthopaedic Surgery

▶ **Surgical techniques.** The use of closed techniques for major long-bone fractures (e.g., intramedullary nailing) is gaining popularity over open reduction and fixation. This reduces blood loss. Similarly, external fixation of unstable pelvic fractures in major trauma reduces transfusion requirements (see also Chapter 4.4) (Morais et al 2014).

▶ **Positioning.** Positioning the patient with the operative site uppermost (e.g., hip replacement in the lateral versus supine position) reduces venous congestion and bleeding (Widman and Isacson 2001). In spine surgery, meticulous attention to the avoidance of abdominal compression also reduces epidural congestion and bleeding.

▶ **Anesthetic technique.** Neuraxial blockade seems to reduce blood loss in comparison with general anesthesia, although the mechanism of action is not well described. Induced hypotension to a mean blood pressure of 55 mmHg may further reduce bleeding in arthroplasty and spine surgery.

▶ **Preoperative autologous blood donation and normovolemic hemodilution.** Both these techniques have face validity and are widely available, albeit only in some countries. Meta-analyses have, however, shown that although their use decreases the exposure to allogeneic RBCs, it increases the need for transfusion overall, and that autologous blood collected is often wasted (Forgie et al 1998, Henry et al 2002). Some health systems (e.g., the National Health Service in the United Kingdom) therefore no longer make routine use of these techniques (see also Chapter 4.3.2) (Boulton and James 2007, Lemaire 2008, Perazzo et al 2013).

> **Note**
>
> The routine use of preoperative autologous blood donation is not indicated any longer.

▶ **Medication management.** The chronic use of nonsteroidal pain killers is common in orthopaedic surgery. Patients presenting for joint replacement also often have cardiac risk factors and take aspirin as a secondary prevention. This author considers blanket advice to discontinue such drugs before surgery to be inappropriate. An individualized patient decision must be made regarding whether to stop or continue these medicines, balancing the risk of exacerbation of bleeding against the need to provide appropriate preoperative analgesia and cardioprotection.

> **Conclusion**
>
> Elective orthopaedic surgery lends itself particularly well to the development of a coordinated institutional PBM program. A narrow range of procedures is responsible for the majority of transfusions required. Consequently, there is opportunity to analyze referral and care pathways, and to audit institutional practice patterns in some detail. These data will be helpful in designing institution-specific policies, protocols, and guidelines that minimize the reliance on allogeneic blood and blood products.
>
> The clinical decisions related to PBM in orthopaedics are relatively simple. The challenge is rather to design systems that ensure the *reliable* application of *all* applicable PBM techniques for individual patients, *without interfering* with the primary goal of safe and expeditious treatment of the orthopaedic problem. Although this is challenging, the potential benefits are great, including reduced risk to the patient as well as public health and financial benefit.

6.6 PBM in Vascular Surgery

B. Clevenger, T. Richards

6.6.1 Introduction

PBM is an evidence-based approach to reduce the risks from anemia and blood transfusion. PBM focuses upon three pillars: the detection and treatment of anemia; the reduction of blood loss; and the optimization of the patient-specific tolerance to anemia, including use of restrictive transfusion triggers.

In vascular surgery this could not be more important for patient welfare and quality of service delivery. Vascular patients commonly have multiple comorbidities. Often, these include cardiac disease and diabetes, both of which are frequently associated with anemia. As with cardiac surgery, vascular surgery relies heavily on RBC transfusion, with most patients receiving antiplatelet agents and with surgical bleeding increased by the use of intraoperative anticoagulants and prolonged operating times.

In large observational cohorts, preoperative anemia in noncardiac surgery is associated with an increased risk of postoperative complications and death (Musallam et al 2011). In cohorts of vascular surgical patients, similar outcomes have been shown (Diehm et al 2007, Dunkelgrun et al 2008). The use of RBC transfusion to treat anemia and bleeding, however, has been shown to increase the morbidity and mortality in a dose-dependent manner (Ferraris et al 2012). Consequently, in high-risk patients undergoing vascular surgery, quality improvement with PBM could not be more appropriate.

> **Note**
>
> In cohorts of vascular surgical patients with preoperative anemia, an increased risk of postoperative complications and death has been shown.

6.6.2 Preoperative Anemia

Preoperative anemia is common in patients undergoing vascular surgery, the prevalence being more than 30% (Diehm et al 2007, Dunkelgrun et al 2008). As hemoglobin concentration decreases below 6 to 10 g/dL, depending upon individual patient characteristics, tissue hypoxia and organ dysfunction become apparent. This is particularly so in patients with cardiovascular disease. Anemia is associated with reduced exercise performance measured by cardiopulmonary exercise testing (Otto et al 2013). A cardiopulmonary exercise test is a routinely utilized marker of perioperative fitness and outcomes in patients undergoing operation for abdominal aortic aneurysm disease.

Vascular patients with severe limb ischemia suffer chronic inflammation and repeated infections, and often require significant intervention. These are all factors associated with functional iron deficiency due to inflammatory-mediated hepcidin activation, leading to iron-restricted erythropoiesis. This can be further compounded in critical illness because of pain and opiate use, and by poor nutrition. In a cohort study of patients admitted with severe limb ischemia, anemia was seen in two-thirds of patients and these were more likely to also be malnourished. Anemia was further associated with an increased hospital length of stay. Routine hematologic markers did not define a cause for the anemia, although a raised C-reactive protein level suggested functional iron deficiency with a trend toward lower mean corpuscular volume levels. Most (90%) patients received RBC transfusion during their hospital stay and most were anemic on discharge (Shah et al 2010). Modern intravenous iron preparations are both efficacious and safe (Lin et al 2013), and their use should be encouraged as a first-line treatment of anemia as part of the preoperative preparation and nutritional support to patients in hospital. Nevertheless, the recognition of anemia in vascular patients should prompt clinicians to consider the need for PBM and the implementation of second- and third-pillar strategies.

Note

Modern intravenous iron preparations should be encouraged as a first-line treatment of anemia as part of the preoperative preparation and nutritional support of vascular patients.

6.6.3 Point-of-care Testing

Point-of-care testing allows a rapid turnaround of results for the management of intraoperative coagulation, bleeding, and transfusion. Conventional tests of full blood count, international normalized ratio, and arterial blood gases using devices located within the theater complex can provide rapid results. The use of viscoelastic tests such as thromboelastography or rotational thromboelas-

tometry allows the global assessment of hemostasis, from speed and strength of clot formation to retraction and fibrinolysis. These tests allow the targeted, algorithm-driven management of coagulation, reducing the risk of bleeding (Görlinger et al 2012), particularly in anticoagulated patients. Platelet function testing can also be used to assess the bleeding risk from antiplatelet drugs preoperatively.

6.6.4 Antifibrinolytic Therapy

Tranexamic acid and ε-aminocaproic acid actively inhibit fibrinolysis. Prophylactic use of tranexamic acid has been shown to be efficacious in reducing blood loss, including a 0.58 relative risk (95% confidence interval, 0.34–0.99) of RBC transfusion in vascular surgery (Ker et al 2012a). A dose of 1 g (15 mg/kg) is recommended in most cases. Concerns remain regarding the risk of thromboembolic complications; large series have shown no increase in thromboembolic events (Poeran et al 2014), but caution should be exercised in high-risk patients.

6.6.5 Cell Salvage

Cell salvage using a double-lumen suction device should be used whenever blood loss of more than 500 mL is possible. A collection reservoir can be set up at the start of surgery, and if sufficient blood is collected, this is processed. This is both cost-effective and efficacious in reducing RBC transfusion (Carless et al 2010b). RBCs from saturated swabs can also be aspirated and processed in the surgical setting.

6.6.6 Restrictive Transfusion Thresholds

Since the 1990s, restrictive transfusion thresholds have been demonstrated to be at least as effective as liberal transfusion strategies (Hébert et al 1999a), and clinical practice has moved toward less liberal transfusion strategies. However, there remains equipoise as to the ideal hemoglobin targets for patients, particular those with cardiovascular disease. Based on evidence from cardiac surgery, a transfusion trigger threshold of 9 g/dL seems to be optimal for those with low cardiovascular reserve (Murphy et al 2015a), which logically extends to vascular surgical patients (Murphy et al 2015b).

6.6.7 Interventional Occlusion Balloons

Advances in, and recognition of, interventional radiological techniques to prevent or control major bleeding have led to occlusion ballons becoming a more commonly used adjunct in vascular surgery. Transcatheter arterial techniques are commonly used for uterine fibroid and tumor embolization. This technology has been developed for the control of emergency bleeding and has gained acceptance and practice in the management of gastrointestinal bleeding and postsurgical bleeding (Beggs et al 2014). Practice can be limited by service provision; these techniques may be more commonly practiced in larger units with more readily available staff and interventional suites. Major

trauma units in the United States and conflict zones have proposed the use of resuscitative endovascular balloon occlusion (REBOA) (Brenner et al 2013). Developed initially to control bleeding in aortic surgery, a soft compliant balloon is placed inside the aorta (where a clamp is difficult) and inflated to control the blood flow and prevent a major hemorrhage. In trauma patients with major hemorrhage, a balloon can be placed over a guide wire from the brachial or, preferably, the femoral artery into the aorta and inflated to prevent exsanguination and allow time for stabilization and definitive treatment in the operating room. In the elective setting, similar techniques can be employed if major hemorrhage is anticipated, such as postpartum hemorrhage (**Fig. 6.5**) or major tumor resection.

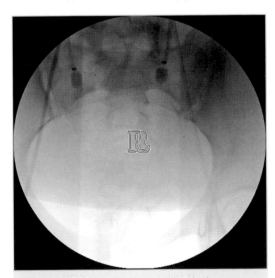

Fig. 6.5 This patient was diagnosed with placenta percreta with serosal invasion of the bladder. Elective cesarean section was planned in the late third trimester; massive blood loss (> 2 L) was anticipated. In preparation, at operation, compliant occlusion balloons were placed in both internal iliac arteries by percutaneous femoral puncture supported by long 6 F sheaths (to allow heparinized saline flush and prevent clot formation). A low-power C-arm was used for guidance. Immediately after delivery of the child, the balloons were inflated under fluoroscopic guidance to stop blood flow into the pelvis and prevent major bleeding. Once hemostasis was obtained, the balloons were deflated and removed. (Courtesy of Dr Jowad Raja, Interventional Radiologist, University College London Hospitals, London, United Kingdom).

Conclusion

Vascular surgery is the second largest user of blood in hospitals, after cardiac surgery. Patients often have significant comorbidities including cardiac disease, diabetes, and malnutrition, and they are frequently anemic. RBC transfusion is common, exacerbated by the prevalence of antiplatelet agent use, prolonged operating times, and the use of intraoperative anticoagulants. Thus, vascular surgery provides an area with the potential for significant benefit from the implementation of PBM.

Preoperative anemia is common. Both chronic inflammation and infection lead to hepcidin-mediated iron-restricted erythropoiesis. Modern intravenous iron preparations are both safe and efficacious in overcoming absolute and functional iron deficiency and should be considered a first-line treatment for anemia in this patient group.

Intraoperative care should include targeted coagulation management using point-of-care tests, antifibrinolytic agents, and routine use of cell salvage to reduce allogeneic blood transfusions. Research into the use of antiplatelet agents and the effects of tranexamic acid on bleeding in surgery is ongoing.

Single-unit transfusion policies should be adopted throughout, and a hemoglobin threshold of 9 g/dL is considered the optimum target postoperatively. Oral iron is not effective postoperatively, and further research is needed on the role of intravenous iron in surgical patients to effect recovery and rehabilitation.

Chapter 7

PBM in Nonsurgical Settings

7.1 Potential for PBM in Intensive Care Medicine

M. Hiesmayr, A. Schiferer

7.1.1 Transfusion Practice in Intensive Care Units

▶ **Transfusion rates.** In intensive care units (ICUs), the transfusion of red blood cells (RBCs) is virtually universal practice. Overall, one in every three patients in intensive care is transfused (Vincent et al 2002, Sakr et al 2010). Among patients whose length of stay in the ICU is longer than 1 week, approximately three in four receive a transfusion (Vincent et al 2002, Corwin et al 2004, Vincent and Piagnerelli 2006). The transfusion rate rises sharply in line with the length of stay (**Fig. 7.1**) and is almost twofold higher for anesthesiology/surgical ICUs than for internal medicine ICUs. More than 70% of all transfused patients receive their first transfusion during the first 2 days in the ICU. The average transfusion volume is 1 unit of RBC concentrate every 3 days.

▶ **Indications for transfusion.** The indication for RBC transfusion is bleeding in 53% to 60% of cases, followed by a low hemoglobin value in association with a reduced physiological reserve (28–29%), impaired perfusion (17%), and coronary heart disease (0.5–8%) (French et al 2002, Vincent et al 2002, Corwin et al 2004, Walsh et al 2004). There appears to be widespread variability between ICUs with regard to the hemoglobin threshold for transfusion. The threshold value is typically between 7 g/dL and 9 g/dL, and it was lower in 2002 than in 1993 (Hébert et al 2005). The transfusion threshold is much higher for patients with myocardial infarction than for patients with trauma, hemorrhage, or severe sepsis. Another important change over the years has been a considerable increase in the transfusion of single units of RBCs. In addition, more restrictive transfusion practices with a lower threshold in the ICU have led to an increase in the rate of post-ICU transfusion. Thus, transfusion decision-making should be considered as a process that requires the concerted action of clinicians from all involved specialties, with the hemoglobin value serving as a basis for discussion rather than as a definitive transfusion trigger.

▶ **Hemoglobin changes over time.** The hemoglobin concentration changes during the course of a patient's stay on the ICU, often depending on the baseline value. Low admission values are usually corrected rapidly by transfusion, whereas high values decline progressively over a period of days provided that there are no acute bleeding events (**Fig. 7.2a, b**) (Nguyen et al 2003). This decline has been attributed to a large volume of blood draws (mean 41 mL/day) (Vincent et al 2002). The daily blood sampling volume may be twice as high for patients with more complex clinical manifestations involving infection, altered coagulation, or invasive treatments such as hemofiltration and extracorporeal membrane oxygenation. Critically ill

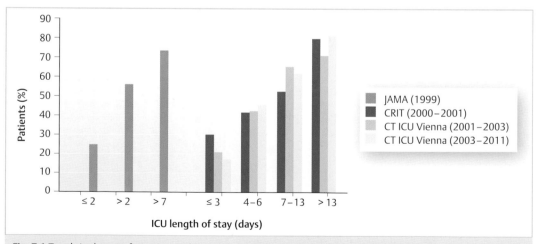

Fig. 7.1 Trends in the transfusion rate in four cohorts. Data sources: JAMA, Vincent et al 2002; CRIT, Corwin et al 2004; CT ICU, Cardiothoracic Intensive Care Unit, Medical University of Vienna, Vienna, Austria.

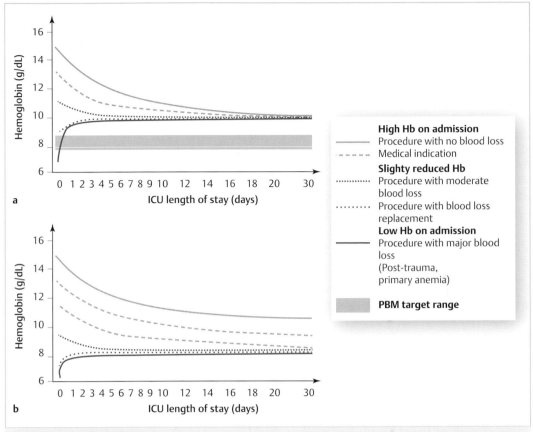

Fig. 7.2 Trends in hemoglobin values during ICU stays; schematic diagram based on data from the Cardiothoracic ICU at the Medical University of Vienna, Vienna, Austria. **(a)** Before the introduction of PBM. **(b)** After the introduction of PBM. Hb, hemoglobin; ICU, intensive care unit.

patients, whose bone marrow function is usually impaired by inflammation, are not able to compensate for blood loss of that magnitude.

Note

Clinicians can make an important contribution to quality improvement and maintenance by regularly appraising the observed average and minimal hemoglobin values, the transfusion rate, and the timing of transfusions against usual practice. Once PBM has been introduced, patients with anemia are only transfused to values slightly above the transfusion threshold, and the steady decline in hemoglobin during a patient's stay on the ICU will be mitigated because of the systematic application of preventive strategies.

7.1.2 Outcome of Anemia

The transfusion thresholds in line with the practice of PBM are markedly lower than the WHO criteria for anemia (WHO 1968). In physiological terms, the body responds to lower hemoglobin values with the stabilization of hypoxia-inducible factor 1α (HIF1α), which is an oxygen-sensitive transcription factor that increases the concentrations of a number of adaptive molecules (Shander et al 2011b). However, even at hemoglobin values that are higher than the transfusion threshold, there are already signs of an adverse effect on certain organ systems. Accordingly, low preoperative hemoglobin values constitute a clear risk factor for cerebral and other complications in the event of a further drop in hemoglobin, e.g., during extracorporeal circulation (Karkouti et al 2008b).

▶ **Tolerance to anemia.** Most observations on the tolerance to anemia have been made in patients who, for logistical or religious reasons, did not receive RBC transfusions. No rise in mortality was observed for patients with a hemoglobin value of around 8 to 8.5 g/dL, whereas patients with a postoperative value of less than 8 g/dL had a higher mortality: around 33% if the hemoglobin value dropped to 4 to 5 g/dL, and 50% to 60% if the value dropped to 3 g/dL (Carson et al 2002b). There was a trend toward increased mortality from cardiovascular disease. In patients with craniocerebral trauma, a worse outcome has repeatedly been observed for mean hemoglobin values below 9 g/dL on admission (Sekhon et al 2012).

7.1.3 Treatment of Anemia (First Pillar of PBM)

In the intensive care setting, two pharmacological strategies for the conservative treatment of anemia are under discussion.

▶ **Erythropoietin.** Corwin et al (2007) conducted a large study on the use of erythropoietin for the stimulation of de novo erythropoiesis. In a mixed cohort of intensive care patients (surgical, medical, trauma), evidence of a statistically nonsignificant trend toward reduced mortality was found for patients treated with erythropoietin, but it was not possible to reduce the need for transfusion by administering erythropoietin. A major side effect was a higher rate of thrombosis among patients who had not received heparin-based antithrombotic treatment or prophylaxis. Apart from its impact on hematopoiesis, erythropoietin may also have a cytoprotective effect at a much higher dose than that customarily used (Hayden et al 2012).

▶ **Iron supplementation.** The second approach to the treatment of anemia is iron supplementation. Whereas treatment strategies based on iron supplementation exist for various patient groups, such as patients with cardiac failure (Anker et al 2009) and those undergoing dialysis, there continues to be a paucity of data on intensive care patients (Corwin et al 2007, Pieracci et al 2009). The conventional method of diagnosing iron deficiency states on the basis of ferritin and transferrin saturation is not suitable in intensive care because the blood iron parameters, which are unrelated to the body's iron stores, fluctuate as part of the acute-phase response. Iron deficiency diagnostic tests tailored to intensive care patients should be able to identify whether individual patients could benefit from iron supplementation. Therefore, diagnostic testing should be investigated in the context of effectiveness studies to allow the definition of meaningful cutoff values and to identify potential treatment side effects, such as infections (Litton et al 2013).

Note

In the intensive care setting, erythropoietin administration and iron supplementation are strategies under discussion for the treatment of anemia. However, it is not yet clear which patients might benefit from these treatment approaches.

7.1.4 Outcome of Transfusion

▶ **Observational studies.** In 42 of 45 observational studies, transfusions in intensive care patients were found to be associated with a 1.5- to 2-fold higher risk of death or infection (Marik and Corwin 2008); the effects of transfusion were neutral in two studies, and they were favorable in one study in patients with acute myocardial infarction and a hematocrit below 30% (Wu et al 2001). However, there was no benefit of transfusion if the hematocrit at admission was higher than 30%. Similar findings were observed in patients with acute coronary syndrome, where a nadir hematocrit of around 25% was associated with the lowest mortality (Rao et al 2004). A randomized pilot study of patients with myocardial infarction revealed that liberal transfusion practices with a target hematocrit of 30% to 33%, compared with 27% to 29%, were associated with a markedly higher rate of complications, e.g., signs of cardiac insufficiency (Cooper et al 2011). Transfusion was associated not only with transfusion-related acute lung injury (TRALI) (Gajic et al 2007), but also with higher rates of positive blood cultures (Shorr et al 2005) and nosocomial pneumonia (Shorr et al 2004).

A number of studies aimed to identify whether transfusion was an independent risk factor for a poor outcome or just a marker for the severity of disease. Based on propensity score matching, transfusions tended to have a neutral or favorable effect. However, it remains unclear why the mortality during the first 5 days was markedly higher in the nontransfused control group than in the transfused group, and why this trend then reversed up to day 30 (Park et al 2012).

▶ **Liberal versus restrictive transfusion strategy.** Several randomized trials compared liberal transfusion practices with hemoglobin target values above 10 g/dL with more restrictive practices based on target values of 7–9 g/dL. In a mixed group of intensive care patients, lower target values did not have a negative effect and reduced the transfusion rate by around one-half (Hébert et al 1999a). The restrictive strategy was beneficial for younger patients and those who were less seriously ill, whereas the implications for patients with myocardial ischemia were unclear. In the second randomized study, it was not possible to identify any benefit for a liberal transfusion strategy in cardiac surgery patients, but the liberal strategy was associated with a markedly higher transfusion rate of 78% versus 47%. In both groups, each single transfusion was associated with a 1.2-fold rise in complications or death after 30 days (Shehata et al 2012). Among patients with septic shock, the mortality at 90 days and the rates of ischemic events and use of life support were similar among those assigned to blood transfusion at a higher hemoglobin threshold and those assigned to blood transfusion at a lower threshold (Holst et al 2014). In another prospective randomized study, a restrictive transfusion threshold after cardiac surgery was not superior to a liberal threshold with respect to morbidity or health care costs (Murphy et al 2015b).

▶ **Cardiac surgery patients.** For the large group of cardiac surgery patients, who account for around 20% of blood consumption, it was demonstrated that transfusion of RBC concentrates did not constitute an independent risk factor if the analysis was adjusted for the amount of blood collected from the chest drains (Dixon et al 2013). The mortality continued to rise in line with the amount of blood in the drains, regardless of whether the patient was transfused or not. The authors inferred that patients with increased bleeding developed subclinical forms of pericardial tamponade, since increased bleeding was accompanied by reduced cardiac output, a greater need for catecholamines, and elevated pulmonary artery pressure, ventila-

tor pressure, and left ventricular filling pressure. The authors concluded that this led to delayed weaning from mechanical ventilation, delayed mobilization, and prolonged ICU stay.

> **Note**
>
> A Cochrane analysis (Carless et al 2010a) recommends a restrictive strategy for all patients without cardiac disease, because this can help to reduce the transfusion rate by around 33% with no increase in the complication rate.

▶ **Recommendations.** The most recent clinical practice guideline (Carson et al 2012b) contains four recommendations:
- Use of a restrictive transfusion strategy (hemoglobin 7–8 g/dL) for stable hospitalized patients.
- Use of a restrictive transfusion strategy (hemoglobin 8 g/dL) for patients with preexisting cardiovascular disease based on clinical symptoms.
- No recommendation with regard to a restrictive or liberal transfusion threshold for patients with acute coronary syndrome.
- Decisions should be influenced by clinical symptoms and hemoglobin values.

7.1.5 Integrative Strategy

Each ICU must devise a strategy that helps to keep the transfusion rate to a minimum. Such a strategy reduces the risk of blood-related side effects and has financial benefits.

The cornerstone of this strategy is an essentially restrictive transfusion policy, which, however, must not lead to a delay in the stabilization of bleeding or trauma patients. Protracted shock phases must definitely be avoided, or at least kept as short as possible.

The *first component* of such an approach must entail the preoperative optimization of all patients prior to large elective surgical procedures. The main focus here is on the appropriate treatment of anemia based on iron supplementation (Litton et al 2013) and, possibly, the administration of erythropoietin (Karkouti et al 2005b). There is evidence to suggest that the transfusion of anemic patients one to two days before surgery could be more beneficial than intraoperative transfusion (Karkouti et al 2012).

The *second component* must involve the timely control of bleeding and meticulous intraoperative hemostasis. The perioperative administration of anticoagulants and platelet inhibitors should only occur on the basis of strict indication criteria and interdisciplinary agreement. Accumulation of low-molecular heparins must be avoided under all circumstances, even in patients with slightly impaired renal function.

The *third component* entails reducing to an absolute minimum the frequency and volume of blood draws for diagnostic and interventional purposes, since even healthy individuals can only produce 20 to 30 mL of new RBCs per day (around 1% of the total RBC volume). The use of smaller sampling tubes and a conservative blood testing strategy helped to reduce diagnostic blood loss by up to 80% (Harber et al 2006, Sanchez-Giron and Alvarez-Mora 2008).

A potential *fourth component* is the promotion of de novo erythropoiesis in the ICU. Although studies to date have not shown any clearly identifiable positive effect of systematic erythropoietin therapy on the transfusion rate, a target group approach could be taken (Hayden et al 2012). Patients exhibiting few signs of active inflammation might show a better response to erythropoietin. The same holds true for the use of iron in the ICU. There is widespread concern that iron might increase the infection rate since iron promotes the growth of several bacterial species (Pieracci and Barie 2005, Weinberg 2009, Auerbach 2014, Auerbach and Macdougall 2014). However, to date there is no evidence that this is an issue in humans, and following cardiac surgery procedures iron reduced the transfusion rate by around one-quarter (Pieracci et al 2009). However, this effect could only be identified in patients who presented with impaired erythropoiesis related to iron deficiency.

Conclusion

The cornerstone of an integrative strategy designed to reduce the transfusion rate in intensive care medicine consists of the use of a restrictive transfusion threshold of 7 to 8 g/dL. However, this must be adapted for patients who have virtually no mechanisms to compensate for ischemia.

Such an integrative strategy should comprise three components: appropriate treatment of anemia based on iron supplementation and, possibly, the administration of iron and/or erythropoietin before major elective surgical proce-

dures; minimization of intra- and perioperative blood loss; and reduction of the frequency and volume of blood drawn for diagnostic purposes to an absolute minimum. A further component may be the promotion of de novo erythropoiesis based on erythropoietin administration or iron supplementation in the ICU.

An integrative strategy can prove successful only if its implementation is regularly assessed by practitioners appraising their own results.

7.2 Potential for PBM in Oncology and Hematology

M. Fridrik

7.2.1 Significance of the Three Pillars

The three pillars of PBM also apply to anemia in the nonsurgical setting, albeit to a varying extent. The cornerstone of the first pillar, which is also the most important pillar in the nonsurgical area, is diagnosis. In patients with iron deficiency anemia, the cause of iron loss (mainly blood loss) must be identified and eliminated. The third pillar plays only a minor role in the nonsurgical setting and is limited to optimization of the individual patient's tolerance to anemia.

7.2.2 Diagnosis of Anemia

Unlike in the surgical setting, where anemia is primarily attributable to perioperative blood loss, anemia in oncology and hematology has a broad variety of causes. Therefore, differential diagnosis of the clinical picture is a prerequisite for effective treatment. A complete blood count, including the differential blood count and the reticulocyte count, gives a general overview. If the differential blood count shows lymphoma cells or blast cells, or if anemia is associated with leukopenia and/or thrombopenia, bone marrow cytology and histology tests should be performed.

Hyperproliferative Anemia

A high reticulocyte count is indicative of active hematopoiesis. This increased activity may be attributable to a regeneration process following blood loss or after supplementation therapy with erythropoietin, iron, vitamin B$_{12}$, or folic acid. However, if the hematocrit does not rise despite a high reticulocyte count, hemolytic anemia is likely to be implicated. The next diagnostic steps include optical examination of a blood smear, Coombs test, test for paroxysmal nocturnal hemoglobinuria, and hemoglobin electrophoresis.

> **Note**
>
> Hemolytic anemia is associated with a high reticulocyte count.

Hypoproliferative Anemia

All other forms of anemia with a low or normal reticulocyte count are classified as hypoproliferative anemia. The mean corpuscular volume (MCV) is another parameter that points to the genesis of anemia. A low MCV is indicative of impaired hemoglobin synthesis, whereas an elevated MCV is suggestive of a nuclear maturation defect (**Fig. 7.3**).

▶ **Low mean corpuscular volume.** Iron deficiency anemia in menstruating women is a classic example of hypoproliferative anemia. At an advanced stage, it is associated with a low MCV, and is diagnosed on the basis of low ferritin. However, a normal ferritin level does not rule out iron deficiency anemia. Also, a low iron level alone is not sufficient for the diagnosis of iron deficiency anemia. A

definitive diagnosis is based on Berlin blue staining of the bone marrow, which is able to identify iron activity in the bone marrow. If one wants to avoid a bone marrow puncture, a rise in the hemoglobin value after a trial of iron therapy for a few weeks also serves to confirm iron deficiency. If iron deficiency anemia is ruled out in the presence of a low MCV and a high reticulocyte count, the only issue to be clarified is thalassemia. Investigation of any form of iron deficiency anemia must include gastrointestinal tests, except in the case of young women.

▶ **High mean corpuscular volume.** A high MCV without reticulocytosis is found most commonly where there is damage to the liver parenchyma, and in myelodysplastic syndromes. The latter are generally associated additionally with leuko- and/or thrombopenia, whereas vitamin B$_{12}$ or folic acid deficiency are rarely implicated as having a causal role. Myelodysplastic syndrome is diagnosed through bone marrow cytology testing.

> **Note**
>
> Bone marrow tests are needed to diagnose macrocytic anemia with low reticulocyte counts and low leukocyte and/or platelet counts.

▶ **Normal mean corpuscular volume.** The diagnosis is more complex if the MCV is normal with

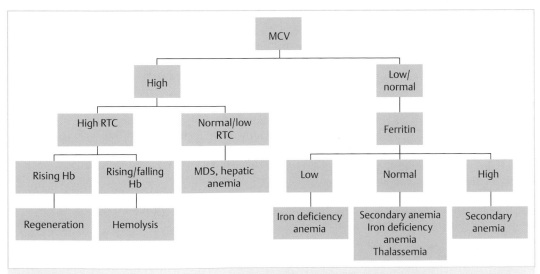

Fig. 7.3 Strategy for the diagnosis of anemia on the basis of the MCV. Hb, hemoglobin; MCV, mean corpuscular volume; MDS, myelodysplastic syndrome; RTC, reticulocyte count.

a low or normal reticulocyte count. This suggests secondary anemia or anemia of chronic disease, and calls for investigation of the thyroid and renal function, screening for chronic infection, and screening for tumors. The ferritin level is generally high and the bone-marrow iron stores are full, but iron is not sufficiently available for erythropoiesis.

7.2.3 Management of Iron Deficiency Anemia

In the Western hemisphere, iron deficiency anemia is almost always caused by acute or chronic blood loss—only rarely is it attributable to malabsorption or an extreme diet. The standard treatment comprises daily oral iron supplementation. The treatment duration is based on the severity of anemia, but treatment must be continued after a normal blood count has been achieved to quickly fill the iron stores. Treatment lasting less than 6 months rarely suffices. To permit their absorption, iron supplements must be taken in a fasting state 1 hour before a meal. Antacids, H_2 blockers, and protein pump inhibitors prevent the absorption. After 3 to 4 weeks of treatment, the blood count should be verified. If the hemoglobin value has not risen, the product is not being absorbed, has not been taken, or the diagnosis was incorrect. The gastrointestinal tolerability of all iron supplements is poor. In such a case, or if the product is not being absorbed, intravenous iron supplementation is justified. A single infusion of ferric carboxymaltose can eliminate anemia and fill the iron stores; the recommended dose with hemoglobin concentrations below 10 g/dL is 1,500 mg (or 1,000 mg for more moderate forms of anemia).

Iron deficiency anemia develops slowly. That is why patients tolerate even a very low hemoglobin value surprisingly well. RBC transfusion is needed to treat iron deficiency anemia only in the event of syncopes. Iron therapy is contraindicated in the presence of iron overload. Iron supplements should also not be administered to treat inflammatory or tumor-associated anemia because they could aggravate the immune status, unless functional iron deficiency is also present. However, the latter is poorly defined (see Chapter 7.2.8).

> **Note**
>
> Iron deficiency anemia is the most common form of anemia in menstruating women, and should be treated with an oral iron supplement for several months.

7.2.4 Management of Vitamin-B_{12} and Folic-acid Deficiency Anemia

An autoimmune process directed against the parietal cells of the stomach causes pernicious anemia. In this situation, parenteral supplementation with vitamin B_{12} is needed. An intramuscular injection of 1 mg of vitamin B_{12} is administered three times weekly until the hematocrit has normalized. Afterward (and also after gastrectomy) 1 mg of vitamin B_{12} is administered every 6 to 8 weeks. Patients with pernicious anemia can tolerate very low hematocrit values and RBC transfusion is not indicated.

Folic-acid deficiency anemia occurs very rarely in Europe and is seen mainly in persons with severe alcohol-related disease. Oral supplementation with 5 mg daily suffices.

7.2.5 Management of Autoimmune Hemolytic Anemia

▶ **Warm-reactive antibodies.** Autoimmune hemolytic anemia caused by warm-reactive autoantibodies produces a positive indirect Coombs test for IgG antibodies. Hemolysis can be generally controlled with prednisolone at 1 mg/kg daily. Alternatively, high-dose dexamethasone can be administered at 40 mg daily for 4 days. If no improvement in hemolysis is seen on prednisolone, or if hemolysis can only be controlled with maintenance treatment of more than 5 mg prednisolone daily, splenectomy should be performed. Alternatively, treatment with rituximab and a glucocorticoid is possible. The required dose is unclear. Instead of the standard intravenous dose of 4×375 mg/m^2 at weekly intervals, doses of 4×100 mg/m^2 are also effective (Lechner and Jäger 2010). RBC transfusion should be avoided in principle since it further aggravates the immune mechanism.

▶ **Cold-reactive antibodies.** Autoimmune hemolytic anemia caused by cold-reactive antibodies is less common. In the Coombs test these antibodies generally only result in complement activation. They are often associated with rheumatologic disease or lymphoma. Apart from treatment of the underlying disease and protection against the cold, treatment is the same as for warm-reactive autoantibodies, but is not as effective. Infusions should be administered at body temperature.

7.2.6 Management of Renal Anemia

There is a loose relationship between the severity of renal anemia and the extent of impaired renal function. Renal anemia is caused by a decline in erythropoietin production. However, iron or vitamin B_{12} deficiency can also be implicated, as can impaired iron utilization due to chronic inflammation or tumor disease. Treatment is based on erythropoietin supplementation therapy, with initial subcutaneous or intravenous injection of 400 IU erythropoietin three times weekly. Then the dose and interval are chosen such that the hemoglobin concentration is between 10 g/dL and 12 g/dL (Palmer et al 2014). Persistent hemoglobin values above 12 g/dL should be avoided. Additional iron supplementation can help to improve anemia and cut back on the need for erythropoietin.

7.2.7 Management of Myelodysplastic Syndromes

Myelodysplastic syndromes are heterogeneous diseases of varying prognosis. The Revised International Prognostic Scoring System classifies the disease on the basis of cytogenetic features, blast percentage, hemoglobin value, platelet count, and neutrophil count into five risk categories (very low, low, intermediate, high, and very high) (Greenberg et al 2012). Although erythropoietin is not licensed in Europe for myelodysplastic syndromes, one-third of the patients with very low and/or low risk respond to high-dose erythropoietin. The initial dose is $3 \times 10,000$ IU/week given subcutaneously. If an adequate (≥ 1 g/dL) rise in hemoglobin is not observed after 6 weeks, the dose can be increased to $3 \times 20,000$ IU. Combination with granulocyte colony-stimulating factor (G-CSF) can help to increase the response rate further. The highest response rates are seen for endogenous erythropoietin levels of less than 100 IU/L. Levels of ≥ 400 IU/L indicate that a response

to erythropoietin is very unlikely (Ludwig and Fritz 1998). If an adequate hemoglobin increase cannot be achieved either with high-dose erythropoietin alone or in combination with G-CSF, erythropoietin must be discontinued. Patients with intermediate or high risk can be treated with 5-azacytidine, leukemia induction therapy, and/or allogeneic stem cell transplantation (Alessandrino et al 2002). Patients who are not suitable candidates for this treatment, or patients who did not respond to treatment, are enrolled in a chronic transfusion program (see Chapter 7.2.10).

7.2.8 Management of Anemia of Chronic Disease

Anemia of chronic disease is characterized by impaired iron utilization. Nonetheless, diagnostic measures should always include tests for iron deficiency, vitamin B_{12} deficiency, and occult blood loss. Typically, serum iron levels are low and ferritin levels are high. This constellation should under no circumstances result in the misguided administration of iron supplements. Apart from the already existing iron overload of the reticuloendothelial system, there is evidence that this would weaken the body's defense against infection. Functional iron deficiency is rare in anemia of chronic disease and difficult to diagnose. A German working group defines functional iron deficiency on the basis of the ferritin index (soluble transferrin receptor divided by the logarithm of ferritin; see Chapter 3.1.2) (Steinmetz et al 2010). The National Comprehensive Cancer Network guidelines use the term *functional iron deficiency* to denote a state where the serum ferritin value is lower than 800 ng/mL and the transferrin saturation is lower than 20% (NCCN 2015). Erythropoietin can improve anemia, but there is evidence that it shortens life expectancy. Erythropoietin is therefore not recommended for the treatment of anemia of chronic disease. Causal therapy must be based on treatment of the underlying disease. If this is not possible, a chronic transfusion program should be initiated (see Chapter 7.2.10).

7.2.9 Management of Anemia during Chemotherapy

Certain cytostatic substances, in particular the platinum derivatives, give rise to anemia through bone marrow suppression and inhibition of erythropoietin production. An Austrian survey carried out in hematology and medical oncology departments identified anemia in 36% of patients (Ludwig et al 2004). It has been unequivocally demonstrated that erythropoietin therapy for tumor patients can reduce the transfusion incidence, improve anemia, and enhance the quality of life. However, a meta-analysis of randomized trials identified a rise in thromboembolic events and a shorter life expectancy among patients with cancer who were treated with erythropoietin (Bohlius et al 2009b). The reason for this finding is not clear. Potential explanations include the association between hemoglobin values above 12 g/dL and thromboembolic events and tumor growth stimulation via erythropoietin receptors on malignant cells. There is no clear proof for either of these two theories. Erythropoietins are therefore only recommended in chemotherapy-induced anemia if treatment does not have a curative intent. Treatment is indicated at a hemoglobin concentration below 10 g/dL and the target range should be 10 to 12 g/dL. This should be achieved with the lowest possible erythropoietin dose. The additional use of iron supplementation is controversial (Rizzo et al 2008). Patients who do not respond to erythropoietin and those who are not suitable candidates for erythropoietin therapy are transfused (see Chapter 7.2.10).

> **Note**
>
> In nephrogenic anemia, myelodysplastic syndromes, and chemotherapy-induced anemia, erythropoietin therapy is indicated for palliative purposes only.

7.2.10 Transfusion Management of Hematologic and Oncologic Diseases

▶ **Individual indication.** In contrast to the transfusion indications in surgical settings, the focus in hematology/oncology is mainly on chronic anemia. Hence, the tolerance to anemia is generally higher, but in multimorbid patients the tolerance can considerably decline again. This is therefore a complex problem. Although anemia is not the sole cause of cancer-related fatigue, there is no disputing that the quality of life increases in line with a rise in hemoglobin. This increase is most pro-

nounced for hemoglobin values in the range of 10 to 12 g/dL. Transfusion gives rise to a rapid increase in hemoglobin and, accordingly, to an immediate improvement in symptoms. However, there are the risks associated with any transfusion, including iron overload, alloimmunization, thrombosis, and a negative impact on the immune status, in addition to the potential occurrence of transfusion incidents. Hematologists and oncologists therefore find themselves in uncertain terrain when making decisions about the indication for transfusion in their patients.

Asymptomatic patients with no comorbidity have a low risk of developing symptoms if they become anemic, so transfusion can be delayed without any concerns. Asymptomatic patients who have comorbidities such as heart failure, coronary heart disease, chronic lung disease, or cerebrovascular disease have a medium risk. The indication for transfusion must be considered at an early stage for such patients. Asymptomatic patients with progressively declining hemoglobin values during intensive chemo- or radiotherapy have a high risk. These patients must receive abundant RBC transfusions. Many anemia symptoms are nonspecific. Anemia that justifies the contemplation of transfusion should include at least one of the following symptoms: tachycardia, tachypnea, chest pain, exertional dyspnea, numbness, syncope, or fatigue that impedes normal work activity.

There are various definitions of what constitutes an indication for transfusion. The European Organization for Research and Treatment of Cancer recommends transfusion for symptomatic patients with a hemoglobin concentration of less than 9 g/dL (Aapro and Link 2008). The American Society of Hematology and the American Society of Clinical Oncology recommend transfusion for symptomatic patients with hemoglobin values below 12 g/dL (Rizzo et al 2010). These guidelines highlight the problem whereby certain patients become oligosymptomatic with hemoglobin values of 7 g/dL or less, whereas others already have major complaints if the hemoglobin concentration is less than 12 g/dL. The indication for transfusion in hematology and oncology patients must therefore always be determined on an individual basis, by weighing up the risks of transfusion against the existing symptoms.

▶ **Number of transfusions.** The number of transfusions depends primarily on the symptoms caused by anemia. The frequent practice to transfuse 2 units of RBCs is not supported by data. It is likely that by slowly raising the hematocrit, more accurate titration of the actual requirements can be obtained and unnecessary transfusions can be avoided (Abraham and Sun 2012).

▶ **Precautionary measures.** Meticulous care must be taken if cardiac risk factors are present. For example, RBC volume overload in patients with cardiac failure can give rise to pulmonary edema. Therefore, a diuretic agent should always be administered before transfusion. If the patient has severe coronary disease, a rapid increase in the hematocrit can trigger stenocardia because of the rise in viscosity. For patients with hyperviscosity syndrome, as seen in Waldenström disease or in multiple myeloma, transfusions may only be administered after successful paraprotein reduction through plasmapheresis or immune absorption, since otherwise hyperviscosity would be further aggravated.

7.2.11 Management of Transfusion Hemosiderosis

Patients who are chronically dependent on RBC transfusion develop iron overload (Mainous et al 2014, Wood 2014). The most reliable way to diagnose this condition is to determine the iron content in a liver biopsy sample. Noninvasive tests, such as MRI or a serum ferritin value of more than 1,000 ng/L, are less reliable. The most insightful data on the consequences of iron overload are obtained from patients with thalassemia. Once the number of transfusions has reached 20, there is irreversible organ damage in the absence of concurrent treatment with chelators. It is unclear at present to what extent this finding can be extrapolated to oncology patients who have a limited life expectancy. Until recently, only parenteral chelate therapy was available, and iron stores could only be effectively reduced with daily infusions at intervals of 12 to 24 hours. However, with the licensing of two oral products, deferasirox and deferiprone, treatment has now been greatly simplified. However, it remains unclear from what projected number of transfusions chelate therapy should be initiated.

Conclusion

Anemia plays a major role in the development of cancer-related fatigue. Initial therapy must whenever possible be aimed at treating the cause of anemia. Anemia developing during palliative chemotherapy can be treated with erythropoietin. A stable hemoglobin concentration between 10 g/dL and 12 g/dL should be targeted. The pros and cons of erythropoietin therapy must be weighed up carefully. Transfusions are the worst treatment option, and their use must be based on very stringent criteria.

7.3 Potential for PBM in Cardiology

R. Goldweit

7.3.1 Introduction

Cardiovascular disease remains a leading cause of death and morbidity around the world despite major advances in understanding disease processes, prevention, and the delivery of improved treatments. The cardiologist or cardiovascular specialist is charged with providing therapy that—in a timely, cost-effective way—improves outcomes for patients who manifest or are at risk for an array of heart and vascular diseases. We have witnessed and will continue to witness paradigm changes in the treatment of cardiovascular disease that only a decade before were unimaginable. They include potentially lifesaving medications, heart surgery, interventional treatments, electrophysiology procedures, and therapies involving cardiac devices such as implantable defibrillators. While progressive, many of these advances are associated with significant bleeding and anemia.

In this vast cardiovascular landscape of vital medical pursuit, transfusion of blood and its related issues have only recently been considered to be a potentially modifiable factor contributing to treatment effectiveness and outcomes (Moscucci et al 2006). Anemia, bleeding, and transfusion have increasingly been shown to be related to adverse events and compromised clinical results (Arant et al 2004, Ndrepepa et al 2008, Goldman 2012, Chhatriwalla et al 2013, LaPar et al 2013, Nicolau et al 2013). This means that the effective management of bleeding and anemia in patients with cardiovascular disease has taken on a new potential of significant clinical importance. Although causality concerning bleeding, anemia, and transfusion on the one hand and outcomes on the other may never be definitively proven, it is of major practical importance that—built on the foundation that bleeding is bad for the cardiovascular patient—the application of PBM in this population has been observed to correlate with improved outcomes (Moskowitz et al 2010, Emmert et al 2011, Cladellas et al 2012, LaPar et al 2013).

Note

Effective management of bleeding and anemia in the patient with cardiovascular disease has taken on a new potential of significant clinical importance.

Medical studies have only recently been designed to include the tracking of major bleeding with major adverse clinical events (Nissenson et al 2003, Sabatine et al 2005, Ndrepepa et al 2008, Levine et al 2011, Chhatriwalla et al 2013, Lau and Lip 2014). This represents a transition away from the old-school or historical approach dealing with bleeding and anemia, which was to "just transfuse packed red blood cells." For decades, bleeding complications were not a priority and were considered a minor side effect of antithrombotic and invasive therapies. Iterations of guidelines and conferences focused on the treatment of heart and vascular disease have only recently covered issues of bleeding and transfusion in the cardiovascular patient but have been limited by a lack of data to support any specific strategy (Carson et al 2012b). Although the WHO supports the multimodal therapeutic concept of PBM (Shander et al 2013), mainstream cardiology has not officially embraced the overarching construct. Perhaps because of ongoing controversy about cause and effect, and despite the recently increased and welcomed attention placed on the association between bleeding, transfusion, and cardiovascular outcomes, clinical recommendations in the major cardiology guidelines have been minimal, scattered, and at best "anemic" (Abraham et al 2010, Levine et al 2011, Siegal et al 2012, Gillebert et al 2013, O'Gara et al 2013, Amsterdam et al 2014).

This identifies a challenge for cardiology that could, if realized, have clinical impact by shifting current cardiovascular care strategies to bring about even better clinical results. Unfortunately, *PBM in cardiology* may not have the public aura or appeal of a newly invented therapy or device. One might assume that front-page headlines trumpeting the next potential paradigm-shifting advance in cardiovascular medicine are likely to describe either an implantable gadget or a pharmaceutical agent. However, as the economics, politics, and structure of the health care environment shift to quality-driven cost-effectiveness, it is time that the potential benefits resulting from the weaving together of modern PBM and cardiology are brought into focus, and that truly advanced modern cardiovascular therapy with optimized outcomes is realized.

7.3.2 The Cardiovascular Specialist's Approach to Anemia and Bleeding: Historical Perspective

Cardiovascular therapeutics and hematologic issues have been linked since ancient times when bloodletting was used as a treatment for dropsy (Ventura and Mehra 2005). The first successful human RBC transfusion was performed almost 200 years ago by an obstetrician for postpartum hemorrhage. Since then, transfusion has evolved, because of the availability and mystique of blood, to the point of indiscriminate overuse and potential harm particularly in the cardiovascular patient. There has been an inspiring evolution of cardiovascular therapeutic advances that have been marred by an increased risk of bleeding, anemia, and transfusion, relentlessly haunting the cardiovascular specialist. As the field evolved from the first diagnostic cardiac catheterization in 1929 to the advent of coronary artery bypass surgery in the 1960s and interventional therapies later, transfusion became the de facto therapy for significant anemia, and cardiac patients became the single biggest demand source for donor blood (Anderson et al 2007). The most recent transformative interventional advance, transcatheter aortic valve replacement (TAVR), first performed in 2002, has also been compromised by a significant incidence of major bleeding that predicts 1-year mortality (Généreux et al 2014).

For decades, the cardiovascular trainee and specialist considered bleeding and anemia as nuisances that were primarily the domain of other specialties or were tolerated as procedural or drug-related side effects and often associated with necessary antithrombotic therapy (Nicolau et al 2013). Anemia was generally considered an innocent bystander of improved disease treatments and low hemoglobin levels were "easily" remedied using allogeneic blood transfusion (Nissenson et al 2003). Bleeding was to be stopped by withdrawing and reversing blood thinners and with mechanical intervention on the bleeding site when possible.

Note

In the past, anemia was generally considered to be an innocent bystander of improved disease treatments and low hemoglobin levels were "easily" remedied using allogeneic blood transfusion.

Especially for the cardiac patient, anemia and bleeding may have immediate clinical implications for hemodynamic stability and cardiac demand (Hall 1993), and this encouraged clinicians to adopt a recipe-based approach with laboratory thresholds—prespecified levels of blood hemoglobin concentration or hematocrit—that could trigger transfusion. Replacing intravascular volume and transfusing blood products were the reflex responses needed to prevent destabilization, steady unstable vital signs, and replete blood counts and factors to prespecified "safe" levels (Barr et al 2011). Although laboratory thresholds may appear to empower the clinician with a sense of clinical control, they were generally derived from simple common sense presumptions about pathophysiology and have not been validated for cardiology or other patients by more rigorous clinical methods (Walsh and Maciver 2009, Barr et al 2011, Curley et al 2014b). Thresholds for transfusion remain a source of debate. Although a recent hemoglobin threshold of 7–8 g/dL was recommended for coronary heart disease patients by the American College of Physicians, it was graded as a weak recommendation based on low-quality evidence (Qaseem et al 2013, Curley et al 2014b).

The development of a bleeding complication in the cardiac patient could delay elective cardiovascular and other procedures, but urgent and emergency procedures were often approached with accelerated levels of blood transfusion and hemodynamic support dictated by clinical circumstances.

Some patients in need of elective procedures were also managed with transfusion-based replacement therapy so that inconvenient delays could be avoided. Stable patients were not infrequently transfused preoperatively as a "safety buffer," for "added security" when blood counts were under perceived threat.

Emphasis was not placed on altering clinical approaches before, during, or after procedures for the goal of reducing bleeding and anemia because replacing volume and transfusing the patient appeared to be expedient, simple enough, and "well tolerated." Early public relations campaigns promoting the donation of blood as a lifesaving endeavor helped to reinforce this mindset. Because of the relative ease of this approach, patients were frequently unnecessarily transfused or even over-transfused (Barr et al 2011). Preventive maneuvers prior to clinical events, strategies for improved hemostasis, and choices and handling of antithrombotic therapy were deployed haphazardly, if at all. The traditional approach to anemia and bleeding outlined above was codified in standard medical manuals and textbooks, and held as the community standard. Peer criticism, institutional review, and potential medicolegal action could be in store for the practitioner who veered off the transfusion-based fix or recipe (Soutoul and Pierre 1988).

7.3.3 Impact of Anemia, Bleeding, and Transfusion on Cardiovascular Disease Outcomes: The Case for PBM in Cardiology

In the last two decades, there has been an increasing evidence base clarifying the association between bleeding, anemia, and transfusion on the one hand and the risk of adverse outcomes on the other for the patient with cardiovascular disease. Studies have demonstrated a significant incidence—higher than previously anticipated—of anemia in this patient population, ranging from 3.4% to 89.45% depending on the subset (Dewilde et al 2014, Shander et al 2014b). Among patients with acute myocardial infarction 15% may be anemic, and among elderly patients the percentage can exceed 40% (Wu et al 2001). The annual bleeding risk can be as high as 45%, depending on the specific combinations of antithrombotic therapy (Dewilde et al 2014). Although the majority of cases of anemia might be the result of iron deficiency, many cardiac patients have anemia compounded by procedural blood loss, blood testing, concomitant medications, another metabolic deficiency, or a chronic disease. Congestive heart failure and renal dysfunction may also play a role along with related erythropoietin deficiency (Vogiatzi et al 2010). More chronic forms of anemia offer an opportunity for earlier detection and proper correction.

Note

Among patients with acute myocardial infarction, 15 % may be anemic, and among elderly patients the percentage can exceed 40 %. The major cause of anemia among cardiac patients is iron deficiency; other causes include procedural blood loss, blood testing, certain medications, another metabolic deficiency, or a chronic disease.

The derangements in physiology caused by bleeding and acute or chronic anemia have special implications for the cardiology patient, and it has been hypothesized that they contribute directly to the observed poorer outcomes; however, the mechanism by which this influence occurs is poorly understood.

Hypovolemia and acute blood loss are associated with hemodynamic compromise, hypotension, and tachycardia. Compensatory mechanisms are activated that are designed to increase the cardiac output and maintain tissue oxygenation. Hemodynamic changes trigger a hyperadrenergic state with catecholamine excess that could destabilize patients with various combinations of cardiomyopathy, valvular disease, and coronary disease. In those with coronary artery atherosclerosis, sheer stress and vasomotion may play a role in the disruption of thin-capped fibroatheromas with associated plaque rupture, clot activation, and vessel thrombosis (Arbab-Zadeh and Fuster 2015). Patients with coronary artery disease can also be destabilized by "demand ischemia." Compromised oxygen carrying capacity can further exacerbate ischemia and cause additional left ventricular dysfunction (Levy et al 1996). With worsening severity of anemia, ischemia and adverse outcomes are observed with increased frequency (Amsterdam et al 2014).

In recent years, the role of transfusion of allogeneic blood has come under considerable scrutiny. A growing literature reveals that there is significant risk and less benefit than traditionally thought from transfusing RBCs (Rao and Sherwood 2014, Velibey et al 2014). While the many potential issues related to the transfusion of blood and blood products are well detailed in other chapters, there are specific blood-product-mediated effects that are particularly salient in the cardiovascular patient who might be a candidate for transfusion. Volume replenishment affects cardiac mechanics via Starling forces and needs to be carefully titrated to provide desirable, and avoid unwanted, results. Hypotension and volume depletion need to be reversed to achieve normovolemia without overshooting appropriate filling pressures as the cardiac patient may be less tolerant than others in handling sudden volume changes. Excessive volume loading with transfusion has not infrequently put patients into acute pulmonary edema, and diuretics and nitrates may need to be given. Patients with diastolic and/or systolic dysfunction appear to be particularly susceptible, as are patients with stenotic or regurgitant valvular disease. Volume-mediated acute pulmonary edema is associated with a potentially dangerous combination of tachycardia, hypertension, increases in sympathetic tone, and hypoxemia. Moreover, the vascular rheology is negatively impacted by increased viscosity and changes in the blood that have been demonstrated to reduce blood flow rates down to capillary vessels. Blood thrombogenicity and platelet activation can be altered with a resultant tendency to thrombotic events (Velibey et al 2014).

Transfusion also alters the blood oxygen dissociation curve, and tissue oxygenation does not change or may actually decrease with transfusion (Shander et al 2011b, Rao and Sherwood 2014, Velibey et al 2014). Intracellular mechanisms within myocytes can cause a downregulation of mechanics, altering relaxation characteristics of the contractile apparatus and compromising systolic and diastolic performance. To date, no adjunctive therapies exist that can reverse these effects.

Although infrequent, other potentially catastrophic problems can pose a significant additional threat to the cardiology patient, who might destabilize with additional stressors. These problems include acute rejection reactions, TRALI, and transfusion-related infections. Acute myocardial infarction that appeared directly mediated by transfusion has been reported, although the mechanism remains to be elucidated (Wang et al 2008).

Standard medications that are known to be useful for treating the cardiac patient may be relatively contraindicated in the patient with acute anemia or bleeding, and their discontinuation can have negative consequences (Liu et al 2012). Antithrombotic therapy with antiplatelet agents, including those used for dual antiplatelet therapy (DAPT), and anticoagulants may need to be avoided. Hypotension or borderline blood pressures may limit the use of diuretics, β-blockers, angiotensin-converting enzyme inhibitors, and other receptor blockers, along with that of nitrates. The withdrawal of these agents can be associated with increased risks of congestive heart failure, vasospasm, ischemia, and thrombosis.

> **Note**
>
> Useful standard medications for the cardiac patient may be relatively contraindicated in patients with acute anemia or bleeding, and their discontinuation can have negative consequences.

7.3.4 Fundamentals of PBM in Cardiology: Algorithm for Optimal Cardiovascular Therapeutics

With the help of programs initially designed to enhance treatment outcomes in patients who are Jehovah's Witnesses, progress has recently been made to replace the traditional strategy for treating bleeding and anemia with the universally applied systematic multimodal approach that is PBM (Moskowitz et al 2010, Emmert et al 2011, McCartney et al 2014).

The basic algorithm for improving cardiology patient outcomes through PBM is shown in **Box 7.1**. The potential for PBM in cardiology is best realized through data-driven approaches derived from well-designed quality studies that confirm proof of concept, and through the avoidance of habit or dogma in making treatment decisions. Strategies that are designed to maintain the hemoglobin concentration while optimizing hemostasis, minimizing blood loss, and preventing unwanted thrombosis are being defined and validated in a growing number of clinical studies (Subherwal et al 2009, Mehran et al 2010, Moskowitz et al 2010,

Shander et al 2011c, Abu-Assi et al 2012, Dewilde et al 2013, Amsterdam et al 2014, Murphy et al 2015b). Although current evidence-based data are limited and the decision tree is often complex, cardiology is in a key position to drive this process with a team approach.

> **Box 7.1 Recommendations for care of the patient with cardiovascular disease**
>
> **Prerequisites**
> - Education: Anemia, bleeding, and transfusion are associated with poor outcomes.
> - Communication: Health care team collaboration.
>
> **Recommendations**
> 1. Screen all patients for bleeding and anemia.
> 2. Correct anemia in all patients (preferably in advance).
> 3. Assess the risk of bleeding and anemia for all patients.
> 4. Prevent and minimize bleeding in all patients.
> 5. Assess and manage all patients for thrombotic and embolic risk, optimize therapy.
> 6. Manage bleeding aggressively in all patients.
> 7. A restrictive approach to RBC transfusion is recommended.
> 8. Understand data and knowledge gaps.
> 9. Recognize special populations with bleeding, anemia, and cardiovascular risk: blood management targets.

As noted, a number of cardiology patient subsets have a high prevalence of anemia and bleeding risk. These problems can be unappreciated and not treated, similar to the situation in other medical specialties. The lack of detection, evaluation, and management often represents an unmet medical need (Qaseem et al 2013). Data have suggested the cardiologist is particularly well suited to address this need (LaPar et al 2013). Regardless of whether the cardiologist is in charge of the patient as the attending physician, or is the consultant to an internist, surgeon, or hospitalist, facilitating optimal blood management can provide clinical rewards and better medical care. The recognition of both anemia and bleeding risk transforms these issues into modifiable factors that need proper management. Important to this role is the communication between the cardiologist and team members, so that care is coordinated and the planned

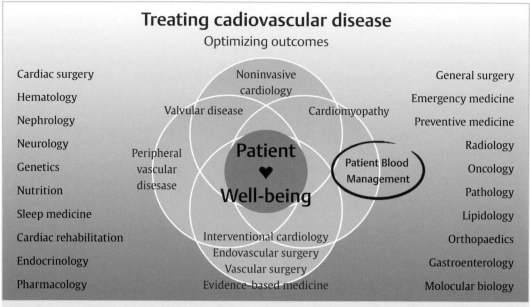

Fig. 7.4 Treating cardiovascular disease: optimizing outcomes.

time line of medical events is optimized. Education of health care team members, including colleagues across other specialties and all members of the heart team, will facilitate achievement of these goals. **Fig. 7.4** is a graphic representation of the multispecialty effort that is needed to provide quality care to the patient with cardiovascular disease. PBM is prominently and centrally displayed. Practicing PBM in cardiology implies the practice of good medicine.

Note

The recognition of anemia and bleeding risk transforms these issues into modifiable risk factors; their management can reduce patient morbidity or even save lives. An important aspect in this context is the communication between the cardiologist and team members, so that care is coordinated and the planned time line of medical events is optimized.

7.3.5 Recommendations for Care of the Patient with Cardiovascular Disease

Recommendation 1: Screen All Patients for Bleeding and Anemia

Although the detection of anemia can be surprisingly easy, i.e., either single hemoglobin determination or complete blood count, it is often ignored completely even in hospitalized patients. There should be a high index of suspicion to make the diagnosis as the individual patient's clinical course evolves. The diagnosis of anemia or bleeding may come to be made despite initial laboratory results that are in the normal range. Some of the challenge relates to undoing bad habits or a past mindset that chose not to emphasize borderline or low hemoglobin values as a significant problem. Not only does the definition of anemia vary for age and gender, as per the WHO guidelines (adult men < 13 g/dL, adult nonpregnant women < 12 g/dL), but women and patients with smaller body mass indexes and low normal hemoglobin can suddenly be found to be anemic after a few days of hospitalization or a series of even minor procedures, with attendant associated risks of allogeneic RBC transfusion and poorer outcomes. An anticipatory and prevention-oriented mindset is strongly recommended. Given the prevalence of anemia, it is reasonable to check hemoglobin measurements routinely in all cardiology patients and sequentially as outpatients, with more frequent laboratory tests through a patient's hospital stay. Judgment should be applied using details of the individual's clinical scenario to determine the optimal frequency of laboratory testing, but less may be more, and a reduced sample size or pediatric tubes might be considered to limit bloodletting. Some guidelines recommend that preadmission testing with hemoglobin measurement be performed as early as 30 days and no less than 2 weeks before all planned surgical or invasive procedures. This time frame allows for corrective therapeutic actions with hematinics (Shander et al 2014b).

Recommendation 2: Correct Anemia in All Patients (Preferably in Advance)

▶ **Treatment of iron deficiency (most common).** Once anemia is detected and the diagnosis is made, the presence of iron deficiency should be assessed as it is the most common cause of anemia. Traditional markers of iron deficiency anemia (MCV, transferrin saturation, and ferritin) may have some limitations for assessing the adequacy of the iron supply for erythropoiesis. The serum transferrin saturation is preferred as the primary index to evaluate the iron status. Oral supplementation with ascorbic acid is recommended to improve absorption and transport if tests suggest an iron deficiency, but this may prove to be ineffective in stressed and hospitalized patients. The decision to use intravenous iron supplementation would guarantee the immediate restoration of iron stores, independent of gut transport. RBC transfusion is not an acceptable treatment for iron deficiency. Referral of patients with iron deficiency anemia and no history of overt bleeding from nongastrointestinal sources should be considered for upper and lower endoscopic investigation of the underlying cause of blood loss. Screening for folate and vitamin B_{12} deficiency should also be considered with supplementation as needed. Specialist referral should be considered for chronic kidney disease with a glomerular filtration rate of less than 60 mL/min and an elevated creatinine level. Hematology/oncology referral

may be indicated for assessing and treating malignancy and myelodysplastic syndrome (Shander et al 2014b).

▶ **Erythropoietin-stimulating agents (cautious use).** Erythropoietin-stimulating agents should be considered in the absence of iron deficiency or following unsuccessful treatment with iron. Erythropoietin-stimulating agents are indicated for anemia of chronic disease and although there have been a few safety concerns, they are well tolerated and effective in the prescribed dose range (Manns and Tonelli 2012). Careful long-term use of erythropoietin may be recommended in selected patients with chronic kidney disease but not in patients with chronic congestive heart failure (correction of iron deficiency is effective) (Roubille et al 2014). In the short term, erythropoietin-stimulating agents have been given preoperatively to anemic patients and have been shown to be safe and effective at reducing the RBC transfusion rate and improving patient outcomes (Cladellas et al 2012, McCartney et al 2014). Care should be taken to avoid an excessive increase in hemoglobin (> 15 g/dL) and overdosage in nonresponders.

> **Note**
>
> With erythropoietin therapy, an excessive increase in hemoglobin and overdosage in nonresponders should be avoided.

▶ **Other corrective measures.** In addition to antiplatelet and anticoagulant medications, certain pharmaceuticals can be associated with different forms of anemia. Medication lists should be reviewed and drugs associated with anemia should be discontinued (Shander et al 2011c).

Attempts to optimize hemoglobin levels in patients having invasive procedures with risk of bleeding are recommended (see Recommendation 5). The invasive or surgical procedure type as well as its urgency and associated bleeding risk should determine the goal for anemia therapy. No firm hemoglobin targets for specific invasive procedures have been determined, but avoiding overtreatment is recommended.

The prevention of additional bleeding is an integral component of correcting anemia (see Recommendation 3). The role of transfusion in correcting anemia is increasingly debated with growing data supporting a restrictive approach (see Recommendation 7).

Recommendation 3: Assess All Patients for Bleeding and Anemia Risk

The concept of risk estimation for a patient's development of bleeding and anemia differs from simple screening (see Recommendation 1) in that it helps to predict the development of future adverse blood-related events, thereby targeting that patient for preventive strategies. A number of scoring systems for risk calculation in cardiology patients have been proposed. Calculation of a bleeding risk score for patients with acute coronary syndromes or atrial fibrillation (Subherwal et al 2009, Mehran et al 2010, Abu-Assi et al 2012, Gombotz and Knotzer 2013) can help to predict the risk and define the aggressiveness of clinical strategies for the maintenance of hemoglobin—the higher the risk the more measures need to be employed. In addition, a focused history of past anemia and bleeding events, including bleeding complicating past invasive procedures, should be detailed along with a review of any current bleeding symptoms. Predisposing comorbidities should also be defined. Other pathology not infrequently coexists with cardiovascular disease that further adds to the risk of anemia and bleeding. These include gastrointestinal, pulmonary, neurologic, nephrologic, urologic, endocrine, rheumatologic, and orthopaedic abnormalities that either directly or indirectly add to the bleeding risk or have related therapies that do. A review of recently taken medications and supplements, antiplatelet therapy, antithrombotic therapy, nonsteroidal anti-inflammatory drugs (NSAIDs), and steroids is recommended even if the patient is not currently anemic or bleeding. Combinations of therapies associated with bleeding risk need to be recognized. Taking a bleeding history and evaluating a broader array of laboratory data is basic to the effort of assessing risk compared with the simple anemia screening mentioned. Complete blood counts, activated partial thromboplastin time, prothrombin time, electrolytes, blood urea nitrogen, liver function tests, and stool guaiacs should be considered part of the clinical assessment. Additional hematology and oncology assessments may uncover an occult malignancy, a coagulopathy, and/or a thrombophilia that directly affects medical therapy and risk management. The bleeding risk associated with these problems can be more than additive.

Recommendation 4: Prevent and Minimize Bleeding in All Patients

▶ **Gastroprotective therapy.** Gastrointestinal prophylaxis should be strongly considered for a broad array of patients with cardiovascular disease, including patients taking nonaspirin NSAIDs and cardiac-dose aspirin (81 mg), patients at risk receiving low-dose aspirin therapy, and patients receiving combined aspirin and anticoagulant therapy (including heparin, low-molecular weight heparin, warfarin, and the new oral anticoagulants [NOACs]). For gastroprotection in patients taking aspirin or NSAIDs, proton pump inhibitors are preferred over misoprostol and H_2 blockers. Proton pump inhibitors should also be prescribed to at-risk patients receiving $P2Y_{12}$ inhibitors, alone or with aspirin, although this therapy may decrease the antiplatelet effects of clopidogrel and its effects on cardiovascular outcomes have been a source of debate (Shah et al 2015). The role of pharmacogenetic testing or platelet function testing in managing therapy with $P2Y_{12}$ inhibitors and proton pump inhibitors has not yet been established. In patients with a history of ulcer disease, testing for and eradicating *Helicobacter pylori* before starting antiplatelet therapy should be considered (Bhatt et al 2008, Abraham et al 2010).

▶ **Drug therapy adjustments.** Unnecessary agents known to be associated with bleeding should be avoided. Any medicines potentially associated with bleeding should be titrated for body weight and renal function. Alertness for drug interactions is required, particularly with concurrent vitamin-K-dependent anticoagulants.

Advance preparation is recommended for all patients having elective or urgent invasive procedures with bleeding risk. This should include the withholding of antiplatelet and/or antithrombotic therapy for an appropriate time interval. A reliable pharmaceutical reference should be checked for guidance because the length of time for appropriate discontinuation can vary with the specific drug, patient characteristics, and type of procedure. A risk–benefit analysis is often needed in making these decisions, along with the decision as to when to safely resume treatment. In a study of aspirin in patients at risk of vascular complications preparing to undergo noncardiac surgery, aspirin had no effect on death or nonfatal myocardial infarction but increased the risk of major bleeding

(Devereaux et al 2014). There are now many anti-platelet and anticoagulant options with over a hundred possible combinations of these medicines, each having their own potential effect on outcomes, and specific pharmacodynamic and bioavailability characteristics. Detailed knowledge is needed to optimize their use to prevent thrombosis while keeping bleeding risks at bay. The best combinations of these agents are not defined to date (Dewilde et al 2014).

Recent data indicate that reduced bleeding is observed in patients undergoing coronary interventions if they are treated with bivalirudin instead of heparin and a glycoprotein IIb/IIIa inhibitor (Palmerini et al 2013). However, there is an ongoing debate related to early thrombotic events with bivalirudin and the bleeding rates of these competing strategies (Palmerini et al 2013, ElGuindy 2014). Bridging anticoagulation strategies should be avoided as they appear to be associated with an increased risk of overall and major bleeding without reducing thromboembolic events, compared with nonbridging (Douketis et al 2015, Siegal et al 2012).

▶ **Preoperative and intraoperative prevention for catheterization and surgical procedures.** All non-essential invasive procedures should be avoided and the risks and benefits of procedures should be carefully weighed. Procedures on patients with active bleeding should be deferred unless there is a suspicion of loss of limb, organ, or life. Elective procedures should be rescheduled to manage anemia first. Anemia is a contraindication for elective procedures, especially if high blood loss is anticipated. A strategy of routine RBC transfusion in stable patients with anemia is not recommended but routine hematinics (e.g., iron, vitamin B_{12}) are.

> **Note**
>
> Anemia is a contraindication for elective procedures, especially if high blood loss is anticipated, and a strategy of routine RBC transfusion in stable anemic patients is not recommended.

Attempts should be made to modify all invasive procedures to reduce the bleeding risk. Proper planning of procedures and preparation for untoward events is recommended. A procedural time-out and a preoperative checklist have been used to reduce error rates with surgical or invasive procedures, and these can also be used to optimize and affect the blood management plan. The time-out and checklist can facilitate the review of comorbidities and bleeding risk; in one study, this strategy changed the management related to anemia and transfusion in 20 % of the patients (Myers et al 2015). Selection of the radial artery instead of the femoral artery as the access site reduces bleeding and improves outcomes in catheterization procedures (Grossman et al 2009, Verheugt et al 2011, Romagnoli et al 2012, Kikkert et al 2014, McDonagh et al 2015). Vessel access should be performed meticulously with the single-wall vessel puncture technique (not transfixion) using small needles, the fewest possible attempts, and imaging or boney landmarks for guidance (to avoid "high" or "low" sticks). Both the catheter and the wound size should be kept as small as posssible. To limit periprocedural blood loss related to blood sampling, unused blood sampling withdrawals should be immediately reinfused before specimen clotting occurs. Attempts should be made to employ a mindset that encourages all drapes to be unstained by blood at the end of the procedure. Also important is the simplification and minimization of intraprocedural antithrombotic therapy. In addition, vascular access sheath removal should be appropriately timed with the offset of discontinued blood thinner effects. Although closure devices have not been shown to reduce access and bleeding site complications, meticulous access site management and closure of arterial wounds with reliable hemostasis, particularly for larger structural heart interventions, is prerequisite (Hamid et al 2015).

In the operating room, techniques to prevent and minimize bleeding (described in detail elsewhere) include meticulous and less traumatic surgical technique, normovolemic hemodilution, proper volume replacement, coagulogram guidance, cell salvage, and use of hemostatic agents (Santos et al 2014). Postprocedure, patients need to be monitored carefully, educated for signs of bleeding, and checked at reasonable intervals for occult bleeding. The family and care providers need education as well.

Recommendation 5: Assess and Manage All Patients for Thrombotic and Embolic Risk, Optimize Therapies

Thrombosis is central to the pathophysiology of atherosclerotic and other cardiovascular disease, and antithrombotic treatment is a mainstay of effective therapy. Preventive therapeutic strategies, directed at risk factor modification, plaque stabilization and regression, deep vein thrombosis, and embolic risk need to be emphasized in at-risk patients. Patients on antithrombotic medications need to be kept on the simplest regimen possible. Prevention of thrombosis is basic to care management because once a thrombotic event occurs, more aggressive therapy with antithrombotics for longer time periods is often warranted. For example, a brief course of enoxaparin for the prophylaxis of deep vein thrombosis may preclude months of vitamin-K-dependent oral anticoagulation or the use of a NOAC. Similarly, aspirin may be appropriate for antiembolic prophylaxis in a young patient with atrial fibrillation and a CHA_2DS_2-Vasc score of less than two, but once a stroke or transient ischemic attack occurs, lifetime anticoagulation is needed.

Evolving device therapies are likely to play a growing role in antithrombotic and antiembolic risk reduction. Controversy surrounds the placement and management of inferior vena cava filters for the treatment of venous thromboembolism in patients in whom anticoagulants are contraindicated or have failed, even when the filters are retrievable (Weinberg et al 2013). The Watchman device (Boston Scientific) is now available for reducing the risk of thromboembolism in patients with nonvalvular atrial fibrillation and an increased risk of stroke, where there is a concern about the risks of long-term anticoagulant agents due to bleeding risk (Alli et al 2015).

Recommendation 6: Manage Active Bleeding Aggressively in All Patients

Aggressive control of bleeding sites is warranted in cardiac patients who are actively bleeding. Volume replacement with appropriate expanders can be critical to maintaining hemodynamic stability. Cardiac medications that could compromise hemodynamics should be given in reduced dosage or held, but tolerating mild hypotension can help

to limit blood loss. When a specific defect in coagulation is known to exist, targeted correction should be considered. Cautious cessation of antithrombotic and antiplatelet therapy needs to be considered. Antithrombotic and antiplatelet therapy should be resumed in a careful but timely manner once stability is achieved and the clinical course becomes clear. The bleeding cardiac patient should be assessed for anemia-related compromised end organ physiology as this could dictate the potential need for transfusion. Serial electrocardiograms, cardiac enzymes, rhythm monitoring, and clinical surveillance are basic to this care. Ultimately, targeted arterial therapy, including mechanical occlusion with ligatures, clips, cautery, or embolization, may need to be employed.

> **Note**
>
> Active bleeding has to be stopped aggressively.

Recommendation 7: A Restrictive Approach to Red Blood Cell Transfusion Is Recommended

Although transfusion is "culturally" embedded as the default therapy, most of the time, anemia can be tolerated by the patient as other corrective measures are pursued. Paradoxically, in most cases it is not the patient but the doctor who does not tolerate the anemia (Santos et al 2014). In stable conditions, reduced hemoglobin levels can be compensated for by a rise in the cardiac output, vasodilation, and an increase in tissue oxygen extraction. End organ function is maintained. As noted, anemia is common in patients with cardiovascular disease, but in most cases it has no immediate clinical impact. For the vast majority of cardiac patients, including those with more severe reductions in hemoglobin, there is no ongoing anemia-mediated derangement in physiology that would be helped by the transfusion of allogeneic blood. In one series of patients with active gastrointestinal bleeding who refused to accept RBCs and had hemoglobin values of less than 3 g/dL, over 50% of the patients survived (Sharma et al 2015). In fact, extremely low hemoglobin levels of less than 2 g/dL can often be tolerated as long as fundamental and supportive therapies are provided. Tolerance to low hemoglobin levels is supported by measures that optimize oxygen delivery while minimizing oxygen consumption. Directed management and continuous reevaluation of supported oxygenation, blood pressure, cardiac output, and circulating blood volume (with titrated crystalloids) should be performed with appropriate analgesia, sedation, maintenance of normothermia, and possibly mechanical ventilation. The hematocrit and hemoglobin are not adequate measures of tissue oxygen delivery, but monitoring for oliguria, reduced renal function, decreased sensorium, lactic acidosis, tachycardia, and myocardial ischemia can provide clues (Santos et al 2014). Patient characteristics, including the medical or surgical context, presence and rate of bleeding, time frame for managing the primary clinical problem, treatability of the primary disease, and presence of comorbidities, along with careful surveillance for evidence of end organ ischemic dysfunction, will determine whether transfusion may be warranted. In the more challenging patients who present with anemia and cardiac instability, including congestive heart failure and acute coronary syndromes, managing the primary cardiac condition while embracing evidenced-based cardiology standards should be the priority along with stopping active bleeding and hematinic therapies. More data are needed on how to modify strategies when anemia is severe or bleeding is ongoing. In patients with cardiovascular disease, the anemia is most often not the sole culprit responsible for the patient's cardiac problems. Transfusion, with its inherent risks and unproven efficacy, could be considered as a last resort when there is ongoing instability in the face of maximal cardiac therapy and no acceptable alternative. The presence or threat of anemia should not disarm the cardiovascular specialist. Instead, it should encourage him or her to utilize appropriate evidence-based tools to craft a safer path for the patient.

The goals of transfusion are to reverse the clinical condition and avoid organ ischemia. In deciding to transfuse, assessment for compromised end organ physiology is paramount, and for each unit of blood a clear indication should exist. The transfusion of blood is not an acceptable form of volume replacement. Avoiding laboratory thresholds should help to limit overtransfusion and inappropriate transfusion. Numerous studies comparing restrictive versus liberal transfusion approaches have shown noninferiority or benefit of the former (Santos et al 2014, Murphy et al 2015). As summarized in recent guidelines, a restrictive transfusion strategy should be used instead of a liberal

transfusion strategy in patients with acute coronary syndromes, and a strategy of routine RBC transfusion in hemodynamically stable patients and hemoglobin levels greater than 8 mg/dL is not recommended (Amsterdam et al 2014).

Recommendation 8: Understand Data and Knowledge Gaps

There has been an exciting accumulation of knowledge concerning the importance and issues related to maintaining the hemoglobin concentration across an array of patients, but much is unknown. Better tools are needed for the detection and risk stratification of bleeding and anemia in the cardiology patient. There is an ongoing need to define the role of confounders on cardiovascular outcomes. Although major bleeding is now more consistently defined, with "universally" accepted definitions, and ranks as a coprimary endpoint in many trials, these issues need ongoing surveillance as advances are released to the health care community. Major bleeding is important when assessing the "net clinical benefit" of a new drug or therapy, but nonmajor bleeding might affect physician and patient behaviors, altering outcomes.

There are knowledge gaps concerning best practices for this patient population with respect to the treatment of anemia, including the roles of intravenous iron and brief courses of erythropoietin. More research is needed that targets optimal therapeutics in different clinical situations involving blood loss and anemia, particularly when combined agents are needed. What role is played by standard medications for different cardiac conditions and how are these medicines adjusted in the anemic or bleeding patient? Can trials be designed to tease out the optimal use in anemic patients of medicines beyond antiplatelet and antithrombotic therapy, including β-blockers, nitrates, calcium channel blockers, ranolazine, and proton pump inhibitors? More data of the type that help to establish guidelines, from randomized double-blind placebo-controlled trials, are needed on how to modify strategies when cardiac disease and anemia are severe or active bleeding is occurring.

Recommendation 9: Recognize Populations with Bleeding, Anemia, and Cardiovascular Risk: Blood Management Targets

▶ **Risk stratification potential.** Even though there are many knowledge gaps concerning the use of PBM in cardiology, there are special subsets of cardiovascular patients that need to be recognized so that full resources can be directed at improving their clinical outcomes. These patients are at significant risk of adverse events and represent the greatest challenge to the cardiologist.

In practical terms, treatments and procedures planned for all patients should take into account the risk of bleeding, anemia, and transfusion and give precedence to treatment approaches known to minimize the risk of blood loss. Bleeding avoidance strategies appear to be of the greatest benefit in higher-risk patients (Chhatriwalla et al 2013). Although more robust risk calculators for different patient presentations are needed, there are some special groups that deserve mention—subsets where outcomes could potentially be most responsive to blood conservation.

▶ **Hospitalized patients.** Inpatients have a high prevalence of bleeding and anemia, which may be hospital-acquired or exacerbated. Although this may be related to underlying disease states, it is compounded by standing orders for blood work, and unnecessary diagnostic testing and blood withdrawal. Not infrequently, blood is withdrawn as a clearing specimen only to be discarded. Various drug therapies and factors associated with the higher-acuity illness of inpatients also contribute to the risk of bleeding and anemia. Stress, antithrombotic therapy, steroids, anti-inflammatory drugs, chemotherapy, and invasive procedures can play a role.

▶ **Elderly patients.** Anemia should not be dismissed as merely the result of aging. This population has a higher incidence of gastrointestinal pathology and related iron deficiency (Abraham et al 2013). Malabsorption, vitamin B_{12} deficiency, chronic kidney disease, malnutrition, and anemia of chronic disease are all more prevalent in elderly patients. Frailty and the higher probability of multiple coexisting diseases also have a negative impact. The problem of frailty may independently contribute to outcomes as has been noted in pa-

tients undergoing TAVR. Quality of life and outcomes have been shown to correlate with anemia (Shander et al 2014b). Transfusion rates appear to increase with age. In addition, in this population, the role of nonmajor bleeding should not be underestimated. Bleeding that is superficial or "nuisance" could lead to the discontinuation of needed antiplatelet or antithrombotic therapy, which could result in subsequent thrombotic complications, such as stent thrombosis.

▶ **Women.** Female gender is associated with anemia and transfusion. Women have been noted for some time by the American Heart Association to have poorer outcomes in cardiovascular disease compared with men. They have more bleeding and poorer outcomes than men with acute coronary syndromes. They have poorer outcomes from cardiac surgery and interventional procedures. Some of these observations may be explained by provider biases in administering care and by a smaller anatomy, body mass, and intravascular volume, but women may also have more advanced age and different clinical presentation morbidities (Rogers et al 2006, Yu et al 2015).

▶ **Chronic kidney dysfunction.** Patients with impaired renal function are known to have a high prevalence of anemia with an increase in bleeding risk and poorer outcomes. Kidney disease is often associated with anemia driven by a decrease in erythropoietin. Coagulopathy in renal disease may contribute to bleeding and anemia (Jalal et al 2010). The RBC mass has been noted to be decreased, and hemodilution can worsen anemia especially in heart failure patients with kidney dysfunction. A cardiorenal syndrome has been proposed to describe the dysfunction associated with congestive heart failure and renal disease. Although accelerated atherosclerosis is seen and ischemic heart disease is the leading cause of death in these patients, there are few studies that define the best plan for optimal medical therapy in these patients.

▶ **Atrial fibrillation.** Patients who have atrial fibrillation or who require chronic oral anticoagulant therapy pose a particular challenge. The need for stroke prophylaxis with chronic oral anticoagulants is defined by the CHA_2DS_2-VASc score or a similar scoring system (Dewilde et al 2014). This population usually consists of older patients with higher rates of comorbidity. The HAS-BLED score has been proposed to measure the bleeding risk in patients with atrial fibrillation (Pisters et al 2010). When patients with atrial fibrillation need interventional, cardiac rhythm, or other procedures, their periprocedural management remains a common but difficult problem, with limited outcome data available (Kosiuk et al 2014). Other patients receiving chronic oral anticoagulant therapy for other indications, including those with a history of mechanical prosthetic valves, thrombophilia, pulmonary embolus, or deep vein thrombosis, are a similar challenge. About 30% to 50% of patients with atrial fibrillation have concomitant coronary artery disease, and in our rapidly aging population the number of people with both conditions is increasing. After percutaneous coronary intervention, these patients often require the addition of DAPT, with aspirin and a $P2Y_{12}$ inhibitor, in combination with ongoing oral anticoagulant therapy for stroke prophylaxis. DAPT and oral anticoagulants, or triple therapy, results in a high annual bleeding risk of 20% to 45% (Dewilde et al 2014). Somewhat controversial data suggest that dual therapy without aspirin but with a $P2Y_{12}$ inhibitor (clopidogrel was mainly studied) and a vitamin-K-dependent antagonist is effective at stroke prevention without an increase in stent thrombosis (Hall 1993, Vogiatzi et al 2010, Dewilde et al 2013).

In contrast, stable patients with coronary artery disease have a low incidence of major bleeding (0.6% per year) and the site of bleeding is most often gastrointestinal (To et al 2009). Despite the low incidence, major bleeding in stable ischemic heart disease is significantly associated with a nearly threefold increased risk of mortality. This risk is associated with the use of vitamin K antagonists and particularly evident if these drugs are combined with antiplatelet therapy. Interestingly, combining aspirin with anticoagulant therapy did not reduce the risk of thrombotic events, including cardiovascular death, myocardial infarction, and nonhemorrhagic stroke (Hamon et al 2014). Combined therapies may appear to be indicated for the treatment of concurrent medical problems, but they carry a bleeding risk that is high and better strategies are needed.

The NOACs, including dabigatran, rivaroxaban, apixaban, and edoxaban, are touted for their safety in patients with nonvalvular atrial fibrillation. Although they have shifted the safety and outcome spectrum compared with warfarin for the prophy-laxis of stroke, concerns have been raised including the lack of readily available means to assess the degree of anticoagulation and the lack of a readily available reversal strategy. The acutely irreversible coagulopathy associated with NOAC therapy can result in life-threatening bleeding complications especially after trauma (Cotton et al 2011, Kosiuk et al 2014), but specific antidotes may soon be available (Pollack et al 2015). Moreover, some of these agents have significant renal clearance, and a decline in renal function can cause an increased risk of drug-related bleeding. Safety data are needed to support the combination of NOACs with aspirin or $P2Y_{12}$ inhibitors for the different clinical scenarios calling for combined agents.

▶ **Percutaneous coronary intervention and acute coronary syndromes.** Patients undergoing coronary intervention and those with acute coronary syndromes, including unstable angina, ST-elevation myocardial infarction, and non-ST-elevation myocardial infarction, have a significant prevalence of anemia- and bleeding-associated untoward events (Amsterdam et al 2014). Scoring systems have been developed for assessing both bleeding and ischemic risk, and the predictors largely overlap (Bassand 2009, Subherwal et al 2009, Mehran et al 2010, Abu-Assi et al 2012). Patients with anemia have more comorbidities, differences in revascularization, and a lower likelihood of receiving medicines that enhance survival. These patients are often subjected to other factors that worsen bleeding and anemia, including blood drawing; interventional therapy; treatment with combinations of aspirin, $P2Y_{12}$ inhibitors, glycoprotein IIb/IIIa inhibitors, and/or antithrombotics; and other invasive procedures including use of an intra-aortic balloon pump or placement of left ventricular assist devices. Female gender, frailty, older age, impaired renal function, heart failure, peripheral artery disease, diabetes mellitus, and instability (heart rate, blood pressure, shock) at admission appear to be independent predictors (Bassand 2009, Yu et al 2015). There are many factors that may contribute to procedure-related bleeding and transfusion risk that are modifiable: choice of guide catheter size (Grossman et al 2009), stent type, adjunctive devices, access site, access technique, antithrombotic regimen, patient preparation, gastrointestinal prophylaxis, approach to transfusion, and use of erythropoietin (Arant et al 2004, Sabatine et al

2005, Bhatt et al 2008, Subherwal et al 2009, Abraham et al 2010, Mehran et al 2010, Levine et al 2011, Nicolau et al 2013). A new rapid onset/offset intravenous $P2Y_{12}$ agent, cangrelor, is now available that will give the interventionalist additional management options (Lhermusier et al 2015).

If bleeding occurs, subsequent antiplatelet therapy use may be compromised. The duration and use of DAPT significantly affects outcome (Wang et al 2008, Dewilde et al 2014, Mauri et al 2014). The optimal duration has not been defined and is a moving target but there may be advantages to continuing DAPT long term (Mauri et al 2014).

New generations of stents, including bioabsorbable platforms that have the potential to return the vessel functionally and anatomically closer to its native state, will require new study so that adjunctive management with respect to thrombosis and bleeding can be optimized.

▶ **Cardiothoracic surgery.** Patients who undergo cardiothoracic surgery, including coronary bypass and/or valve surgery, are at extreme risk of anemia, bleeding, and transfusion but therapeutic options exist (Santos et al 2014). The management of hemoglobin levels improves outcome in cardiothoracic surgery (Moskowitz et al 2010). New technologies are now being used to replace heart valves percutaneously with reduced but still substantial bleeding complications. Patients undergoing TAVR have bleeding complications that predict mortality to a lesser degree than bleeding complications in patients undergoing surgical aortic valve replacement (Binder et al 2014, Généreux et al 2014). Given these observations, transfusion has been recommended as a quality indicator in cardiac surgery (Shander and Goodnough 2010).

▶ **Other cardiology subsets.** Patients with congestive heart failure have an increased risk of venous and arterial thromboembolism, and often require treatment with antiplatelet and antithrombotic medication. In chronic heart failure, the incidence of anemia can vary from 15% to 70%. The prognosis in patients with congestive heart failure has been linked to anemia (Roubille et al 2014). Associated chronic or acute kidney disease, as fully manifested in cardiorenal syndromes, may decrease the production of erythropoietin and independently cause significant disorders of hemostasis (Jalal et al 2010).

Other subsets of patients who have a potential for enhanced outcomes with the application of PBM principles include cardiac patients undergoing noncardiac surgery, electrophysiology patients, patients with cerebrovascular disease, patients in critical care, and patients who meet newly established criteria for frailty.

Conclusion

Invasive strategies and antithrombotic therapy remain at the core of treatment for cardiovascular disease and have reduced the frequency of death and untoward events in patients with cerebrovascular disease, acute coronary syndromes, and peripheral vascular disease. Moreover, the coupling of invasive procedures with the increasing use of combinations of more potent pharmaceuticals, including aspirin, $P2Y_{12}$ platelet inhibitors, heparin or low-molecular weight heparin, glycoprotein IIb/IIIa inhibitors, direct thrombin inhibitors, vitamin-K-dependent anticoagulants, and NOACs, has been associated with an increased risk of bleeding.

In this chapter, the importance of anemia and bleeding for an array of cardiology patients, often related to their antithrombotic regimens and invasive surgical or interventional procedures, was reviewed with an emphasis on strategies for improving outcomes. The evidence base for improving outcomes in cardiology patients through medical and surgical management concepts designed to maintain the hemoglobin concentration while optimizing hemostasis, minimizing blood loss, and preventing unwanted thrombosis was reviewed for key areas of cardiovascular care. Available data-driven evidence was synthesized to present a reasonable algorithm to realize the potential for PBM in cardiology.

The cardiology team's cognizance of blood-related issues along with optimized management strategies for achieving the correct balance between anti-ischemic benefits and the bleeding risk of antithrombotic drugs and procedures is key to caring for patients with cardiovascular issues and improving their survival. More quality clinical studies pointed at cardiovascular PBM issues are needed. The evidenced-based data directing management decisions for attaining optimal outcomes will continue to expand for the benefit of our patients. That said, this chapter could be retitled "Potential for Cardiology in PBM."

Chapter 8

Practical Implementation of PBM and Outlook

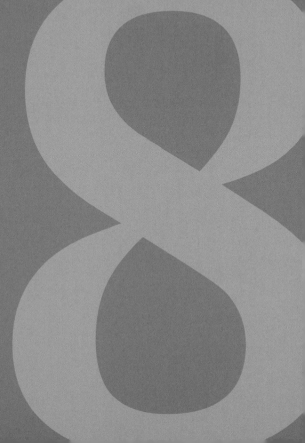

8.1 PBM and Outcome

D. R. Spahn

8.1.1 Outcome after the Implementation of First-pillar Measures

In 2010, the WHO adopted PBM as one of the most important aspects of transfusion safety (WHO 2010b). This is important because preoperative anemia is frequent (Kulier and Gombotz 2001, Guralnik et al 2004) and it independently increases the postoperative morbidity and mortality (Musallam et al 2011, Jans et al 2014), increases the 90-day readmission rate (Jans et al 2014), and prolongs hospitalization (Williams et al 2013, Jans et al 2014). This is true even for mild anemia (hemoglobin concentration of 10–13 g/dL in men; hemoglobin concentration of 10–12 g/dL in women) (Musallam et al 2011). In addition, preoperative anemia is a highly significant risk factor for perioperative red blood cell (RBC) transfusion (Gombotz et al 2007, Williams et al 2013, Jans et al 2014). RBC transfusions increase the postoperative mortality and morbidity further (Bernard et al 2009, Ferraris et al 2012) and they are associated with high costs (Shander et al 2010, Ferraris et al 2012).

The treatment of preoperative anemia (first pillar of PBM) (Goodnough and Shander 2012, Spahn and Goodnough 2013) lowers the RBC transfusion rate (Spahn 2010, Yoo et al 2011, Muñoz et al 2014b), the frequencies of acute kidney injury (Yoo et al 2011) and nosocomial infection (Muñoz et al 2014b), and the hospital length of stay (Muñoz et al 2014b). Interestingly, most benefits were also observed after very-short-term administration of intravenous iron and erythropoietin (Yoo et al 2011, Muñoz et al 2014b).

So-Osman et al (2014) assessed the effect of preoperative erythropoietin administration using a highly complex treatment protocol in patients undergoing hip or knee arthroplasty. Despite the fact that 34% of the patients randomized to the erythropoietin group did not even receive one of the four planned erythropoietin injections, the RBC transfusion rate decreased significantly from 26% to 16% in this group; the number of RBC units transfused per patient also decreased, from 0.7 units to 0.5 units, but the difference was not statistically significant. However, when the analysis was restricted to include only patients who had been treated per protocol, the proportion of transfused patients decreased significantly by 70% and the number of RBC units transfused per patient decreased by 62% (So-Osman et al 2014). Preoperative anemia treatment is therefore generally recommended prior to surgery (Gombotz 2011, Goodnough et al 2011, Goodnough and Shander 2012, Shander et al 2012b, Spahn and Goodnough 2013).

> **Note**
>
> The treatment of preoperative anemia is generally recommended prior to surgery.

8.1.2 Outcome after the Implementation of Second-pillar Measures

The avoidance of excessive blood loss (second pillar of PBM) is beneficial since high blood loss in itself—independently of preoperative anemia and allogeneic RBC transfusion—increases the mortality and morbidity. This has been demonstrated in patients undergoing cardiac surgery (Vivacqua et al 2011, Ranucci et al 2013). In the study by Vivacqua et al (2011), patients with high blood loss resulting in reoperation had an approximately threefold increased mortality and a twofold increased rate of major complications. In the study by Ranucci et al (2013), patients with major bleeding had a 3.5-fold increased mortality irrespective of whether they had received RBC transfusions.

In addition to meticulous surgical technique aimed at perfect local hemostasis, an important measure of the second pillar is the avoidance of perioperative coagulopathy by closely monitoring the patient's coagulation status using viscoelastic techniques and by providing targeted, individualized coagulation therapy (Spahn and Ganter 2010, Weber et al 2012, Bolliger and Tanaka 2013, Haas et al 2014). In a prospective randomized study of cardiac surgery patients with coagulopathy after heparin reversal, Weber and colleagues (2012) demonstrated that an algorithm based on rotational thromboelastometry and treatment with coagulation factor concentrates was effective in reducing the need for allogeneic blood products, with significant declines in the consumption of RBCs (median 5 units versus 3 units), fresh frozen plasma (FFP; median 5 units versus 0 units), and platelets (median 2 units versus 2 units. Postoperative blood loss was also reduced and the 6-month survival improved substantially (Weber et al 2012). Interestingly, the costs of hemotherapy were reduced by approximately 50%, from €3,109 to €1,658 per patient (Weber et al 2012). Similarly, Haas and colleagues (2014) found in children undergoing surgery for craniosynostosis that the introduction of an algorithm based on rotational thromboelastometry and treatment with coagulation factor concentrates significantly decreased the need for allogeneic blood products while the total costs of hemotherapy were decreased.

8.1.3 Outcome after the Implementation of Third-pillar Measures

The use of a restrictive hemoglobin transfusion threshold (third pillar of PBM) also results in better patient outcomes. In a study of more than 14,000 patients undergoing cardiac surgery, LaPar and colleagues (2013) found that the introduction of a restrictive transfusion regimen resulted in a reduction in RBC transfusions from 24% to 18% intraoperatively and from 39% to 33% postoperatively; the mortality was reduced from 1.8% to 1.0% and the rate of major postoperative complications was reduced from 15% to 13%. In addition, the total costs decreased from $30,500 to $26,200 (LaPar et al 2013). Villanueva and colleagues (2013a) showed in a prospective randomized multicenter study in patients with upper gastrointestinal bleeding that a restrictive transfusion regimen improved the survival, decreased the rate of complications, and reduced the hospital length of stay by approximately 2 days. A Cochrane meta-analysis including 19 prospective randomized studies and 6,264 patients indicated that the use of a restrictive transfusion strategy decreased RBC transfusions, in-hospital mortality, and infections (Carson et al 2012a).

> **Note**
>
> The use of a restrictive transfusion strategy does not only decrease the volume of RBC transfusions but also the in-hospital mortality and the rate of infections.

Another meta-analysis including 18 prospective randomized studies and 7,593 patients confirmed the reduction in RBC transfusions when using a restrictive hemoglobin transfusion threshold; moreover, the analysis showed that a restrictive strategy resulted in 30% fewer infections, particularly serious infections, and that this benefit was particularly relevant in orthopaedic surgery (Rohde et al 2014). A very interesting finding of this meta-analysis was that the benefit in lowering the incidence of postoperative infections was fully maintained when the analysis was limited to studies using leukocyte-reduced RBC transfusions.

8.1.4 Outcome after the Implementation of a Full PBM Program

In addition to studies showing the benefit of individual PBM measures, there are also reports on the outcomes after implementing a full PBM program (Moskowitz et al 2010, Kotze et al 2012, Leahy et al 2014, Theusinger et al 2014b). Moskowitz and colleagues (2010) demonstrated that the implementation of a PBM program in cardiac surgery resulted in reductions in the rate of RBC transfusions (from 43% to 11%), the rate of complications (from 26% to 11%), and the mortality (from 2.5% to 0.8%). Subsequently, Kotze and colleagues (2012) reported on the success of implementing PBM in orthopaedic surgery. They were able to reduce the rate of RBC transfusions from 23% to 7% in hip arthroplasty and from 7% to 0% in knee arthroplasty. In addition, the length of hospitalization decreased from 6 days to 5 days in hip arthroplasty and from 6 days to 4 days in knee arthroplasty, and the overall 90-day readmission rate decreased from 14% to 8% (Kotze et al 2012). In 2014, Leahy and colleagues reported on the success of implementing PBM in Western Australia; the mean number of RBC units used per admission declined by 26%, the use of FFP transfusions decreased by 38%, and the use of platelet transfusions decreased by 16%. Finally, Theusinger and colleagues (2014b) reported the results of implementing PBM in orthopaedic surgery; they focused on treating preoperative anemia, improving surgical technique, and lowering the hemoglobin threshold for transfusion to 8 g/dL. In a total of 8,871 patients undergoing major hip, knee, or spine surgery, this program decreased the transfusion rate from 20% to 10%.

Despite the great overall success of these PBM programs, it is interesting to note that they all implemented selected PBM measures only, while other measures were not implemented. This clearly indicates that the full potential of PBM has not yet been achieved in any of these centers.

PBM programs are not only beneficial in terms of the outcome of surgical patients; they also reduce the treatment costs substantially (Kotze et al 2012, Spahn et al 2012, Weber et al 2012, Cohn et al 2014, Haas et al 2014). Calculation of the total hospital costs for the population of orthopaedic surgery patients studied by Kotze et al (2012)—accounting for the reductions in RBC transfusion, length of hospitalization, and readmission—revealed that a net cost saving of at least £160,000 was achieved (Spahn et al 2012).

Conclusion

The combination of reduced transfusion rates, outcome benefits, and cost savings (**Box 8.1**) makes PBM programs highly attractive not only for patients but also for physicians and hospitals—a real win–win situation (Spahn et al 2012). As a consequence, PBM programs should be introduced as a matter of urgency.

Box 8.1 Outcome benefits of PBM

- Lower mortality
- Fewer complications
- Reduced hospital length of stay
- Lower costs

8.2 Establishment of PBM in Teaching and Practice

A. Hofmann, H. Gombotz

8.2.1 Establishment of PBM in the Literature, Teaching, and Continuing Education

A PubMed search for "Patient Blood Management [All Fields]" shows that this phrase was first used in 2007 in a publication by the Australian hematologist and transfusion specialist James Isbister (Isbister 2007). As early as 1988, Isbister advocated a paradigm shift in the use of RBC transfusion in clinical practice (Isbister 1988). In 2005, together with international colleagues and representatives of various medical societies, he coined the term *Patient Blood Management* during preparations for a symposium. The main intention was to enable a distinction between the new term and *Blood Management,* a term that mainly refers to activities related to blood banks and transfusion (Farmer et al 2013a). In 2008, the term *Patient Blood Management* first appeared in the title of a medical publication (Spahn et al 2008). From November 2012 to July 2015, the number of papers listed in PubMed and Embase that addressed the topic of PBM increased to 174. The articles appeared in journals from the fields of anesthesiology, intensive care medicine, general surgery, cardiac surgery, gynecology and obstetrics, internal medicine, hemotherapy, transfusion medicine, and oncology. Moreover, PBM has been featured in some of the major general medical journals. This unusually broad spectrum of journals reflects the fact that PBM is a multidisciplinary approach that has the potential to affect the treatment and outcome of millions of patients in the coming years.

The growing interest in PBM is also borne out by the increasing number of national and international societies that organize lectures on this subject and offer block sessions on PBM at conferences and symposia. Furthermore, several multidisciplinary medical societies exist that deal specifically with PBM and with hemotherapy strategies designed to improve patient outcome by avoiding and preempting the use of allogeneic blood products. Since 2012, the American Association of Blood Banks has also focused on this topic (www.aabb.org/pbm), albeit their definition of PBM does not in all respects concord with the definitions used in the literature or by specialist societies (SABM 2012).

Note

The concept of PBM is becoming ever more broadly established in the literature from various medical disciplines, and the topic is increasingly covered at symposia and conferences held by national and international professional societies.

8.2.2 Establishment of PBM as the Standard of Care in Australia

Australia has played a pioneering role in the implementation of PBM as the standard of care (Spahn et al 2008, Hofmann et al 2012, Leahy and Mukhtar 2012). In 2007, the Department of Health in Western Australia launched an initiative that became known as the *Western Australia PBM Program*. It was the world's first PBM program to be implemented across the public health system of an entire state or jurisdiction and has won widespread support among local, national, and international experts and clinicians.

▶ **Aims of the project.** The Western Australia PBM Program was launched to sustainably implement evidence-based PBM as the new standard of care in public hospitals and, with the involvement of general practitioners, in the preoperative management of anemia (www.health.wa.gov.au/blood-management). According to the 2011 Executive Summary, the initiative aims to improve patient outcomes by optimizing blood utilization and reducing inappropriate transfusions while at the same time delivering substantial cost savings. The program has also been described as an initiative focusing on quality, safety, and effectiveness with resource and financial implications (DHWA 2011). This rare combination of achieving improved treatment outcomes while using fewer resources is, of course, attractive and bolsters the implementation of PBM. To promote the implementation of PBM, the Western Australia Department of Health made increasingly more personnel available; it launched postgraduate training courses under the leadership of a multidisciplinary faculty; it ran training courses on surgical hemostasis in cooperation with the University of Western Australia; it helped create an IT infrastructure to support continuous benchmarking of transfusion and outcome; and it produced patient information on PBM.

▶ **Favorable structural conditions.** Favorable structural conditions continue to have a positive impact on the Western Australia PBM Program and enable the rapid implementation of PBM throughout Australia:
- The supply of blood and blood products at the national and state/territory level is managed and coordinated by the National Blood Authority

(NBA). In 2006, this government agency established a Clinical Advisory Council, which recommended the replacement of the then existing product-focused transfusion guidelines ("Guidelines on the Use of Blood and Blood Products" from 2001) with patient-focused guidelines. PBM was seen as the ideal clinical framework for these new guidelines. Subsequently, the NBA made sufficient funds available for the development of six comprehensive, evidence-based PBM guideline modules. These modules were developed under the direction of a national PBM Steering Committee with the support of an Expert Working Group (a multidisciplinary group of representatives from 14 professional societies in Australia/New Zealand), a Clinical Reference Group (hospital representatives), and a Consumer Reference Group (patient representatives) (NBA 2014; http://www.blood.gov.au). The six modules focus on PBM in the following areas: (1) Critical Bleeding/Massive Transfusion; (2) Perioperative Setting; (3) Medical; (4) Critical Care; (5) Obstetrics and Maternity; and (6) Pediatrics and Neonatology. At the time of writing, five of the six modules had been published, with publication of the sixth module expected in the near future (www.blood.gov.au/pbm-guidelines). The introduction to each module clearly states that PBM helps to improve outcomes by avoiding unnecessary RBC transfusions. Special emphasis is placed on the three-pillar model, highlighting the role of PBM in treating the potential reasons for transfusion with the implication that transfusion can be avoided in many clinical scenarios and is no longer the default decision.
- The national PBM guidelines refer to the Western Australia PBM Program as a model to be emulated at the transnational level.
- The Australian Commission on Safety and Quality in Health Care (ACSQHC), which was set up to drive the implementation of safety and quality systems in health care in Australia, considers PBM to be an important contributor to patient safety and treatment quality. The implementation of PBM is therefore an important criterion for the accreditation of hospitals to the blood and blood product standard developed by the ACSQHC (ACSQHC 2012).
- The Australian Red Cross Blood Service, which—under the supervision of the NBA—is responsible for the supply of all blood products in Australia, has supported all Australian PBM initiatives from

the start through continuing education programs and information materials for clinicians and patients covering PBM, the management of anemia, and related topics (ARCBS 2014a, ARCBS 2014b, Raison 2012).

• BloodSafe eLearning Australia—an amalgamation of statutory agencies and other qualified organizations—runs web-based training courses for clinicians that focus on transfusion medicine and PBM. By the middle of 2012, 135,000 clinicians and more than 700 hospitals had registered with this program, which includes training modules on the management of anemia and bleeding (https://bloodsafelearning.org.au).

In the meantime, private hospital organizations in Western Australia have also started to implement PBM on a large scale (Hollywood Private Hospital 2012).

Note

Australia has played a pioneering role in the implementation of PBM on a broad scale. Government authorities in Australia have created favorable conditions to promote this development. For example, previous transfusion guidelines in Australia were replaced with PBM guidelines. PBM enjoys the support of a large and growing number of clinicians from various disciplines and of the Australian Red Cross Blood Service.

8.2.3 PBM Programs in Other Countries

▶ **Austria.** The situation in Austria deserves particular mention. A benchmark study funded by the Austrian Federal Ministry of Health investigated the variability in blood transfusion practices before elective procedures at 18 public hospitals. The study revealed that PBM led to a significant reduction in the consumption of blood products while assuring a similar, or even better, outcome (Gombotz et al 2007). These results were confirmed by a second benchmark study, also funded by the Ministry of Health (see Chapter 1.6) (Gombotz et al 2012). In parallel to the first study, process cost analysis of the total expenditure for RBC transfusions was carried out, for example at Linz General Hospital (Austria's fourth largest hospital) (Shander et al 2010). Following

publication of the results of the First Austrian Benchmark Study, Linz General Hospital implemented a comprehensive PBM program. From 2005 to 2011, the number of RBCs transfused per hospital admission dropped from 14,000 to less than 6,000 (see **Fig. 1.9**, Chapter 1.6). In 2014, the total transfusion index at Linz General Hospital was at 0.16, which represents the lowest figure among the eight largest public hospitals in the country (H. Gombotz, oral communication, July 2015).

▶ **European Union and Switzerland.** In 2014, the Consumers, Health, Agriculture and Food Executive Agency of the European Commission announced a pilot program for the implementation of PBM in five European teaching hospitals (www.europe-pbm.eu). The main objectives of the project are (AIT 2014):

• To assess blood use in various medical specialties.
• To identify regional and national differences in terms of blood use and PBM strategies.
• To identify good practice in the field of PBM.
• To develop EU guidance on good practice related to PBM.

In addition, the Joint United Kingdom Blood Transfusion and Tissue Transplantation Services Professional Advisory Committee offers continuing support for the implementation of PBM.

According to Shander et al (2012b), efforts to implement PBM are undertaken in the Netherlands, Spain, Switzerland, and the United Kingdom. The authors also identified a number of obstacles to the widespread implementation of PBM, such as lack of awareness regarding the clinical impact of anemia on patient outcome, limited understanding of transfusion and adverse outcomes, behavioral issues, and misperceptions regarding the cost-effectiveness of transfusion. Shander et al (2012b) also issued recommendations for tackling these obstacles. Similar hurdles were encountered when the Western Australia PBM Program was introduced, but these were successfully overcome in most cases.

▶ **Canada.** Also noteworthy are the PBM-related initiatives launched in Canada. These include the Transfusion Ontario programs organized by the Ontario Ministry of Health and the Ontario Blood System Reference Group. In addition to providing continuing education and quality control in transfusion medicine, the Transfusion Ontario programs are aimed at promoting the sustainable implementation of treatment modalities to reduce blood consumption in the entire province of Ontario. One of the programs, Ontario Transfusion Coordinators (ONTraC), was initiated with the participation of 25 hospitals (www.ontracprogram. com). During the first 12 months of continuous benchmarking, and also subsequently, marked improvements were noted in most hospitals in terms of both the transfusion rate and the transfusion index. Significant reductions were also seen in the rate of postoperative infections and the hospital length of stay (Freedman et al 2005, Freedman 2005, Freedman et al 2008).

▶ **USA.** It was in the United States, almost 20 years ago, that the first measures for blood conservation in surgery and internal medicine (the precursors of modern PBM) were introduced, in particular at Englewood Hospital and Medical Center in Englewood, NJ (IPBMBMS 2012). Despite this fact, PBM has to date been implemented in only around 200 hospitals in the United States. However, the Joint Commission, the country's most important organization for the accreditation and certification of hospitals and health care establishments, has acknowledged PBM as an important quality measure. The Joint Commission's most recent PBM performance measures to evaluate transfusion practice at U.S. hospitals were published in 2011 (JC 2011).

Furthermore, the U.S. Department of Health and Human Services took the first steps toward the nationwide promotion of PBM in 2011 (see Chapter 8.2.4). The SABM, with members comprising of clinicians from multiple disciplines, focuses with increasing success on matters related to PBM in the United States and abroad (Wald 2014).

> **Note** !
>
> Compared with the progress, prominence, and acceptance of PBM in Australia, North America and many European countries are still lagging behind in terms of implementing PBM; some other countries have not even taken initial steps to develop PBM. In light of the potential implications in terms of better patient outcomes accompanied by other benefits including cost savings, concerted action should be taken at the international level to incorporate PBM into teaching and practice.

8.2.4 Prioritization of PBM by the WHO

▶ **WHO resolution.** Given that to date no multidisciplinary PBM programs have been set up, apart from the initiative in Australia and isolated projects in a few European countries, Canada, and the United States, it is all the more important that the WHO Executive Board recognized the opportunities for and the significance of PBM, and advocated its implementation. In view of the safety risks associated with blood transfusion and the growing bottlenecks in the supply of blood and blood products, the topic of PBM was placed on the provisional agenda of the 126th Executive Board meeting (WHO 2009). The final agenda was expanded to accommodate a few additional items, two of which again related to PBM. At the 126th Executive Board meeting held at the WHO headquarters in Geneva on January 22, 2010, it was decided to recommend to the World Health Assembly—the highest WHO decision-making body—the adoption of a resolution on the "Availability, Safety and Quality of Blood Products" (WHO 2010a). The resolution contains the following passages:

...patient blood management means that before surgery every reasonable measure should be taken to optimize the patient's own blood volume, to minimize the patient's blood loss and to harness and optimize the patient-specific physiological tolerance of anemia following WHO's guide for optimal clinical use (three pillars of patient blood management).

The Sixty-third World Health Assembly...urges Member States...to establish or strengthen systems for the safe and rational use of blood products and to provide training for all staff involved in clinical transfusion, to implement potential solutions in order to minimize transfusion errors and promote patient safety, to promote the availability of transfusion alternatives including, where appropriate, autologous transfusion and patient blood management.

The Sixty-third World Health Assembly...requests the Director-General...to provide guidance, training and support to Member States on safe and rational use of blood products to support the introduction of transfusion alternatives including, where appropriate, autologous transfusion, safe transfusion practices and patient blood management.

At the 63rd meeting of the World Health Assembly in Geneva in May 2010, the resolution was adopted in all its points, including explicit reference to the three-pillar concept as an important element of modern health care systems (WHO 2010b). This decision brought PBM to the official attention of all 193 WHO Member States.

▶ **WHO expert meeting.** The following year, the WHO, in collaboration with the Sharjah Blood Transfusion and Research Center and co-sponsored by the government of the United Arab Emirates, organized its first multinational PBM expert meeting entitled "Global Forum for Blood Safety: Patient Blood Management" (WHO 2011b). Below are some of the priorities for action that were identified at the meeting:

- *Benchmark transfusion prescription and practices. ...*
- *Collect a minimum set of data on patient transfusion outcomes. ...*
- *Identify major national clinical needs and, based on these, develop and implement national guidelines on blood use including PBM. ...*
- *Conduct multicentric studies on:*
  - *Patient outcomes [using PBM].*
  - *Alternatives [to the transfusion of allogeneic blood components].*
- *Conduct benchmarking studies to compare practices in different hospitals and clinicians. ...*
- *Focus on outcome research.*
- *Translate – Make available current evidence through desk research – Meta-analysis.*
  - *Move forward on randomized controlled trials (RCTs).*
  - *Need more funding for RCTs in PBM.*

▶ **U.S. Department of Health and Human Services and Advisory Committee on Blood Safety and Availability.** Having regard to Resolution WHA63.12, the U.S. Department of Health and Human Services convened its first expert meeting on PBM in 2011. Based on the information presented by the experts, the Advisory Committee on Blood Safety and Availability compiled a document setting out recommendations for the national implementation of PBM (USDHHS 2011). The document includes the following statements:

- *Blood transfusion carries significant risk that may outweigh its benefits in some settings and add unnecessary costs.*

- *Wide variability, in the use of transfusions, indicates that there is both excessive and inappropriate use of blood transfusions.*
- *Medical advances and aging of the population are expected to drive demands for transfusions that could exceed supplies in one to two decades.*
- *Programs of patient-oriented blood management at some hospitals have demonstrated significant reduction in blood use, without increase in patient harm, based on expert decision-making.*

Based on these acknowledgements, the Committee recommended that the authorities:

- *Identify mechanisms to obtain data on PBM, utilization of transfusion, and clinical outcomes.*
- *Support development and promulgation of national standards for blood use recognizing the value of patient management, blood conservation, and conservative blood use. ...*
- *Establish metrics for good practices of blood use and PBM.*
- *Advise the Office of National Coordination of Healthcare Information Technology (ONC HIT) on the need to integrate PBM and blood utilization into electronic health records.*
- *Promote education of medical students and practitioners on optimizing PBM and use of transfusion and elevate awareness of the essential role of blood management in the quality and cost efficiency of clinical care.*
- *Promote patient education about the risks, benefits, and alternatives of transfusion...*
- *Support demonstration projects on PBM...*

Note

On adopting Resolution WHA63.12, the World Health Assembly, in its capacity as the highest WHO decision-making body, officially recognized PBM—including the three-pillar concept—as an important element of modern health care systems and expects its implementation by the 193 Member States.

Conclusion

There is a burgeoning literature on the adverse effects of allogeneic RBC transfusion on patient outcomes and the attendant costs (Isbister et al 2011, Vamvakas 2011, Hofmann et al 2013). At the same time, a growing number of publications attest to the benefits and cost-effectiveness of PBM (Moskowitz et al 2010, Weltert et al 2010, Yoo et al 2011, Kotze et al 2012, Spahn et al 2012, Frank et al 2014b). These issues are increasingly addressed in postgraduate training and continuing education programs.

As demonstrated in Australia, the constructive cooperation between main stakeholders, such as statutory authorities, practitioners, patient groups, and the blood services, makes it possible to implement PBM in clinical practice on a large scale in the space of a few years. Besides, Resolution WHA63.12 provides a global framework for the implementation of PBM, and leading accreditation and certification bodies have begun to define quality criteria.

8.3 The Australian PBM Concept—a Success Story

S. L. Farmer, S. Towler, A. Hofmann

8.3.1 Introduction

The ACSQHC has declared the National PBM Collaborative a top national priority (ACSQHC 2015b). The collaborative is being undertaken in consultation with the NBA Australia, states and territories, and public and private health care providers. Its aim is that PBM be the standard of care applied by all clinicians for patients facing a medical or surgical intervention who are at high risk of significant blood loss. The ACSQHC stated that the best and safest blood for patients is their *own* circulating blood, and that this valuable and unique natural resource should therefore be conserved and managed in the same way as all other body systems. This includes the assessment and management of conditions that might lead to a blood transfusion, so that transfusions are undertaken only when clinically appropriate. The ACSQHC, with its key role in the accreditation of public and private hospitals, sees the following benefits from PBM: improved patient outcomes (including fewer complications, faster recovery, and shorter hospital stay), reduced patient exposure to the potential risks (including allergic and immunologic complications) from receiving allogeneic blood components, reduced risk of infection, and reduced transfusion of incorrect blood (blood meant for someone else).

A national competent authority aiming to implement PBM as a new standard of care across the Australian health care system and declaring it a top national priority marks the latest development in a success story that goes back a quarter of a century and is the result of consistent and considered work on all elements of the Australian health system.

8.3.2 Key Historical Developments

▶ **1980s.** In 1988, Sydney hematologist and transfusion medicine specialist James Isbister, who in 2005 coined the term *Patient Blood Management* (Farmer et al 2013a), highlighted the need for a paradigm shift in transfusion practice (Isbister 1988).

▶ **1990s.** Practical application of this paradigm shift began in 1990, when one of the authors, Shannon Farmer, and hospital administrator Mel Jeisman co-founded Australia's first comprehensive Blood Conservation Program at Kaleeya Hospital, a private health care facility in Western Australia with links to Fremantle Hospital, a nearby tertiary care teaching institution. Although Australia prided itself on having one of the safest transfusion services in the world (in terms of the transmission of infections), the hospital's administration was concerned about a newly added blood bag label containing a warning that the product may transmit infectious agents. They had also become interested in techniques to avoid transfusion and in reports from the United States about Bloodless Medicine and Surgery programs indicating that this approach could improve patient outcomes (Farmer and Webb 2000).

The hospital's Medical Advisory Committee and Board of Directors envisaged this approach as the way of the future for medicine and surgery. While they saw that there was an ethics element to the program with the opportunity to provide good medical and surgical care for patients declining blood transfusions for personal reasons, they believed that this approach should be the standard of care for all patients. Therefore, from its inception the program was implemented hospital-wide. A multidisciplinary team of surgeons, anesthesiologists, critical care physicians, hematologists, pathologists, gynecologists, primary care physicians, and pharmacists committed to the program. Shannon Farmer was appointed Coordinator of the program and an anesthesiologist, Vladimir Martyn, worked as Medical Director. Services at the hospital included orthopaedic, general, vascular, urologic, plastic, head and neck, and pediatric surgery, hematology, and general medicine. The perioperative approach to patient care included the assessment and optimization of a patient's bleeding risk, hemoglobin level, and iron status prior to surgery; the application of surgical, anesthetic, pharmacological, and laboratory techniques to reduce iatrogenic blood loss; the use of restrictive transfusion thresholds; and the postoperative optimization of hemoglobin recovery with intravenous iron and other hematinics (Martyn et al 2002). This resulted in significant reductions in blood loss and blood transfusions with positive patient outcomes. A retrospective review of all patients undergoing total hip replacement (primary and revision) at Kaleeya Hospital in 1989 (pre-Blood Conservation Program) and 1996 revealed that transfusion use decreased from 97.7% of patients to 16.0%. The average estimated intraoperative blood loss decreased from 1,783 mL (range, 400–5,000 mL) to 833 mL (range, 100–2,000 mL). During the same period, the hospital length of stay decreased from an average of 19.23 days (range, 10–55 days) in 1989 to 14.32 days (range, 8–24 days) in 1996. Although these are long lengths of stay by today's standards, the program's average length of stay was 0.6 days shorter than the 1995–1996 Australian national private-hospital weighted average of 14.9 days (Kaleeya Hospital Publication 2004, AABC 2006). Although many factors likely contributed to the observed reduction in hospital stay, this experience was consistent with similar initiatives outside Australia reported at the time and with studies showing that, after adjustment for risk factors, this approach is associated with reduced morbidity and hospital length of stay (Ott and Cooley 1977, Rosengart et al 1997, Helm et al 1998, Farmer and Webb 2000, Moskowitz et al 2010, Kotze et al 2012).

Simon Towler, an anesthesiologist and intensive care specialist, was appointed to the hospital's Board of Directors in 2002 providing additional executive and clinical support for the program. In time, the successful program at Kaleeya Hospital resulted in collaborations with clinicians across all tertiary hospitals in the state of Western Australia.

▶ **2000.** In 2000, the Australian Health Ministers' Advisory Committee endorsed a *Review of the Alternatives to Homologous Blood Donation* (Blood and Blood Products Committee 2000). Recommendations included the "minimization of blood loss as the first priority," "minimization of the use of all blood products, homologous and autologous," and "implementation of a transfusion protocol... The protocol should apply to all blood products, whether homologous or autologous, and potential alternatives."

Given the growing interest in blood conservation nationally, Kaleeya Hospital founded the Australasian Association for Blood Conservation (AABC) in January 2000 to bring about collaboration between clinicians across the country with an interest in the field. A peer-review journal was launched entitled *Updates in Blood Conservation and Transfusion Alternatives: Journal of the Australasian Association for Blood Conservation.*

Later that year, Vladimir Martyn was invited to present the Kaleeya Hospital Blood Conservation Program experience at the joint Annual Scientific Meeting of the Haematology Society of Australia and New Zealand, the Australian and New Zealand Society of Blood Transfusion, and the Australasian Society of Thrombosis and Haemostasis (later known as HAA). This presentation introduced the concept and results of a comprehensive hospital-wide blood conservation program to the Australian transfusion community.

▶ **2001.** In parallel, a 2001 report with terms of reference on governance, organization, administration, and expenditure in the blood sector prepared by a committee chaired by Sir Ninian Stephen (referred to as the Stephen's report) was presented to the Commonwealth Minister for Health and Aged Care (Stephen 2001). The report indicated that real clinician-led change was needed in hospitals. Its recommendations included the establishment of national safety and quality standards, the strengthening of hospital governance arrangements, the engagement of clinicians, the development of guidelines, and the inclusion of practice in this area in accreditation and national hemovigilance systems. The report stated: "Opportunities for significant public health and safety gains lie in the better use of blood and blood products and alternatives... This will include the adoption of guidelines, policy and program development, data collection, audit, and patient and staff education." The Stephen's report became a focal point for change and elements were effectively written into legislation that resulted, in time, in the formation of the NBA with the endorsement of all Australian governments.

With the time appearing to be right, the AABC, in association with Kaleeya Hospital, organized Australia's first international multidisciplinary conference on blood conservation for October 8–9, 2001. A faculty of national and international experts in blood conservation was organized. One month out, the conference had to be cancelled because of insufficient registrations. The organizers were devastated and experienced considerable financial loss. It appeared Australia was not yet ready for a broad paradigm shift. The cancellation, however, sparked unexpected interest resulting over time in broad national uptake.

▶ **2002.** What in hindsight has been recognized as a watershed was reached in 2002. Disappointed in the cancellation of what they saw as an important meeting, the conveners of the 2002 HAA Annual Scientific Meeting invited Shannon Farmer to arrange a cut-down version of the AABC conference program for their meeting. The program included representatives of the Australian Red Cross Blood Service and the Australian regulatory body, the Therapeutic Goods Administration, as well as local and international experts in what would soon become known as *Patient Blood Management*. This meeting engaged hematology and transfusion medicine specialists in Australia.

The Western Australia branch of the Australian Medical Association, also disappointed at the cancellation of the AABC conference, devoted their entire 2003 Continuing Medical Education meeting to blood conservation. This meeting was oversubscribed, indicating the growing interest in the field.

▶ **2003–2005.** The HAA subsequently devoted entire sessions to blood conservation at their 2003 and 2005 Annual Scientific Meetings. At the 2003 meeting, Aryeh Shander was invited to present results from the formal Blood Conservation Program at Englewood Hospital and Medical Center in Englewood, NJ, and Simon Towler spoke on the need for formal hospital-wide programs in Australia. Axel Hofmann, an expert from Austria with a focus on health economics and outcomes research, was invited to speak on the cost-effectiveness of hemotherapies and blood conservation at the 2005 meeting.

▶ **2006.** By 2006, James Isbister had coined the term *Patient Blood Management* to capture the patient-centered nature of the approach. In that year, the Australian Red Cross Blood Service devoted its entire 3-day Course in Transfusion Medicine to PBM with a lineup of national and international experts in PBM and formal PBM programs. It attracted a multidisciplinary audience and was the best attended meeting in the more than 20 years it had been run. A broad base of understanding was growing in Australia of the cost benefits of PBM and the clinical benefits of a programmatic approach to its implementation in health care services.

In the same year, Simon Towler was appointed Chief Medical Officer in Western Australia. By then, a large body of evidence on adverse transfusion outcomes across many different patient populations had accumulated and the evidence for benefit was scant (Spiess 2004b, Jackson et al 2006, Tinmouth et al 2006, Spiess 2007, Rawn 2008).

Although improved test assays and technologies were available for a number of disease agents, blood safety remained an ongoing challenge because of newly emerging pathogens as well as known and re-emerging pathogens for which no assays were available (Alter et al 2007, Blajchman and Vamvakas 2006). Additionally, the results of the first multidisciplinary consensus conference on a standard methodology to account for the cost of blood transfusion were published, showing that previous cost studies may have underestimated both the direct and the indirect costs of transfusion (Shander 2005). In light of the accumulating clinical evidence and in response to the precautionary principle, supported by the financial argument and his positive experience with the local Blood Conservation Program at Kaleeya Hospital, Towler saw an urgent need for a system-wide practice change.

Against this backdrop, Shannon Farmer, Axel Hofmann, and Dan Friedman, another expert in the field of blood conservation/PBM—at the time all members of the multidisciplinary, multiprofessional SABM—were invited by the Western Australia State Health Executive Forum to submit a proposal for the design and implementation of a comprehensive sustainable state-wide PBM program. Friedman had already established more than 90 PBM programs in U.S. hospitals. Hofmann, by now a regularly invited speaker to Australia, conducted international research on the cost of hemotherapies and was one of the investigators of the Austrian Benchmark Study on blood use in elective surgery, a study commissioned by the Austrian federal government to prospectively analyze transfusion practice in public hospitals, identify predictors of transfusion, and develop strategies to optimize practice (Gombotz et al 2007, Shander et al 2007, Hofmann et al 2009, Shander et al 2010, Hofmann et al 2013).

▶ **2007.** In December 2007, with professional help and support from national and international key opinion leaders (making up a Clinical Consulting Group) in the fields of surgery, anesthesiology, intensive care, and hematology,[1] the expert group submitted a comprehensive, evidence-based proposal for the implementation of PBM as the standard of care in Western Australia's public health system. This unique document contained the most collective and exhaustive experience in PBM and PBM program implementation at the time. It included a comprehensive business case, baseline assessment and projections, budget methodology, program design, project management, quality control, data requirements for continuous benchmarking, staffing requirements, job descriptions,

leadership models, committee roles and responsibilities, work resource allocation, work breakdown structure, timetables, stakeholder identification, consumer engagement, communication strategies and tools, education models and target audience profiles, clinical compliance with national standards and guidelines, and very importantly, SWOT (strengths, weaknesses, opportunities, and threats) analysis and proven culture change methodology in relation to PBM (Woodward and Roper 1950, Kotter and Schlesinger 1979, Kotter 1996, Kotter and Cohen 2002).

▶ **2008–2015.** In mid-2008, the State Health Executive Forum approved the proposal for a 5-year project to implement a sustainable program in Western Australia's public health system and the Department of Health contracted the expert group to facilitate this. In 2008, the *Western Australia PBM Program 2008–2012* was launched under the guiding vision and mission to improve patient outcomes while reducing costs. The Executive Summary described the project as a quality, safety, and effectiveness initiative with resource and financial implications (DHWA 2011).

One of the early project tasks was the establishment of a multidisciplinary Clinical Reference Group (CRG) to secure clinical engagement and provide leadership within the various institutions. By means of Expressions of Interest forms and personal communications, a 71-member CRG was assembled from universities, all tertiary hospitals, and a number of private hospitals with representation from leading physicians of all disciplines, nurses, pharmacists, and transfusion scientists; a number brought their PBM expertise from their previous clinical work at the Kaleeya Hospital program. They would serve as PBM champions at the institution/clinical practice level. The project was officially launched by the Department of Health in November 2008 at an educational symposium conducted by members of the PBM project faculty (national and international experts in PBM). An introductory series of presentations was made to hospital executives and executive committees, and symposia were held by the international faculty at all tertiary hospitals.

Multiple education initiatives were employed to promote a change in culture. Members of the Clinical Consulting Group and other local and visiting experts facilitated nine PBM workshops and six

---

[1] A faculty of national and international experts served as a clinical consulting group in the development and initiation of the project. These included: James Isbister, hematology and transfusion medicine, Australia; Aryeh Shander, critical care and anesthesiology, United States; Manuel Estioko, cardiothoracic surgery, United States; Jochen Erhard, visceral and liver transplantation surgery, Germany; Donat Spahn, anesthesiology, Switzerland; Hans Gombotz, anesthesiology and critical care, Austria; Peter Rehak, statistics and data analysis, Austria; Julie McMorrow, pharmacy, Australia; Irwin Gross, pathology, United States.

symposia.[2] Local surgeons from different specialties including general, trauma, cardiothoracic, gynecologic, and neurosurgery participated in two surgical hemostasis/PBM workshops at the Clinical Training and Evaluation Centre, The University of Western Australia.[3] The expert group, along with CRG members, conducted educational roadshows in more than 60 departments including surgery, anesthesia, critical care, obstetrics, gynecology, trauma/emergency, hematology, oncology, cardiology, gastroenterology, general medicine, and pediatrics. Presentation topics included the drivers for urgent change, evidence-based guidelines, clinical implementation of the PBM nine-field matrix (see **Fig. 1.2**), and department-specific benchmarking (Hofmann et al 2011, Farmer et al 2013b). Evaluation forms showed an overwhelmingly positive response to the presentations: 69% of the participants stated they would change their clinical practice based on what was presented while 13% said they would not change their practice; the main reason provided was that the information reinforced their already conservative practice. Other educational initiatives included the production of an informative website with materials for clinicians and patients (www.health.wa.gov.au/bloodmanagement), development of an email mailing list to provide regular updates from the literature, and ongoing one-on-one meetings with department heads and key clinicians.

The program design included appointments of positions to provide clinical leadership including executive sponsorship by the Chief Medical Officer of the time, Simon Towler, a State PBM Medical Director (hematologist Michael Leahy was appointed to this position in November 2009), and a State PBM Nurse Coordinator (Trudi Gallagher, an experienced PBM coordinator from the USA, was appointed to this position in September 2011), along with a PBM Medical Director and a PBM Nurse Coordinator in each major hospital and health service. However, in the first few months of the implementation phase, the global financial crisis struck bringing about a freeze on staff appointments. Hiring of PBM clinical nurse consultants, PBM medical directors, and other staff was either deferred or cancelled and access to important IT resources was suddenly limited. However, the project passed this unexpected stress test with many of the CRG members continuing their support pro bono, the contracted experts taking on additional work, and a PBM team within the Department of Health also providing support.

The Centre for Population Health Research at Curtin University, Western Australia, with support from James Semmens and Aqif Mukhtar, was instrumental in developing the initial software modules to measure and continuously benchmark transfusion rates, transfusion indices, and demographic, clinical, and other parameters in relation to PBM (Mukhtar et al 2013). Later in the change management process, benchmark analyst Kevin Trentino and data management specialist Stuart Swain, supported by hospital administrators and executives, took the development of these tools to the next level by linking transfusion data to patient outcomes data (Tynan 2013). With support from clinical costing, this group was then able to analyze the hospital costs associated with RBC transfusions. The findings were helpful to prioritize areas to reduce RBC transfusion rates and further promote PBM activities (Trentino et al 2015).

The role of Fremantle Hospital, one of the five tertiary care centers in Western Australia, was pivotal for the overall success. From 2009, it served as a pilot site for the Western Australia PBM Program. Led by clinical hematologist Michael Leahy, a multiprofessional PBM team undertook major system re-engineering to implement PBM. With preoperative clinics assessing and optimizing hemoglobin

---

[2] Experts included: Benny Sorensen, hematology, Denmark and United Kingdom; Klaus Görlinger, anesthesiology, Germany; Herbert Schöchl, trauma, Austria; Trudi Gallagher, PBM coordinator, United States; Ivor Cavill, hematology, United Kingdom; Amanda Thomson, hematology, Australia; Kathryn Robinson, hematology, Australia; John Olynyk, gastroenterology, Australia; Bernd Froessler, anesthesiology, Australia; Neil Gordon, Laboratory Medicine and Medical Science, Australia; Jeffrey Hamdorf, School of Surgery, Australia; Paul Moroz, General Surgery, Australia; Chris Hogan, Hematology, Australia; Larry McNicol, Anesthesiology, Australia; Darryl Teague, Orthopaedic Surgery, Australia; Craig French, Critical Care/Anesthesiology, Australia; David Roxby, Transfusion Science, Australia; Roger Browning, Anesthesiology, Australia; Julie Tovey, Nursing, Australia; Toby Richards, Vascular Surgery, United Kingdom.

---

[3] Facilitated by Jeffrey Hamdorf, Head of School of Surgery, The University of Western Australia.

levels and iron stores, improved perioperative hemostasis, reduced blood sample volumes, pop-up alerts with electronic blood ordering, the implementation of individualized and restrictive transfusion thresholds, and a single-unit transfusion policy, the RBC use per admission dropped by 26% within 3 years despite a 22% increase in admissions (Leahy et al 2014). Fremantle Hospital became the first tertiary hospital in Australia with a fully embedded PBM program. In November 2013, it received the Western Australia Health Excellence Award in the category of Health Promotion and Early Intervention for their PBM program.

Another important success factor was the full endorsement and support of the Australian Red Cross Blood Service, both at the jurisdictional and at the national level. With the announcement of the program in 2008, the then Chief Executive Officer of the Australian Red Cross Blood Service's Board of Directors, Robert Hetzel, wrote to the Australian Health Minister's Advisory Council indicating the Board's utmost support for the project and highlighting that, with early indications of success, other states may want to adopt a similar approach. From the outset of the Western Australia program, Lynn Aston (Transfusion Medicine Specialist at the Australian Red Cross Blood Service, Western Australia) and Anne McNae and Julianne Lefante (Transfusion Nurses for the Australian Red Cross Blood Service in Western Australia and Northern Territory) took proactive roles in both independent and collaborative PBM education at the various hospitals. The official website of the Australian Red Cross Blood Service features PBM as the timely application of evidence-based medical and surgical concepts designed to maintain hemoglobin concentration, optimize hemostasis, and minimize blood loss in an effort to improve patient outcome (ARCBS 2014b). Together with the Clinical Excellence Commission of New South Wales and other stakeholders, the Australian Red Cross Blood Service developed a series of "myth-busting" posters, addressing myths with titles such as "Blood, it's safer than it's ever been," "A blood transfusion will get my patient home sooner," "Blood transfusions improve healing," and "Blood, it's free anyway" (CEC 2015).

Other Australian jurisdictions (states) have also developed PBM programs and activities to reduce blood utilization. The Department of Health and Human Services in Victoria runs the Blood Matters Program for improving the quality and safety of hospital transfusion care to patients (DHHS 2015). The Government of South Australia runs the BloodSafe program, a blood transfusion safety and quality improvement collaborative between SA Health, the Australian Red Cross Blood Service, SA public and private hospitals, and their transfusion service providers (SA Health 2015). The BloodSafe eLearning courses are now referred to as Australia's most recognized online courses relating to PBM and clinical transfusion practice (BloodSafe eLearning Australia 2015). Queensland Health has a blood and blood product management program (Queensland Government 2014).

▶ **Development of PBM guidelines.** In 2008, the NBA Australia commenced the development of six evidence-based PBM guidelines modules covering (1) Critical Bleeding/Massive Transfusion, (2) Perioperative, (3) Medical, (4) Critical Care, (5) Obstetrics and Maternity, and (6) Pediatrics and Neonatology. At the time of writing, modules 1–5 were completed and approved by the National Health and Medical Research Council (www. blood.gov.au/pbm-guidelines). Based on the exhaustive review of the literature to produce the guidelines, module 2 contains an evidence-based recommendation that "health-care services should establish a multidisciplinary, multimodal perioperative patient blood management program" (NBA 2012). The NBA also established a national PBM Steering Committee to assist with the implementation of PBM nationally and to improve intergovernmental coordination and cooperation in jurisdictional PBM initiatives. This collaboration has resulted in the development of various PBM implementation tools (www.blood.gov.au/implementing-pbm).

▶ **Establishment of quality standards.** Implementation of a PBM program and the national PBM guidelines assists hospitals in Australia to attain accreditation against National Safety and Quality Health Service standards (Standard 7: Blood and Blood Products) developed by the ACSQHC (ACSQHC 2012, ACSQHC 2015a). As of January 1, 2013 these standards are mandatory for hospitals and services providing day procedures. Consequently, the ACSQHC has declared the National PBM Collaborative a top national priority (ACSQHC 2015b).

8.3.3 Results of the Western Australia PBM Program in the Australian Context

The Western Australia PBM Project was the world's first comprehensive program requested by the public sector to benefit patients statewide who are at risk of severe bleeding and/or who have anemia, with the concomitant risk of allogeneic blood transfusion. As shown in **Figs. 8.1–8.3**, when the program implementation began in 2008, Western Australia already had the lowest transfusion rate of the five large jurisdictions. Due to the successful history of the early Blood Conservation Program at Kaleeya Hospital, a comprehensive evidence-based PBM implementation strategy with a strong guiding vision and mission, an implementation team coupled with a faculty of nationally and internationally recognized and well-published multidisciplinary key clinical opinion leaders, a large CRG with local champions, committed intellectual and IT support from professional benchmark and data analysts, and employment of proven change management principles, the Western Australia PBM Program succeeded in shifting the paradigm from default transfusion to PBM. It has significantly reduced blood component utilization and is now reporting the lowest transfusion index per 1,000 population of all countries with a high Human Development Index.

The NBA PBM guidelines refer to the Western Australia Program as a pilot model for Australia (NBA 2012). In 2014, under the theme "PBM as a standard of care in Australia: Past, Present and Future," the NBA in association with the Western Australia Department of Health organized Australia's inaugural national PBM conference at the Perth Convention Centre in Western Australia. The program showcased PBM successes to date and addressed future opportunities and challenges.

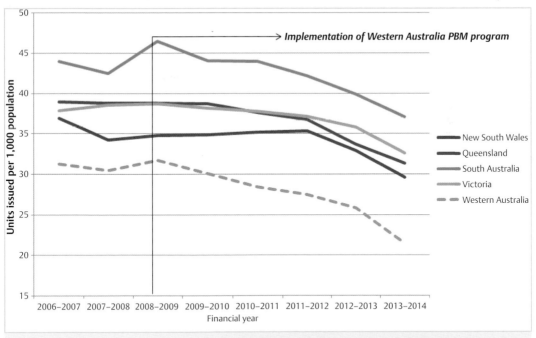

Fig. 8.1 Comparison of red blood cell issuance between Australia's five largest jurisdictions, 2006–2014. (Data sources: NBA Annual Reports and NBA written communication, December 2014; data printed with permission).

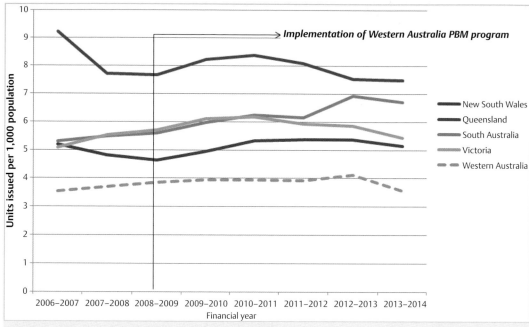

Fig. 8.2 Comparison of platelet issuance between Australia's five largest jurisdictions, 2006–2014. (Data sources: NBA Annual Reports and NBA written communication, December 2014; data printed with permission).

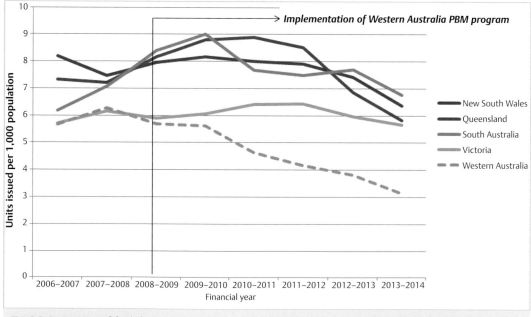

Fig. 8.3 Comparison of fresh frozen plasma issuance between Australia's five largest jurisdictions, 2006–2014. (Data sources: NBA Annual Reports and NBA written communication, December 2014; data printed with permission).

8.3.4 How Health Systems Worldwide Could Benefit from the Australian PBM Success

Figs. 8.4–8.6 compare blood component issuance for RBCs, platelets, and FFP in Western Australia, Australia, and Germany, the largest EU member state. In absence of a system-wide PBM program, the German health system is one of the world's highest per capita users of blood products. Issuance per 1,000 inhabitants in 2013 was 53.3 RBC units, 6.6 platelet units, and 12.1 FFP units. Total use in 2013 was approximately 4.30 million RBC units, 0.53 million platelet units, and 0.98 million FFP units (Paul-Ehrlich-Institut 2015, Eurostat 2015).

Note

Germany would issue 42.7% fewer blood components when matching the Australian benchmark and 60.9% when matching the Western Australian benchmark.

When using the 2013 to 2014 Australian and Western Australian issuance rates per 1,000 inhabitants (30.2 and 21.5 RBC units, 5.6 and 3.6 platelet units, 5.7 and 3.1 FFP units, respectively; NBA written communication, December 2014) as target rates for Germany, utilization would drop to 2.44 and 1.73 million RBC units, 0.45 and 0.29 million platelet units, and 0.46 and 0.25 million FFP units, respectively. Overall, Germany would issue 42.7% fewer blood components when matching the Australian benchmark and 60.9% when matching the Western Australian benchmark.

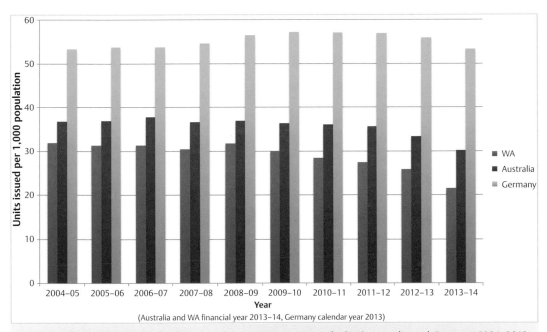

Fig. 8.4 Comparison of red blood cell issuance between Western Australia (WA), Australia, and Germany, 2004–2013. Data sources: NBA Annual Reports; NBA written communication, December 2014, data printed with permission; Paul-Ehrlich-Institut 2015; Eurostat 2015.)

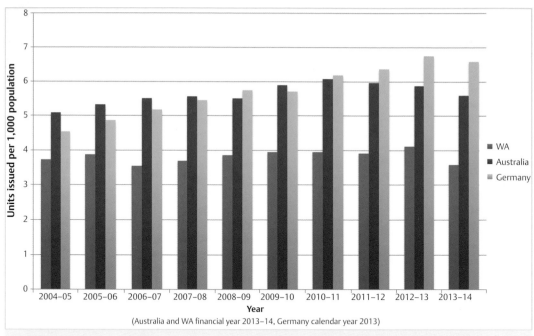

Fig. 8.5 Comparison of platelet issuance comparison between Western Australia (WA), Australia, and Germany, 2004–2013. (Data sources: NBA Annual Reports; NBA written communication, December 2014, data printed with permission; Paul-Ehrlich-Institut 2015; Eurostat 2015.)

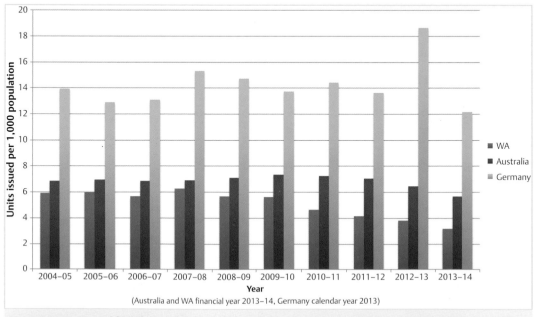

Fig. 8.6 Comparison of fresh frozen plasma issuance between Western Australia (WA), Australia, and Germany, 2004–2013. (Data sources: NBA Annual Reports; NBA written communication, December 2014, data printed with permission; Paul-Ehrlich-Institut 2015; Eurostat 2015.)

Conclusion

As the Western Australia PBM Program has demonstrated, the reduction in product expenditures alone would justify the implementation of a country-wide PBM program (Towler 2014). Greater justification is demonstrated when taking into account activity-based cost savings from the reduced transfusion incidence (Shander et al 2007, Shander et al 2010) and improved patient outcomes including reduced average hospital length of stay, reduced morbidity, and reduced mortality (Hofmann et al 2013, Trentino et al 2015).

The ACSQHC has declared PBM a top national priority. The Western Australia PBM Program does not only serve as a template for implementing PBM programs in Australia, but it is also a reference model for modern health systems around the globe.

8.4 Landmark Studies and Current Clinical Trials in the Field of PBM

P. Meybohm, K. Zacharowski

8.4.1 Introduction

The level of implementation of PBM varies widely across the world. To date, not a single country has successfully run a PBM program that covers all aspects of the three-pillar model. Although some hospitals have adopted the full three-pillar approach with various different PBM strategies for a decade, most hospitals in most countries have adopted very few, if any, PBM measures. This is particularly interesting in view of the fact that the WHO passed a resolution in favor of PBM as early as May 2010.

Note

While some hospitals have adopted the full three-pillar model of PBM for a decade, using various different PBM strategies, most hospitals in most of countries have adopted very few, if any, PBM measures.

Several factors hamper the successful implementation of PBM, including a lack of standards and inadequacy of financial and personnel resources. Most importantly, the results of clinical studies are needed to enable evidence-based practice in the field of PBM. In this respect, it is worthwhile to mention a German study that includes more than 100,000 patients seen during 2012–2015 (NCT 0 182 0949; see also **Table 8.4**). The results from this trial may help to underline the importance of implementing a PBM program to improve patient outcome.

The current chapter summarizes published studies and ongoing clinical trials that focus on the implementation of a PBM program.

8.4.2 Trials Focusing on the Management of Preoperative Anemia

Preoperative anemia, even in its mild form, is independently associated with an increased risk of morbidity and mortality in patients undergoing major surgery.

▶ **The Netherlands (Leiden)** In a prospective RCT by So-Osman and colleagues (2014), adult elective hip- and knee-surgery patients with hemoglobin levels of 10 to 13 g/dL were randomly allocated to an erythropoietin group (n = 339) or a control group (n = 344). With erythropoietin, the mean use of RBCs was 0.50 units per patient and the transfusion rate was 16%; the respective figures in the control group were 0.71 units per patient and 26%. Consequently, erythropoietin treatment resulted in a 29% nonsignificant reduction in mean RBC use (odds ratio [OR], 0.71; 95% confidence interval [CI], 0.42–1.13) and a 50% reduction in the transfusion rate (OR, 0.5; 95% CI, 0.35–0.75). Erythropoietin treatment increased costs by €785 (95% CI, €262–€1,309) per patient, translating into costs of €7,300 per avoided transfusion.

▶ **United Kingdom (Steeton)** In a before-and-after comparison, Kotze and colleagues (2012) analyzed data for a prospective cohort of 317 consecutive patients with primary hip or knee arthroplasty after the implementation of a PBM program and those for a historical cohort of 717 patients at Airedale General Hospital.

The PBM program was based on two pillars: (1) preoperative identification and management of anemia, and (2) intraoperative blood conservation methods comprising spinal anesthesia rather than general anesthesia, antifibrinolytic drug treatment with tranexamic acid (1 g), cell salvage if the intraoperative blood loss was anticipated to exceed 1,000 mL or if there was significant unexpected hemorrhage, and induced hypotension (mean arterial pressure 55 mmHg).

Regarding the first pillar (management of preoperative anemia), 52 of 73 anemic patients were treated with oral iron (n = 19), parenteral iron (n = 11), or erythropoietin plus oral iron (n = 22). Interestingly, in those treated for anemia, there was an inverse relationship between the baseline hemoglobin value and the hemoglobin response to treatment.

The prevalence of anemia in the post-implementation group decreased from 25.9% (73/281) at listing to 10.3% (29/281) after treatment (p < 0.001). The implementation of PBM was associated with lower transfusion rates for hip arthroplasty (23% versus 7.6%; p < 0.001) and knee arthroplasty (6.7% versus 0%; p < 0.001). The length of stay decreased from 6 days (range, 5–8 days) to 5 days (range, 3–7 days) for total hip replacement and to 4 days (range, 3–6 days) for total knee replacement (p < 0.001 for both comparisons).

Table 8.1 shows currently recruiting trials that focus on the management of preoperative anemia.

8.4.3 Trials Focusing on the Minimization of Blood Loss

Measures to minimize blood loss include management of the bleeding risk; minimization of iatrogenic blood loss; use of blood-sparing surgical techniques; cell salvage/retransfusion; and management of hemostasis/anticoagulation. Several studies have been published on each of these topics. This chapter focuses on published meta-analyses and currently recruiting trials.

▶ **Management of the bleeding risk, minimization of iatrogenic blood loss.** Henry and colleagues (2011) published a Cochrane update on the use of antifibrinolytic drugs and their effects on blood loss, need for transfusion, and need for reoperation; the update included 252 RCTs with over 25,000 participants. In general, antifibrinolytic drugs provided reductions in blood loss and allogeneic RBC transfusion. Aprotinin appeared to be slightly more effective than lysine analogues (tranexamic acid or ε-aminocaproic acid) in reducing blood loss and RBC transfusion. However, head-to-head comparisons showed a lower risk

of death with lysine analogues than with aprotinin.

▶ **Blood-sparing surgical techniques, cell salvage/ retransfusion, management of hemostasis/anticoagulation.** Wang and colleagues (2009) determined the overall safety and efficacy of cell salvage in cardiac surgery in a meta-analysis of 31 RCTs involving 2,282 patients. The use of an intraoperative cell saver reduced the rates of exposure to any allogeneic blood product (OR, 0.63; 95% CI, 0.43–0.94; p = 0.02) and to RBCs (OR, 0.60; 95% CI, 0.39–0.92; p = 0.02), and decreased the mean volume of total allogeneic blood products transfused per patient (– 256 mL; 95% CI, – 416 mL to – 95 mL; p = 0.002). However, there were no differences in hospital mortality, postoperative stroke or transient ischemia attack, atrial fibrillation, renal dysfunction, and infection between the groups with and without cell salvage. Bolliger and Tanaka (2013) conducted a meta-analysis to assess the effects of thrombelastography/thromboelastometry-guided therapy on the use of allogeneic blood products in patients undergoing cardiac surgery. Twelve trials including 6,835 patients were analyzed; seven of these trials were RCTs with a total of 749 patients. In an analysis including all trials, thrombelastography/thromboelastometry-guided therapy resulted in fewer transfusions of RBCs, FFP, and platelets with ORs of 0.62 (95% CI, 0.56–0.69; p < 0.001), 0.28 (95% CI, 0.24–0.33; p < 0.001), and 0.55 (95% CI, 0.49–0.62; p < 0.001), respectively. However, more than 50% of the patients in this analysis came from a single retrospective study. In an analysis that included RCTs only, the ORs for the transfusion of RBCs, FFP, and platelets were 0.54 (95% CI, 0.38–0.77; p < 0.001), 0.36 (95% CI, 0.25–0.53; p < 0.001), and 0.57 (95% CI, 0.39–0.81; p = 0.002), respectively.

Table 8.2 shows currently recruiting trials that focus on the minimization of blood loss.

8.4.4 Evidence-based RBC Transfusion Trigger

The main question in this context is whether patients can tolerate a restrictive transfusion strategy, with the threshold for RBC transfusion set at a hemoglobin concentration of 7 g/dL.

Hopewell and colleagues (2013) reviewed large observational studies (> 1,000 patients) that

Table 8.1 Currently recruiting trials focusing on the management of preoperative anemia. (Data source: ClinicalTrials.gov [accessed July 14, 2015])

Study	ClinicalTrials.gov Identifier	Hospital/location	Estimated completion date	Patients	Intervention group	Control group
The Benefits of a Preoperative Anemia Management Program (PAMP)	NCT 0188 8003	Birmingham, AL	2015	n = 51 patients undergoing total hip/knee replacement Anemia defined as Hb <13.0 g/dL and MCV <100 fL, with an Hct between 30% and 39%	Anemia treatment group: epoetin α and IV iron preoperatively	Conventional treatment group: current standard of care (without management of anemia) Non-anemia group: current standard of care
Impact of Preoperative Treatment of Anemia and Iron Deficiency in Cardiac Surgery on Outcome	NCT 0203 1289	Zurich, Switzerland	December 2016	n = 1,000 patients undergoing cardiac surgery Anemia or iron deficiency	Erythropoietin/ferric carboxymaltose/vitamin B_{12}/folic acid) given 1–2 days prior to surgery in patients with iron deficiency and a maximum of 3 days prior to surgery in patients with anemia	Placebo
Intravenous Iron in Colorectal Cancer Associated Anaemia (IVICA)	NCT 0170 1310	Nottingham, United Kingdom	2015	n = 116 patients with nonmetastatic colorectal adenocarcinoma	A minimum of 1 dose of 1,000 mg ferric carboxymaltose, at least 14 days prior to surgery	Ferrous sulfate 200 mg twice a day for a minimum of 2 weeks
Preoperative Intravenous Iron to Treat Anemia in Major Surgery (PREVENTT)	NCT 0169 2418	London, United Kingdom	August 2017	n = 500 patients undergoing elective major open abdominal surgery Anemia defined as Hb 9.0–12.0 g/dL	1,000 mg of ferric carboxymaltose	Placebo
The Use of Iron Therapy for Patients With Anemia After Surgery (VITAPOP)	NCT 0197 5272	Maastricht, The Netherlands	Not yet recruiting; December 2015	n = 120 patients undergoing gynecological surgery Anemia defined as Hb 8–11 g/dL	1,000 mg of ferric carboxymaltose, 1 day after surgery	200 mg ferrous fumarate twice a day starting 24–48 hours after surgery, or placebo

Continued ▶

Table 8.1 Continued

Study	ClinicalTrials.gov Identifier	Hospital/location	Estimated completion date	Patients	Intervention group	Control group
Active Preoperative Anemia Management in Patients Undergoing Cardiac Surgery (APART)	NCT 0 218 9889	University of Texas Southwestern Medical Center, Dallas, TX	April 2016	n = 50 patients scheduled for elective cardiac surgery (coronary artery bypass graft±heart valve) • Diagnosed with preoperative anemia, defined as Hb <13.0 g/dL	300 U/kg EPO plus 510 mg ferumoxytol IV 7–28 days before surgery (first dose); 300 U/kg EPO plus 510 mg ferumoxytol IV 1–7 days before surgery (second dose), 300 U/kg EPO 2 days after surgery (third dose)	No preoperative intervention for anemia; exception: iron deficiency anemia found during baseline If laboratory values indicate iron deficiency, oral iron will be recommended to take until surgery
Trial Comparing Ferric(III) Carboxymaltose Infusion With Oral Iron Supplementation as Treatment of Anemia (FIT)	NCT 0 224 3735	Multicenter trial in the Netherlands	June 2016	n = 198	Ferric carboxymaltose (dose according to Summary of Product Characteristics depending on body weight and Hb value; administered in one or two infusions with 1 week in between; maximum dose 1,000 mg or 15 mg/kg per week)	200 mg ferrous fumarate daily from randomization until day before surgery

Abbreviations: EPO, erythropoietin; Hb, hemoglobin; Hct, hematocrit; IV, intravenous; MCV, mean corpuscular volume.

Table 8.2 Currently recruiting trials focusing on the minimization of blood loss. (Data source: ClinicalTrials.gov [accessed July 14, 2015])

Study	ClinicalTrials.gov Identifier	Hospital/location	Estimated completion date	Patients	Intervention group	Control group
World Maternal Antifibrinolytic Trial (WOMAN)	NCT 0 087 2469	Worldwide multicenter trial	May 2016	n = 20,000 women with postpartum hemorrhage following vaginal or cesarean delivery	Tranexamic acid (1–2 g)	Placebo
Point-of-Care Testing in Coagulopathic Patients Undergoing Cardiac Surgery: a Multicenter Study (MultiPOC)	NCT 0 182 6123	Multicenter trial in Germany and Austria	December 2015	n = 160 patients undergoing complex cardiothoracic surgery with a bleeding complication	POC testing (hemostatic therapy based on POC measures obtained by viscoelastic tests [ROTEM] and aggregometry tests [Multiplate device])	Conventional coagulating testing (hemostatic therapy based on conventional standard coagulation analyses such as INR, aPTT, fibrinogen and platelet concentration, or ACT)
Trial of Feedback on Blood Use (TOFU)	NCT 0 223 2568	Brigham and Women's Hospital, Boston, MA	December 2015	n = 40 hip surgery patients in the postoperative period	Feedback arm: orthopaedic surgeons receive monthly reports providing individualized data on compliance with the FOCUS trial RBC transfusion guideline (pretransfusion Hb < 8 g/dL); feedback data are anonymized, but surgeons are able to see their own data in comparison with their peers	Control arm: orthopaedic surgeons do not receive any feedback on their use of RBC transfusion

Abbreviations: ACT, activated clotting time; aPTT, activated prothrombin time; Hb, hemoglobin; INR, international normalized ratio; POC, point of care; RBC, red blood cell; ROTEM, rotational thromboelastometry.

investigated the effect of RBC transfusion versus no RBC transfusion from 2006 until the end of 2010. They found an increased mortality rate following RBC transfusion in most studies, even after adjustment for confounding factors such as age and comorbidities. However, it is very difficult to completely eliminate the impact of confounding in observational studies; prospective RCTs provide a higher quality of evidence.

Goodnough and colleagues (2013) summarized four large high-quality trials, which were conducted in the settings of critical care, cardiac surgery, hip fracture, and acute upper gastrointestinal hemorrhage. The hemoglobin thresholds varied slightly. Of importance, there was good separation of the mean hemoglobin value in the restrictive and liberal transfusion groups. These trials found that the clinical outcomes with a restrictive hemoglobin trigger of 7 g/dL were similar to those in patients transfused to a hemoglobin concentration of more than 9 g/dL.

The most recent study investigating a restrictive versus a liberal transfusion threshold recruited 2,007 adult patients with a postoperative hemoglobin level of less than 9 g/dL who had undergone nonemergency cardiac surgery at one of 17 centers in the United Kingdom (Murphy et al 2015b). The patients were randomly assigned to a restrictive transfusion threshold (hemoglobin < 7.5 g/dL) or a liberal transfusion threshold (hemoglobin < 9 g/dL). The transfusion rates in the two groups were 53.4% and 92.2%, respectively. The primary outcome—serious infection (sepsis or wound infection) or an ischemic event (permanent stroke, myocardial infarction, infarction of the gut, or acute kidney injury) within 3 months after randomization—occurred in 35.1% of patients in the restrictive transfusion group and 33.0% of patients in the liberal transfusion group (OR, 1.11; 95% CI, 0.91–1.34; p = 0.30). The 90-day mortality was higher with the restrictive transfusion strategy than with the liberal strategy (4.2% versus 2.6%; hazard ratio, 1.64; 95% CI, 1.00–2.67; p = 0.045).

Table 8.3 shows currently recruiting trials that focus on the hemoglobin trigger for transfusion.

> **Note**
>
> The transfusion trigger should serve as a discussion point and not as a strict indication for transfusion (Koch 2014).

8.4.5 Trials Focusing on the Implementation of a Multimodal PBM Program

Many hospitals worldwide have implemented a multimodal PBM program in recent years, but only a few groups have published research data on this topic.

▶ **Austria.** Funded by the federal government, Gombotz and colleagues (2007) conducted the first prospective, observational Austrian Benchmark Study on blood utilization in elective surgery in 18 randomly selected hospitals. It was the first study ever to show that transfusions in elective settings is highly predictable (97.4%) based on:
• The level of anemia prior to surgery.
• The volume of perioperative blood loss.
• The transfusion threshold.

The publication of these findings paved the way for a broader acceptance of PBM: based on the understanding that anemia, blood loss, and a liberal transfusion threshold are three independent risk factors for adverse outcomes, and that the three pillars of PBM specifically address each of these risk factors, clinicians recognized the broad potential benefit of PBM. The preemption of anemia, the minimization of blood loss, and the use of physiological transfusion thresholds can lead to substantial reductions in allogeneic RBC transfusion and potentially to improved outcomes, along with reduced costs for the health care system.

The study group then conducted a second prospective, observational benchmark study on blood utilization that included most of the hospitals that had been randomly selected for the first study (Gombotz et al 2014). The second study confirmed the high variability in RBC transfusions, blood loss, and preoperative anemia (Gombotz et al 2014). However, the investigators observed improvements in blood utilization, blood loss, and management of anemia, most likely following the implementation of some PBM measures. In one of Austria's largest public hospitals, the use of allogeneic blood products dropped by almost 70% during a 5-year PBM implementation period (see **Fig. 1.3**, Chapter 1.1). Despite this success, public authorities in Austria have not pursued the country-wide implementation of PBM.

Table 8.3 Currently recruiting trials focusing on transfusion triggers. (Data source: ClinicalTrials.gov [accessed July 14, 2015])

Study	Clinical Trials.gov Identifier	Hospital/location	Estimated completion date	Patients	Intervention group	Control group
Clinic Trial for Perioperative Transfusion Trigger Score (POTTS)	NCT 0 159 7232	Multicenter trial in West China	December 2015	n = 3,000; Hb <10 g/dL	Transfusion trigger: based on POTTS	(1) Transfusion trigger: Hb >10 g/dL (2) Transfusion trigger: based on experience
Transfusion Requirements in Cardiac Surgery (TRICSII)	NCT 0 148 4639	Multicenter trial in Canada	2016/2017	n = 208 high-risk cardiac surgery patients (euroSCORE ≥6)	Restrictive transfusion trigger: Hb ≤7.5 g/dL intraoperatively and postoperatively	Liberal transfusion trigger: Hb ≤9.5 g/dL intraoperatively and postoperatively in the ICU, and Hb <8.5 g/dL on the ward

Abbreviations: euroSCORE, European System for Cardiac Operative Risk Evaluation; Hb, hemoglobin; Hct, hematocrit; ICU, intensive care unit; POTTS, Perioperative Transfusion Trigger Score.

► **United States (Englewood, NJ).** Moskowitz and colleagues (2010) compared a PBM cohort (n = 588) with a propensity-score-matched control cohort (n = 586) undergoing isolated coronary artery bypass graft surgery (CABG). The PBM program included:
- Preoperative optimization of hemoglobin.
- Intraoperative acute normovolemic hemodilution.
- Autotransfusion.
- Tolerance to perioperative anemia (hemoglobin 6–7 g/dL).
- Meticulous surgical technique.
- Endovascular vein harvest.
- On-site coagulation monitoring (thromboelastography and determination of the heparin concentration).
- Targeted pharmacotherapy (antifibrinolytic agents and desmopressin acetate).

In the PBM cohort, fewer patients were transfused (10.6% versus 42.5%; $p < 0.001$), fewer patients experienced perioperative complications (11.1% versus 18.7%; $p < 0.001$), and the hospital mortality was significantly reduced (0.8% versus 2.5%; $p = 0.02$).

► **Western Australia (Fremantle).** Leahy and colleagues (2014) retrospectively assessed the effects of a PBM program that had been introduced at Fremantle Hospital in 2009; this program was a pilot for the state-wide PBM program launched by the Western Australian Department of Health. The authors analyzed the data of more than 250,000 surgical patients.

The PBM program included:
- Preoperative clinics.
- Management of perioperative anemia.
- Perioperative hemostasis.
- Reduced blood sample volumes.
- Restrictive transfusion triggers.
- A single-unit transfusion policy.

Between the implementation of PBM in 2009 and the year 2011, the mean number of RBC units transfused per admission declined by 26%. The use of FFP and platelets declined by 38% and 16%, respectively. Among elective admissions, the largest decline in the RBC transfusion rate was seen in patients undergoing cardiothoracic surgery (from 27.5% to 12.8%). The frequency of single-unit RBC transfusions increased from 13% to 28% ($p < 0.001$), and the frequency of double-unit transfusions decreased from 48% to 37% ($p < 0.001$). The frequency of RBC transfusions among patients with a pretransfusion hemoglobin value of more than 10 g/dL decreased from 16% to 12%. Continuing education and feedback to specialists helped to maintain the program, improve patient outcomes, and decrease the transfusion rate.

► **Switzerland (Zurich).** Theusinger and colleagues (2014b) introduced a PBM program at the Department of Orthopedics, Balgrist Hospital, in 2009. In this retrospective before-and-after study, a pre-PBM cohort (year 2008) was compared with a post-PBM cohort (years 2009–2011) of orthopaedic patients (hip, n = 3,062; knee, n = 2,953; and spine, n = 2,856).

The PBM program included:
- Management and treatment of preoperative anemia.
- Reduction of intraoperative blood loss by surgical, anesthesiological, and pharmacological techniques.
- Lowering of the transfusion trigger to a hemoglobin level of ≤ 8 g/dL.

In patients undergoing hip surgery, the frequency of immediate preoperative anemia decreased from 17.6% to 12.9% ($p < 0.001$), whereas the loss of RBC mass was unchanged (626 ± 434 mL versus 635 ± 450 mL; $p = 0.974$). The transfusion rate decreased from 21.8% to 15.7% ($p < 0.001$). There was no change in the number of RBC units transfused ($p = 0.761$).

In knee surgery patients, the prevalence of immediate preoperative anemia dropped from 15.5% to 7.8% ($p < 0.001$) and the loss of RBC mass declined from 573 ± 355 mL to 476 ± 365 mL ($p < 0.001$). The transfusion rate decreased from 19.3% to 4.9% ($p < 0.001$), and the number of RBC units transfused decreased from 0.53 ± 1.27 units to 0.16 ± 0.90 units ($p < 0.001$).

In patients undergoing spine surgery, there was no change in the prevalence of immediate preoperative anemia ($p = 0.113$). The loss of RBC mass dropped from 551 ± 421 mL to 404 ± 337 mL ($p < 0.001$), the transfusion rate decreased from 18.6% to 8.6% ($p < 0.001$), and the number of RBC units transfused was reduced from 0.66 ± 1.80 units to 0.22 ± 0.89 units ($p = 0.008$).

Table 8.4 Currently recruiting trials focusing on a multimodal PBM strategy. (Data source: ClinicalTrials.gov [accessed July 14, 2015])

Study	Clinical Trials.gov Identifier	Hospital/location	Estimated completion date	Patients	Intervention group	Control group
Safety and Effectiveness of a PBM Program in Surgical Patients	NCT 0182 0949	Multicenter trial in Germany (Frankfurt, Bonn, Kiel, Münster)	October 2015	n > 100,000 surgical patients	PBM program includes (1) management of preoperative anemia, (2) rational transfusion trigger, and (3) a perioperative checklist for different blood-sparing techniques (e.g., cell salvage, normothermia, reduced blood samples, POC testing for bedside coagulation management)	Current standard of care

Abbreviations: POC, point of care.

► **Canada (Ontario).** Freedman (2014) summarized the outcomes of the ONTraC PBM program from its inception in 2002 until 2011. This PBM program includes:

- Provision of salaries (plus benefits) for transfusion coordinators at 25 hospitals in Ontario. These coordinators act as a "clinical bridge" between the Transfusion Service and the rest of the hospital; their tasks include:
  - Management of a blood conservation program (50% of the time).
  - Patient, family, and staff education (25% of the time).
  - Program data management (20% of the time).
  - Local institutional/regional activities (5% of the time).
- Preadmission clinic visits (3–5 weeks before surgery).
- Diagnosis and treatment of anemia through the family doctor, surgeon, anesthetist, or hematologist.
- Erythropoietin and/or iron therapy.
- Identification of patients at risk of transfusion ahead of surgery.
- Informed consent and discussion of transfusion alternatives.
- Cell salvage.

The mean transfusion rate decreased significantly from 2002 to 2011 (knee surgery: 24.5% versus 10.1%; primary CABG surgery: 60.2% versus 25.2%). Among patients specifically seen for preoperative anemia by the coordinators, the frequency of treatment with erythropoietin and intravenous iron was twofold higher than among those not seen by the coordinators. The proportion of hospitals meeting an arbitrary benchmark—transfusion rate of less than 30% in CABG surgery—increased from 0% in 2002 to 80% in 2011.

► **United States (Birmingham, AL).** Oliver and colleagues (2014) compared data for a pre-PBM cohort (6 months in 2007; n = 9,519) and a post-PBM cohort (same months in 2011; n = 9,261) to investigate why RBC transfusions were given and whether there was a change in the mean number of units transfused per patient.

The PBM program included:

- Formation of a Blood Utilization and Management Committee.
- Restrictive transfusion trigger (hemoglobin level of 7 g/dL) in nonbleeding patients.

- "Transfuse and assess" strategy (transfusion of single units).
- Retrospective review of the appropriateness of RBC transfusion.
- Reduction of blood wastage for tests and procedures.
- Perioperative blood conservation by decreasing extracorporeal volumes and hemodilution.

The total number of RBC units transfused decreased from 19,888 units pre-PBM (mean of 0.96 units per patient discharged) to 14,472 units post-PBM (mean of 0.55 units per patient discharged). Interestingly, the number of patients receiving a double unit of RBCs per transfusion episode significantly decreased from 48% to 33%, whereas the number of patients receiving a single unit increased from 22% to 51% ($p < 0.0001$ for both comparisons).

Table 8.4 shows currently recruiting trials that focus on a multimodal PBM program.

Conclusion

Several large clinical trials have demonstrated the effectiveness of multimodal PBM programs. The studies have consistently shown a lower incidence of immediate preoperative anemia, a reduction in blood loss, and a lower transfusion rate.

However, several questions remain, the major questions being:

- Which combinations of PBM measures are most effective in different clinical scenarios?
- Does the implementation of a PBM program have an impact on patient safety?
- Is PBM cost-effective in general, and if yes, which combinations of PBM measures are most cost-effective?

At the time of writing, several promising trials are under way to address these questions.

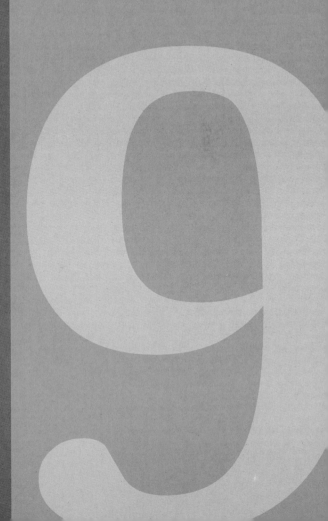

Chapter 9

Appendix

9.1 References

Aapro MS, Link H. September 2007 update on EORTC guidelines and anemia management with erythropoiesis-stimulating agents. Oncologist 2008;13(Suppl 3):33–36

Abholz HH, Donner-Banzhoff N. Epidemiologische und biostatistische Aspekte der Allgemeinmedizin. In: Kochen MM, ed. Allgemeinmedizin und Familienmedizin. 3 rd ed. Stuttgart: Thieme; 2006

Abraham I, Sun D. The cost of blood transfusion in Western Europe as estimated from six studies. Transfusion 2012;52 (9):1983–1988

Abraham NS, Hartman C, Richardson P, Castillo D, Street RL Jr, Naik AD. Risk of lower and upper gastrointestinal bleeding, transfusions, and hospitalizations with complex antithrombotic therapy in elderly patients. Circulation 2013;128(17):1869–1877

Abraham NS, Hlatky MA, Antman EM, et al. ACCF/ACG/AHA 2010 expert consensus document on the concomitant use of proton pump inhibitors and thienopyridines: A focused update of the ACCF/ACG/AHA 2008 expert consensus document on reducing the gastrointestinal risks of antiplatelet therapy and NSAID use. A Report of the American College of Cardiology Foundation Task Force on Expert Consensus Documents. J Am Coll Cardiol 2010;56(24):2051–2066

Abu-Assi E, Raposeiras-Roubin S, Lear P, et al. Comparing the predictive validity of three contemporary bleeding risk scores in acute coronary syndrome. Eur Heart J Acute Cardiovasc Care 2012;1(3):222–231

Acheson AG, Brookes MJ, Spahn DR. Effects of allogeneic red blood cell transfusions on clinical outcomes in patients undergoing colorectal cancer surgery: a systematic review and meta-analysis. Ann Surg 2012;256(2):235–244

AIT Austrian Institute of Technology. European Patient Blood Management (PBM) Project started [press release]. March 21, 2014. http://www.pressetext.com/news/2 014 032 1006. Accessed July 7, 2015

Alberius P, Klinge B, Sjögren S. Effects of bone wax on rabbit cranial bone lesions. J Craniomaxillofac Surg 1987;15(2): 63–67

Alessandrino EP, Amadori S, Barosi G, et al; Italian Society of Hematology. Evidence- and consensus-based practice guidelines for the therapy of primary myelodysplastic syndromes. A statement from the Italian Society of Hematology. Haematologica 2002;87(12):1286–1306

Alizadeh Ghavidel A, Mirmesdagh Y, Samiei N, Gholampour Dehaki M. Haemostatic role of TachoSil surgical patch in cardiac surgery. J Cardiovasc Thorac Res 2014;6(2):91–95

Alli O, Asirvatham S, Holmes DR Jr. Strategies to incorporate left atrial appendage occlusion into clinical practice. J Am Coll Cardiol 2015;65(21):2337–2344

Allison RT. Foreign body reactions and an associated histological artefact due to bone wax. Br J Biomed Sci 1994;51 (1):14–17

Al-Refaie WB, Parsons HM, Markin A, Abrams J, Habermann EB. Blood transfusion and cancer surgery outcomes: a continued reason for concern. Surgery 2012;152(3):344–354

Alshryda S, Mason J, Sarda P, et al. Topical (intra-articular) tranexamic acid reduces blood loss and transfusion rates following total hip replacement: a randomized controlled trial (TRANX-H). J Bone Joint Surg Am 2013;95 (21):1969–1974

Alter HJ, Stramer SL, Dodd RY. Emerging infectious diseases that threaten the blood supply. Semin Hematol 2007;44 (1):32–41

Aly Hassan A, Lochbuehler H, Frey L, Messmer K. Global tissue oxygenation during normovolaemic haemodilution in young children. Paediatr Anaesth 1997;7(3):197–204

Amato A, Pescatori M. Perioperative blood transfusions for the recurrence of colorectal cancer. Cochrane Database Syst Rev 2006;(1):CD 005 033

American Association of Blood Banks (AABB). Standards for Blood Banks and Transfusion Services. 29th ed. Behesda, MD: AABB; 2014

American Society of Anesthesiologists Task Force on Perioperative Blood Management (ASATF). Practice guidelines for perioperative blood management: an updated report by the American Society of Anesthesiologists Task Force on Perioperative Blood Management*. Anesthesiology 2015;122(2):241–275

Amsterdam EA, Wenger NK, Brindis RG, et al. AHA/ACC Guideline for the Management of Patients with Non-ST-Elevation Acute Coronary Syndromes: a report of the American Heart Association Task Force on Practice Guidelines. J Am Coll Cardiol 2014;64(24):e139–e228

Anastasiadis K, Asteriou C, Antonitsis P, et al. Enhanced recovery after elective coronary revascularization surgery with minimal versus conventional extracorporeal circulation: a prospective randomized study. J Cardiothor Vasc Anesth 2013;27:859–864

Anderson SA, Menis M, O'Connell K, Burwen DR. Blood use by inpatient elderly population in the United States. Transfusion 2007;47(4):582–592

Anglin CO, Spence JS, Warner MA, et al. Effects of platelet and plasma transfusion on outcome in traumatic brain injury patients with moderate bleeding diatheses. J Neurosurg 2013;118 (3):676–686

Anker SD, Comin Colet J, Filippatos G, et al; FAIR-HF Trial Investigators. Ferric carboxymaltose in patients with heart failure and iron deficiency. N Engl J Med 2009;361(25):2436–2448

Apelseth TO, Molnar L, Arnold E, Heddle NM. Benchmarking: applications to transfusion medicine. Transfus Med Rev 2012;26(4):321–332

Arant CB, Wessel TR, Olson MB, et al; National Heart, Lung, and Blood Institute Women's Ischemia Syndrome Evaluation Study. Hemoglobin level is an independent predictor for adverse cardiovascular outcomes in women undergoing evaluation for chest pain: results from the National Heart, Lung, and Blood Institute Women's Ischemia Syndrome Evaluation Study. J Am Coll Cardiol 2004;43(11):2009–2014

Arbab-Zadeh A, Fuster V. The myth of the "vulnerable plaque": Transitioning from a focus on individual lesions to atherosclerotic disease burden for coronary artery disease risk assessment. J Am Coll Cardiol 2015;65(8):846–855

Archer C, Levy AR, McGregor M. Value of routine preoperative chest x-rays: a meta-analysis. Can J Anaesth 1993;40 (11):1022–1027

Arnaud F, Parreño-Sadalan D, Tomori T, et al. Comparison of 10 hemostatic dressings in a groin transection model in swine. J Trauma 2009;67(4):848–855

Arshad F, Lisman T, Porte RJ. Hypercoagulability as a contributor to thrombotic complications in the liver transplant recipient. Liver Int 2013;33(6):820–827

Arya VK, Nagdeve NG, Kumar A, Thingnam SK, Dhaliwal RS. Comparison of hemodynamic changes after acute normovolemic hemodilution using Ringer's lactate versus 5% albumin in patients on beta-blockers undergoing coronary artery bypass surgery. J Cardiothorac Vasc Anesth 2006;20(6):812–818

Ashworth A, Klein AA. Cell salvage as part of a blood conservation strategy in anaesthesia. Br J Anaesth 2010;105 (4):401–416

Association of Anaesthetists of Great Britain and Ireland (AAGBI). Safety Guideline: Blood Transfusion and the Anaesthetist: Intraoperative Cell Salvage. Published 2009. http://www.aagbi.org/ sites/default/files/cell%20_salvage_2009 _amended.pdf. Accessed March 12, 2015

Athibovonsuk P, Manchana T, Sirisabya N. Prevention of blood transfusion with intravenous iron in gynecologic cancer patients receiving platinum-based chemotherapy. Gynecol Oncol 2013;131 (3):679–682

Attali M, Barel Y, Somin M, et al. A cost-effective method for reducing the volume of laboratory tests in a university-associated teaching hospital. Mt Sinai J Med 2006;73(5):787–794

Aubron C, Reade MC, Fraser JF, Cooper DJ. Efficacy and safety of fibrinogen concentrate in trauma patients—a systematic review. J Crit Care 2014;29:e11–e17

AuBuchon JP, Herschel L, Roger J, et al. Efficacy of apheresis platelets treated with riboflavin and ultraviolet light for pathogen reduction. Transfusion 2005;45(8):1335–1341

Audet AM, Andrzejewski C, Popovsky MA. Red blood cell transfusion practices in patients undergoing orthopedic surgery: a multi-institutional analysis. Orthopedics 1998;21(8):851–858

Auerbach M, Goodnough LT, Picard D, Maniatis A. The role of intravenous iron in anemia management and transfusion avoidance. Transfusion 2008;48 (5):988–1000

Auerbach M, Macdougall IC. Safety of intravenous iron formulations: facts and folklore. Blood Transfus 2014;12:296–300

Auerbach M. Intravenous iron in the perioperative setting. Am J Hematol 2014;89(9):933 10 1002/ajh.23 793

Australasian Association for Blood Conservation (AABC). Comprehensive Patient Blood Management: A Strategy to Reduce Blood Usage and Costs and Improve Clinical Outcomes. Proposal to the National Blood Authority. Perth: Australasian Association for Blood Conservation; 2006

Australian Commission on Safety and Quality in Health Care (ACSQH). Accreditation and the NSQHS Standards. Updated April 2015a. http://www.safetyandquality.gov.au/our-work/accreditation-and-the-nsqhs-standards. Accessed July 24, 2015

Australian Commission on Safety and Quality in Health Care (ACSQHC). National Priorities. 2015b. http://www. safetyandquality.gov.au/national-priorities. Accessed July 24, 2015

Australian Commission on Safety and Quality in Health Care (ACSQH). Safety and Quality Improvement Guide Standard 7: Blood and Blood Products (October 2012). Sydney: ACSQHC; 2012. http://www.safetyandquality.gov. au/wp-content/uploads/2012/10/Standard7_Oct_2012_WEB.pdf. Accessed July 24, 2015

Australian Red Cross Blood Service (ARCBS). Anaemia and haemostasis overview. Updated September 2014a. http://www.transfusion.com.au/transfusion_practice/anaemia_haemostasis_-management. Accessed March 12, 2015

Australian Red Cross Blood Service (ARCBS). Patient Blood Management. Updated October 2014b. http://www. transfusion.com.au/transfusion_practice/patient_blood_management. Accessed March 12, 2015

Axford TC, Dearani JA, Ragno G, et al. Safety and therapeutic effectiveness of reinfused shed blood after open heart surgery. Ann Thorac Surg 1994;57(3):615–622

Azmoon S, Demarest C, Pucillo AL, et al. Neurologic and cardiac benefits of therapeutic hypothermia. Cardiol Rev 2011;19(3):108–114

Baele P, Beguin C, Waterloos H, et al. The Belgium BIOMED Study about transfusion for surgery. Acta Anaesthesiol Belg 1998;49(4):243–303

Baele PL, De Bruyère M, Deneys V, et al. Results of the SAnGUIS study in Belgium. A concerted action of the Commission of the European Communities IVth Medical and Health Research Programme. The Belgium SAnGUIS Study Group. Safe AND Good Use of blood In Surgery. Acta Chir Belg 1994a;94 (Suppl):1–61

Baele PL, De Bruyère M, Deneys V, et al. The SANGUIS Study in Belgium: an overview of methods and results. Safe and good use of blood in surgery. Acta Chir Belg 1994b;94(2):69–74

Baikoussis NG, Papakonstantinou NA, Apostolakis E. The "benefits" of the mini-extracorporeal circulation in the minimal invasive cardiac surgery era. J Cardiol 2014;63(6):391–396

Banbury MK, Brizzio ME, Rajeswaran J, Lytle BW, Blackstone EH. Transfusion increases the risk of postoperative infection after cardiovascular surgery. J Am Coll Surg 2006;202(1):131–138

Barker LF, Gerety RJ. The clinical problem of hepatitis transmission. Prog Clin Biol Res 1976;11:163–182

Baron DM, Hochrieser H, Posch M, et al; European Surgical Outcomes Study (EuSOS) group for Trials Groups of European Society of Intensive Care Medicine; European Society of Anaesthesiology. Preoperative anaemia is associated with poor clinical outcome in non-cardiac surgery patients. Br J Anaesth 2014;113(3):416–423

Barr PJ, Donnelly M, Cardwell CR, Parker M, Morris K, Bailie KEM. The appropriateness of red blood cell use and the extent of overtransfusion: right decision? Right amount? Transfusion 2011;51 (8):1684–1694

Bassand JP. Acute Coronary Syndromes and Percutaneous Coronary Interventions: impact of bleeding and blood transfusion. Hamostaseologie 2009;29 (4):381–387

Bateman ST, Lacroix J, Boven K, et al; Pediatric Acute Lung Injury and Sepsis Investigators Network. Anemia, blood loss, and blood transfusions in North American children in the intensive care unit. Am J Respir Crit Care Med 2008;178(1):26–33

Baxi AC, Josephson CD, Iannucci GJ, Mahle WT. Necrotizing enterocolitis in infants with congenital heart disease: the role of red blood cell transfusions. Pediatr Cardiol 2014;35(6):1024–1029

Beale E, Zhu J, Chan L, Shulman I, Harwood R, Demetriades D. Blood transfusion in critically injured patients: a prospective study. Injury 2006;37(5):455–465

Beattie WS, Karkouti K, Wijeysundera DN, Tait G. Risk associated with preoperative anemia in noncardiac surgery: a single-center cohort study. Anesthesiology 2009;110(3):574–581

Beggs AD, Dilworth MP, Powell SL, Atherton H, Griffiths EA. A systematic review of transarterial embolization versus emergency surgery in treatment of major nonvariceal upper gastrointestinal bleeding. Clin Exp Gastroenterol 2014;7:93–104

Belatti DA, Phisitkul P. Trends in orthopedics: an analysis of Medicare claims, 2000-2010. Orthopedics 2013;36(3): e366 –e372

Belda FJ, Aguilera L, García de la Asunción J, et al; Spanish Reduccion de la Tasa de Infeccion Quirurgica Group. Supplemental perioperative oxygen and the risk of surgical wound infection: a randomized controlled trial. JAMA 2005;294(16):2035–2042

Bell WR, Braine HG, Ness PM, Kickler TS. Improved survival in thrombotic thrombocytopenic purpura-hemolytic uremic syndrome. Clinical experience in 108 patients. N Engl J Med 1991;325(6):398–403

Bellamy MC. Wet, dry or something else? Br J Anaesth 2006;97(6):755–757

Bennett-Guerrero E, Zhao Y, O'Brien SM, et al. Variation in use of blood transfusion in coronary artery bypass graft surgery. JAMA 2010;304(14):1568–1575

Berend K, Levi M. Management of adult Jehovah's Witness patients with acute bleeding. Am J Med 2009;122 (12):1071–1076

Berger MD, Gerber B, Arn K, Senn O, Schanz U, Stussi G. Significant reduction of red blood cell transfusion requirements by changing from a double-unit to a single-unit transfusion policy in patients receiving intensive chemotherapy or stem cell transplantation. Haematologica 2012;97(1):116–122

Beris P, Muñoz M, García-Erce JA, Thomas D, Maniatis A, Van der Linden P. Perioperative anaemia management: consensus statement on the role of intravenous iron. Br J Anaesth 2008;100 (5):599–604

Bernard AC, Davenport DL, Chang PK, et al. Intraoperative transfusion of 1 U to 2 U packed red blood cells is associated with increased 30-day mortality, surgical-site infection, pneumonia, and sepsis in general surgery patients. J Am Coll Surg 2009;208:931–937.e2

Bernard SA, Gray TW, Buist MD, et al. Treatment of comatose survivors of out-of-hospital cardiac arrest with induced hypothermia. N Engl J Med 2002;346(8):557–563

Berséus O, Hervig T, Seghatchian J. Military walking blood bank and the civilian blood service. Transfus Apheresis Sci 2012;46(3):341–342

Beutler E, Waalen J. The definition of anemia: what is the lower limit of normal of the blood hemoglobin concentration? Blood 2006;107(5):1747–1750

Bhatt DL, Scheiman J, Abraham NS, et al; American College of Cardiology Foundation Task Force on Clinical Expert Consensus Documents. ACCF/ACG/AHA 2008 expert consensus document on reducing the gastrointestinal risks of antiplatelet therapy and NSAID use: a report of the American College of Cardiology Foundation Task Force on Clinical Expert Consensus Documents. Circulation 2008;118(18):1894–1909

Bierbaum BE, Callaghan JJ, Galante JO, Rubash HE, Tooms RE, Welch RB. An analysis of blood management in patients having a total hip or knee arthroplasty. J Bone Joint Surg Am 1999;81 (1):2–10

Bilecen S, Peelen LM, Kalkman CJ, Spanjersberg AJ, Moons KG, Nierich AP. Fibrinogen concentrate therapy in complex cardiac surgery. J Cardiothorac Vasc Anesth 2013;27(1):12–17

Bilgin YM, van de Watering LM, Versteegh MI, van Oers MH, Vamvakas EC, Brand A. Postoperative complications associated with transfusion of platelets and plasma in cardiac surgery. Transfusion 2011;51(12):2603–2610

Binder RK, Barbanti M, Ye J, et al. Blood loss and transfusion rates associated with transcatheter aortic valve replacement: recommendations for patients who refuse blood transfusion. Catheter Cardiovasc Interv 2014;83(6):E221–E226

Binhas M, Salomon L, Roudot-Thoraval F, Armand C, Plaud B, Marty J. Radical prostatectomy with robot-assisted radical prostatectomy and laparoscopic radical prostatectomy under low-dose aspirin does not significantly increase blood loss. Urology 2012;79(3):591–595

Birg H. Die demographische Zeitenwende. 3rd ed. Munich: C.H. Beck; 2003:105

Biscoping J, Götz E, Biermann E. Gewinnung und Anwendung von Eigenblut unter den Vorgaben des Transfusionsgesetzes. Published November 2013. http://www.bda.de/docman/619-gewinnung-und-anwendung-von-eigenblut-unter-den-vorgaben-des-transfusionsgesetzes.html. Accessed March 12, 2015

Blair SD, Janvrin SB, McCollum CN, Greenhalgh RM. Effect of early blood transfusion on gastrointestinal haemorrhage. Br J Surg 1986;73(10):783–785

Blajchman MA, Beckers EAM, Dickmeiss E, Lin L, Moore G, Muylle L. Bacterial detection of platelets: current problems and possible resolutions. Transfus Med Rev 2005;19(4):259–272

Blajchman MA, Goldman M. Bacterial contamination of platelet concentrates: incidence, significance, and prevention. Semin Hematol 2001;38(4 Suppl 11):20–26

Blajchman MA, Vamvakas EC. The continuing risk of transfusion-transmitted infections. N Engl J Med 2006;355 (13):1303–1305

Blood and Blood Products Committee. Review of the Alternatives to Homologous Blood Donation: A Report by the Blood and Blood Products Committee, Australian Health Ministers' Advisory Council. Canberra: Department of Health and Aged Care; 2000

BloodSafe eLearning Australia. Website. 2015. https://bloodsafelearning.org.au. Accessed July 24, 2015

Blumberg N, Heal JM, Liesveld JL, Phillips GL, Rowe JM. Platelet transfusion and survival in adults with acute leukemia. Leukemia 2008;22(3):631–635

Bochicchio GV, Napolitano L, Joshi M, Bochicchio K, Meyer W, Scalea TM. Outcome analysis of blood product transfusion in trauma patients: a prospective, risk-adjusted study. World J Surg 2008;32(10):2185–2189

Boehm K, Beyer B, Tennstedt P, et al. No impact of blood transfusion on oncological outcome after radical prostatectomy in patients with prostate cancer. World J Urol 2014 Epub 2014 Jul 3

Boffard KD, Riou B, Warren B, et al; NovoSeven Trauma Study Group. Recombinant factor VIIa as adjunctive therapy for bleeding control in severely injured trauma patients: two parallel randomized, placebo-controlled, double-blind clinical trials. J Trauma 2005;59(1):8–18

Bohlius J, Schmidlin K, Brillant C, et al. Erythropoietin or darbepoetin for patients with cancer–meta-analysis based on individual patient data. Cochrane Database Syst Rev 2009a;(3): CD007303

Bohlius J, Schmidlin K, Brillant C, et al. Recombinant human erythropoiesis-stimulating agents and mortality in patients with cancer: a meta-analysis of randomised trials. Lancet 2009b;373 (9674):1532–1542

Bojang KA, Palmer A, Boele van Hensbroek M, Banya WA, Greenwood BM. Management of severe malarial anaemia in Gambian children. Trans R Soc Trop Med Hyg 1997;91(5):557–561

Bolliger D, Tanaka KA. Roles of thrombelastography and thromboelastometry for patient blood management in cardiac surgery. Transfus Med Rev 2013;27(4):213–220

Bolton-Maggs PHB (ed), Poles D, Watt A, Thomas D, Cohen H, on behalf of the Serious Hazards of Transfusion (SHOT) Steering Group. The 2012 Annual SHOT Report. Published 2013. http://www.shotuk.org/wp-content/uploads/2013/08/SHOT-Annual-Report-2012.pdf. Accessed March 12, 2015

Boralessa H, Goldhill DR, Tucker K, Mortimer AJ, Grant-Casey J. National comparative audit of blood use in elective primary unilateral total hip replacement surgery in the UK. Ann R Coll Surg Engl 2009;91(7):599–605

Boulton FE, James V; British Committee for Standards in Haematology, Transfusion Task Force. Guidelines for policies on alternatives to allogeneic blood transfusion. 1. Predeposit autologous blood donation and transfusion. Transfus Med 2007;17(5):354–365

Bowley DM, Barker P, Boffard KD. Intraoperative blood salvage in penetrating abdominal trauma: a randomised, controlled trial. World J Surg 2006;30 (6):1074–1080

Bracey AW, Radovancevic R, Riggs SA, et al. Lowering the hemoglobin threshold for transfusion in coronary artery bypass procedures: effect on patient outcome. Transfusion 1999;39(10):1070–1077

Bräuer A, English MJ, Steinmetz N, et al. Efficacy of forced-air warming systems with full body blankets. Can J Anaesth 2007;54(1):34–41

Branco BC, Inaba K, Doughty R, et al. The increasing burden of phlebotomy in the development of anaemia and need for blood transfusion amongst trauma patients. Injury 2012;43(1):78–83

Brenner ML, Moore LJ, DuBose JJ, et al. A clinical series of resuscitative endovascular balloon occlusion of the aorta for hemorrhage control and resuscitation. J Trauma Acute Care Surg 2013;75 (3):506–511

Brohi K, Cohen MJ, Ganter MT, et al. Acute coagulopathy of trauma: hypoperfusion induces systemic anticoagulation and hyperfibrinolysis. J Trauma 2008;64 (5):1211–1217

Brohi K, Cohen MJ, Ganter MT, Matthay MA, Mackersie RC, Pittet JF. Acute traumatic coagulopathy: initiated by hypoperfusion: modulated through the protein C pathway? Ann Surg 2007;245(5):812–818

Bruhn C. Patient blood management - fewer transfusions, lower costs [article in German]. Dtsch Med Wochenschr 2013;138(36):1752

Brunskill SJ, Millette SL, Shokoohi A, et al. Red blood cell transfusion for people undergoing hip fracture surgery. Cochrane Database Syst Rev 2015;(4): CD 009 699

Bundesärztekammer (BAEK). Cross-Sectional Guidelines for Therapy with Blood Components and Plasma Derivates. 4th revised edition. Published 2009, updated 2011a. www.bundesaerztekammer.de/downloads/Querschnittsleitlinie_Gesamtdokument-englisch_0 703 2011.pdf. Accessed July 24, 2015

Bundesärztekammer (BAEK). Revision of the "Guideline of the German Medical Association on Quality Assurance in Medical Laboratory Examinations – Rili-BAEK" (unauthorized translation). J Lab Med 2015;39(1):26–69. http://www.degruyter.com/view/j/labm.2015.39.issue-1/labmed-2014-0046/labmed-2014-0046.xml?format=INT. Accessed May 11, 2015

Bundesärztekammer (BAEK). Richtlinien zur Gewinnung von Blut und Blutbestandteilen und zur Anwendung von Blutprodukten (Hämotherapie). Zweite Richtlinienanpassung 2010. Köln: Deutscher Ärzte-Verlag; 2010

Bundesärztekammer (BAEK). Struktur der Ärzteschaft 2011. 2011b. http://www.bundesaerztekammer.de/downloads/Stat11Abb01.pdf. Accessed March 12, 2015

Bundesministeriums für Gesundheit und Soziale Sicherung (BGSS). Mitteilung des Arbeitskreises Blut. 2005. http://www.bda.de/docman/alle-dokumente-fuer-suchindex/oeffentlich/empfehlungen/621-aktuelle-empfehlungen-zur-autologen-haemotherapie/file.html. Accessed March 12, 2015

Bundgaard-Nielsen M, Ruhnau B, Secher NH, Kehlet H. Flow-related techniques for preoperative goal-directed fluid optimization. Br J Anaesth 2007;98(1):38–44

Burns DL, Mascioli EA, Bistrian BR. Parenteral iron dextran therapy: a review. Nutrition 1995;11(2):163–168

Bursi F, Barbieri A, Politi L, et al. Perioperative red blood cell transfusion and outcome in stable patients after elective major vascular surgery. Eur J Vasc Endovasc Surg 2009;37(3):311–318

Busch MP, Dodd RY. NAT and blood safety: what is the paradigm? Transfusion 2000;40(10):1157–1160

Buser A, Sigle J, Halter J. Blood transfusions in the treatment of chronic anemia [in German]. Ther Umsch 2010;67:265–269

Butwick AJ, Aleshi P, Fontaine M, Riley ET, Goodnough LT. Retrospective analysis of transfusion outcomes in pregnant patients at a tertiary obstetric center. Int J Obstet Anesth 2009;18(4):302–308

Cabral KP, Fraser GL, Duprey J, et al. Prothrombin complex concentrates to reverse warfarin-induced coagulopathy in patients with intracranial bleeding. Clin Neurol Neurosurg 2013;115 (6):770–774

Cabrales P, Martini J, Intaglietta M, Tsai AG. Blood viscosity maintains microvascular conditions during normovolemic anemia independent of blood oxygen-carrying capacity. Am J Physiol Heart Circ Physiol 2006;291(2):H581–H590

Cabrales P, Nacharaju P, Manjula BN, Tsai AG, Acharya SA, Intaglietta M. Early difference in tissue pH and microvascular hemodynamics in hemorrhagic shock resuscitation using polyethylene glycol-albumin- and hydroxyethyl starch-based plasma expanders. Shock 2005a;24(1):66–73

Cabrales P, Tsai AG. Plasma viscosity regulates systemic and microvascular perfusion during acute extreme anemic conditions. Am J Physiol Heart Circ Physiol 2006;291(5):H2445–H2452

Cabrales P, Tsai AG, Intaglietta M. Is resuscitation from hemorrhagic shock limited by blood oxygen-carrying capacity or blood viscosity? Shock 2007;27 (4):380–389

Cabrales P, Tsai AG, Intaglietta M. Microvascular pressure and functional capillary density in extreme hemodilution with low- and high-viscosity dextran and a low-viscosity Hb-based O2 carrier. Am J Physiol Heart Circ Physiol 2004;287(1):H363–H373

Cabrales P, Tsai AG, Winslow RM, Intaglietta M. Extreme hemodilution with PEG-hemoglobin vs. PEG-albumin. Am J Physiol Heart Circ Physiol 2005b;289 (6):H2392–H2400

Calderon-Margalit R, Mor-Yosef S, Mayer M, Adler B, Shapira SC. An administrative intervention to improve the utilization of laboratory tests within a university hospital. Int J Qual Health Care 2005;17(3):243–248

Camp RC. Benchmarking: The Search for Industry Best Practices that Lead to Superior Performance. Milwaukee: ASQ Quality Press; 1989:xv,299

Card R, Sawyer M, Degnan B, et al. Institute for Clinical Systems Improvement. Perioperative Protocol. Updated March 2014. https://www.icsi.org/_asset/0c2xkr/Periop.pdf. Accessed June 10, 2015

Carless PA, Henry DA, Anthony DM. Fibrin sealant use for minimizing peri-operative allogeneic blood transfusion. Cochrane Database Syst Rev 2003;(2): CD 004 171

Carless PA, Henry DA, Carson JL, et al. Transfusion thresholds and other strategies for guiding allogeneic red blood cell transfusion. Cochrane Database Syst Rev 2010a;(10):CD 002 042

Carless PA, Henry DA, Moxey AJ, et al. Cell salvage for minimising perioperative allogeneic blood transfusion. Cochrane Database Syst Rev 2010b;(3): CD 001 888

Carless PA, Henry DA, Moxey AJ, et al. Desmopressin for minimising perioperative allogeneic blood transfusion. Cochrane

Database Syst Rev 2004b;(1): CD 001 884

Carless P, Moxey A, O'Connell D, Henry D. Autologous transfusion techniques: a systematic review of their efficacy. Transfus Med 2004a;14(2):123–144

Carrascal Y, Maroto L, Rey J, et al. Impact of preoperative anemia on cardiac surgery in octogenarians. Interact Cardiovasc Thorac Surg 2010;10(2):249–255

Carson JL. Blood transfusion and risk of infection: new convincing evidence. JAMA 2014;311(13):1293–1294

Carson JL, Altman DG, Duff A, et al. Risk of bacterial infection associated with allogeneic blood transfusion among patients undergoing hip fracture repair. Transfusion 1999;39(7):694–700

Carson JL, Brooks MM, Abbott JD, et al. Liberal versus restrictive transfusion thresholds for patients with symptomatic coronary artery disease. Am Heart J 2013;165(6):964–971.e1

Carson JL, Carless PA, Hébert PC. Transfusion thresholds and other strategies for guiding allogeneic red blood cell transfusion. Cochrane Database Syst Rev 2012a;(4):CD 002 042

Carson JL, Duff A, Poses RM, et al. Effect of anaemia and cardiovascular disease on surgical mortality and morbidity. Lancet 1996;348(9034):1055–1060

Carson JL, Grossman BJ, Kleinman S, et al; Clinical Transfusion Medicine Committee of the AABB. Red blood cell transfusion: a clinical practice guideline from the AABB*. Ann Intern Med 2012b;157 (1):49–58

Carson JL, Hill S, Carless P, Hébert P, Henry D. Transfusion triggers: a systematic review of the literature. Transfus Med Rev 2002a;16(3):187–199

Carson JL, Noveck H, Berlin JA, Gould SA. Mortality and morbidity in patients with very low postoperative Hb levels who decline blood transfusion. Transfusion 2002b;42(7):812–818

Carson JL, Poses RM, Spence RK, Bonavita G. Severity of anaemia and operative mortality and morbidity. Lancet 1988;1 (8588):727–729

Carson JL, Terrin ML, Noveck H, et al; FOCUS Investigators. Liberal or restrictive transfusion in high-risk patients after hip surgery. N Engl J Med 2011;365(26):2453–2462

Casati V, D'Angelo A, Barbato L, et al. Perioperative management of four anaemic female Jehovah's Witnesses undergoing urgent complex cardiac surgery. Br J Anaesth 2007;99(3):349–352

Castillo JJ, Dalia S, Pascual SK. Association between red blood cell transfusions and development of non-Hodgkin lymphoma: a meta-analysis of observational studies. Blood 2010;116(16):2897–2907

Cataldi S, Bruder N, Dufour H, Lefevre P, Grisoli F, François G. Intraoperative autologous blood transfusion in intracranial surgery. Neurosurgery 1997;40 (4):765–772

Cattaneo M. Desmopressin in the treatment of patients with defects of platelet function. Haematologica 2002;87 (11):1122–1124

Cauwenberghs S, van Pampus E, Curvers J, Akkerman JW, Heemskerk JW. Hemostatic and signaling functions of transfused platelets. Transfus Med Rev 2007;21(4):287–294

Centers for Medicare & Medicaid Services (CMS). National Health Expenditures by type of expenditure and source of funds, calendar years 1960–2013. http://www.cms.gov/Research-Statistics-Data-and-Systems/Statistics-Trends-and-Reports/NationalHealthExpendData/Downloads/NHE2013.zip. Accessed July 24, 2015

Chaiwat O, Lang JD, Vavilala MS, et al. Early packed red blood cell transfusion and acute respiratory distress syndrome after trauma. Anesthesiology 2009;110 (2):351–360

Chan R, Leniger-Follert E. Effect of isovolemic hemodilution on oxygen supply and electrocorticogram in cat brain during focal ischemia and in normal tissue. Int J Microcirc Clin Exp 1983;2(4):297–313

Chang CH, Chang Y, Chen DW, Ueng SW, Lee MS. Topical tranexamic acid reduces blood loss and transfusion rates associated with primary total hip arthroplasty. Clin Orthop Relat Res 2014a;472 (5):1552–1557

Chang H, Hall GA, Geerts WH, Greenwood C, McLeod RS, Sher GD. Allogeneic red blood cell transfusion is an independent risk factor for the development of postoperative bacterial infection. Vox Sang 2000;78(1):13–18

Chang HW, Nam J, Cho J-H, Lee J-R, Kim Y-J, Kim W-H. Five-year experience with mini-volume priming in infants ≤5 kg: safety of significantly smaller transfusion volumes. Artif Organs 2014b;38(1):78–87

Chapler CK, Cain SM. The physiologic reserve in oxygen carrying capacity: studies in experimental hemodilution. Can J Physiol Pharmacol 1986;64(1):7–12

Chaplin H Jr, Mollison PL, Vetter H. The body/venous hematocrit ratio: its constancy over a wide hematocrit range. J Clin Invest 1953;32(12):1309–1316

Charles A, Shaikh AA, Walters M, Huehl S, Pomerantz R. Blood transfusion is an independent predictor of mortality after blunt trauma. Am Surg 2007;73(1):1–5

Chassot PG, Kern C, Ravussin P. Hemorrhage and transfusion: the case of Jehovah's witnesses [article in French]. Rev Med Suisse 2006;2(88):2674–2679

Chatpun S, Cabrales P. Cardiac mechano-energetic cost of elevated plasma viscosity after moderate hemodilution. Biorheology 2010;47(3-4):225–237

Chatterjee S, Wetterslev J, Sharma A, Lichstein E, Mukherjee D. Association of blood transfusion with increased mortality in myocardial infarction: a meta-analysis and diversity-adjusted study sequential analysis. JAMA Intern Med 2013;173(2):132–139

Chelemer SB, Prato BS, Cox PM Jr, O'Connor GT, Morton JR. Association of bacterial infection and red blood cell transfusion after coronary artery bypass surgery. Ann Thorac Surg 2002;73(1):138–142

Chhatriwalla AK, Amin AP, Kennedy KF, et al; National Cardiovascular Data Registry. Association between bleeding events and in-hospital mortality after percutaneous coronary intervention. JAMA 2013;309(10):1022–1029

Chudy M, Weber-Schehl M, Pichl L, et al. Blood screening nucleic acid amplification tests for human immunodeficiency virus Type 1 may require two different amplification targets. Transfusion 2012;52(2):431–439

Churchhouse AM, Mathews TJ, McBride OM, Dunning J. Does blood transfusion increase the chance of recurrence in patients undergoing surgery for lung cancer? Interact Cardiovasc Thorac Surg 2012;14(1):85–90

Ciesla DJ, Moore EE, Johnson JL, Burch JM, Cothren CC, Sauaia A. A 12-year prospective study of postinjury multiple organ failure: has anything changed? Arch Surg 2005;140(5):432–440

Cladellas M, Farré N, Comín-Colet J, et al. Effects of preoperative intravenous erythropoietin plus iron on outcome in anemic patients after cardiac valve replacement. Am J Cardiol 2012;110 (7):1021–1026

Claridge JA, Sawyer RG, Schulman AM, McLemore EC, Young JS. Blood transfusions correlate with infections in trauma patients in a dose-dependent manner. Am Surg 2002;68(7):566–572

Clinical Excellence Commission (CEC). Posters. 2015. http://www.cec.health.nsw.gov.au/resources/posters. Accessed July 24, 2015

Cohn CS, Welbig J, Bowman R, Kammann S, Frey K, Zantek N. A data-driven approach to patient blood management. Transfusion 2014;54(2):316–322

Collins SR, Blank RS, Deatherage LS, Dull RO. Special article: the endothelial glycocalyx: emerging concepts in pulmonary edema and acute lung injury. Anesth Analg 2013;117(3):664–674

Cooper HA, Rao SV, Greenberg MD, et al. Conservative versus liberal red cell transfusion in acute myocardial infarction (the CRIT Randomized Pilot Study). Am J Cardiol 2011;108(8):1108–1111

Corwin HL. Blood transfusion: first, do no harm! Chest 1999;116(5):1149–1150

Corwin HL, Carson JL. Blood transfusion—when is more really less? N Engl J Med 2007;356(16):1667–1669

Corwin HL, Gettinger A, Fabian TC, et al; EPO Critical Care Trials Group. Efficacy and safety of epoetin alfa in critically ill patients. N Engl J Med 2007;357(10):965–976

Corwin HL, Gettinger A, Pearl RG, et al. The CRIT Study: Anemia and blood transfusion in the critically ill—current clinical practice in the United States. Crit Care Med 2004;32(1):39–52

Cotton BA, McCarthy JJ, Holcomb JB. Acutely injured patients on dabigatran. N Engl J Med 2011;365(21):2039–2040

Cox ED, Schreiber MA, McManus J, Wade CE, Holcomb JB. New hemostatic agents in the combat setting. Transfusion 2009;49(Suppl 5):248S– 255S

Croce MA, Tolley EA, Claridge JA, Fabian TC. Transfusions result in pulmonary morbidity and death after a moderate degree of injury. J Trauma 2005;59(1):19–24

Crystal GJ, Kim SJ, Salem MM, Abdel-Latif M. Myocardial oxygen supply/demand relations during phenylephrine infusions in dogs. Anesth Analg 1991;73(3):283–288

Crystal GJ, Salem MR. Beta-adrenergic stimulation restores oxygen extraction reserve during acute normovolemic hemodilution. Anesth Analg 2002;95(4):851–857 table of contents

Curley A, Venkatesh V, Stanworth S, et al. Platelets for neonatal transfusion - study 2: a randomised controlled trial to compare two different platelet count thresholds for prophylactic platelet transfusion to preterm neonates. Neonatology 2014a;106(2):102–106

Curley GF, Shehata N, Mazer CD, Hare GM, Friedrich JO. Transfusion triggers for guiding RBC transfusion for cardiovascular surgery: a systematic review and meta-analysis. Crit Care Med 2014b;42(12):2611–2624

Curry N, Stanworth S, Hopewell S, Dorée C, Brohi K, Hyde C. Trauma-induced coagulopathy—a review of the systematic reviews: is there sufficient evidence to guide clinical transfusion practice? Transfus Med Rev 2011;25(3):217–231.e2

Cywinski JB, Alster JM, Miller C, Vogt DP, Parker BM. Prediction of intraoperative transfusion requirements during orthotopic liver transplantation and the influence on postoperative patient survival. Anesth Analg 2014;118(2):428–437

Dai J, Tu W, Yang Z, Lin R. Case report: intraoperative management of extreme hemodilution in a patient with a severed axillary artery. Anesth Analg 2010;111(5):1204–1206

Dallman PR. In: Hallberg L, Asp NG, eds. Iron Nutrition in Health and Disease. London: John Libbey; 1996:65–74

Dalrymple-Hay MJ, Pack L, Deakin CD, et al. Autotransfusion of washed shed mediastinal fluid decreases the requirement for autologous blood transfusion following cardiac surgery: a prospective randomized trial. Eur J Cardiothorac Surg 1999;15(6):830–834

Dangsuwan P, Manchana T. Blood transfusion reduction with intravenous iron in gynecologic cancer patients receiving chemotherapy. Gynecol Oncol 2010;116(3):522–525

Darby S, Hill D, Deo H, et al. Residential radon and lung cancer—detailed results of a collaborative analysis of individual data on 7148 persons with lung cancer and 14,208 persons without lung cancer from 13 epidemiologic studies in Europe. Scand J Work Environ Health 2006;32(Suppl 1):1–83

Davenport R. Pathogenesis of acute traumatic coagulopathy. Transfusion 2013;53(Suppl 1):23S– 27S

David O, Sinha R, Robinson K, Cardone D. The prevalence of anaemia, hypochromia and microcytosis in preoperative cardiac surgical patients. Anaesth Intensive Care 2013;41(3):316–321

de Araújo Azi LM, Lopes FM, Garcia LV. Postoperative management of severe acute anemia in a Jehovah's Witness. Transfusion 2014;54(4):1153–1157

de Boer MT, Boonstra EA, Lisman T, Porte RJ. Role of fibrin sealants in liver surgery. Dig Surg 2012;29(1):54–61

de Calignon A, Polydoro M, Suárez-Calvet M, et al. Propagation of tau pathology in a model of early Alzheimer's disease. Neuron 2012;73(4):685–697

de Gast-Bakker DH, de Wilde RBP, Hazekamp MG, et al. Safety and effects of two red blood cell transfusion strategies in pediatric cardiac surgery patients: a randomized controlled trial.

Intensive Care Med 2013;39(11):2011–2019

De Hert S, Imberger G, Carlisle J, et al; Task Force on Preoperative Evaluation of the Adult Noncardiac Surgery Patient of the European Society of Anaesthesiology. Preoperative evaluation of the adult patient undergoing non-cardiac surgery: guidelines from the European Society of Anaesthesiology. Eur J Anaesthesiol 2011;28(10):684–722

de Jong KP, Wertenbroek MW. Liver resection combined with local ablation: where are the limits? Dig Surg 2011;28(2):127–133

de Korte D. 10 years experience with bacterial screening of platelet concentrates in the Netherlands. Transfus Med Hemother 2011;38(4):251–254

de Korte D, Curvers J, de Kort WL, et al. Effects of skin disinfection method, deviation bag, and bacterial screening on clinical safety of platelet transfusions in the Netherlands. Transfusion 2006;46(3):476–485

de Korte D, Marcelis JH, Verhoeven AJ, Soeterboek AM. Diversion of first blood volume results in a reduction of bacterial contamination for whole-blood collections. Vox Sang 2002;83(1):13–16

De Santo L, Romano G, Della Corte A, et al. Preoperative anemia in patients undergoing coronary artery bypass grafting predicts acute kidney injury. J Thorac Cardiovasc Surg 2009;138(4):965–970

Del Vecchio L, Locatelli F. Erythropoietin and iron therapy in patients with renal failure. In: Maniatis A, Van der Linden P, Hardy JF, eds. Alternatives to Blood Transfusion in Transfusion Medicine. 2nd ed. Oxford: Blackwell Publishing; 2011:357–367

Delgado-Corcoran C, Bodily S, Frank DU, Witte MK, Castillo R, Bratton SL. Reducing blood testing in pediatric patients after heart surgery: a quality improvement project. Pediatr Crit Care Med 2014;15(8):756–761

Department of Health and Human Services (DHHS), State Government of Victoria, Australia. Blood Matters Program. Updated July 2015. http://www.health.vic.gov.au/bloodmatters/index.htm. Accessed July 24, 2015

Department of Health of Western Australia (DHWA). Patient Blood Management—Executive Summary. Perth: Department of Health of Western Australia; 2011

Deutsche Gesellschaft für Anästhesiologie und Intensivmedizin (DGAI). Gemeinsame Empfehlung der Deutschen Gesellschaft für Anästhesiologie und Intensivmedizin (DGAI), der Deutschen Gesellschaft für Chirurgie (DGC) und

233

der Deutschen Gesellschaft für Innere Medizin (DGIM). Präoperative Evaluation erwachsener Patienten vor elektiven, nicht kardiochirurgischen Eingriffen. Anästh Intensivmed 2010;57:788–797

Deutsche Gesellschaft für Anästhesiologie und Intensivmedizin (DGAI). Leitlinie für ambulantes Operieren bzw. Tageschirurgie. Nürnberg: DGAI; 1999

Devereaux PJ, Mrkobrada M, Sessler DI, et al; POISE-2 Investigators. Aspirin in patients undergoing noncardiac surgery. N Engl J Med 2014;370(16):1494–1503

Devine DV, Serrano K. The platelet storage lesion. Clin Lab Med 2010;30(2):475–487

Devon KM, McLeod RS. Pre and peri-operative erythropoietin for reducing allogeneic blood transfusions in colorectal cancer surgery. Cochrane Database Syst Rev 2009;(1):CD 007 148

Dewilde WJ, Janssen PW, Verheugt FWA, et al. Triple therapy for atrial fibrillation and percutaneous coronary intervention: a contemporary review. J Am Coll Cardiol 2014;64(12):1270–1280

Dewilde WJ, Oirbans T, Verheugt FW, et al; WOEST study investigators. Use of clopidogrel with or without aspirin in patients taking oral anticoagulant therapy and undergoing percutaneous coronary intervention: an open-label, randomised, controlled trial. Lancet 2013;381(9872):1107–1115

Dexter F, Witkowski TA, Epstein RH. Forecasting preanesthesia clinic appointment duration from the electronic medical record medication list. Anesth Analg 2012;114(3):670–673

Diehm N, Benenati JF, Becker GJ, et al. Anemia is associated with abdominal aortic aneurysm (AAA) size and decreased long-term survival after endovascular AAA repair. J Vasc Surg 2007;46(4):676–681

Dietrich W, Spannagl M, Boehm J, et al. Tranexamic acid and aprotinin in primary cardiac operations: an analysis of 220 cardiac surgical patients treated with tranexamic acid or aprotinin. Anesth Analg 2008;107(5):1469–1478

Divers SG, Kannan K, Stewart RM, et al. Quantitation of CD 62, soluble CD 62, and lysosome-associated membrane proteins 1 and 2 for evaluation of the quality of stored platelet concentrates. Transfusion 1995;35(4):292–297

Dixon B, Reid D, Collins M, et al. The operating surgeon is an independent predictor of chest tube drainage following cardiac surgery. J Cardiothorac Vasc Anesth 2014;28(2):242–246

Dixon B, Santamaria JD, Reid D, et al. The association of blood transfusion with

mortality after cardiac surgery: cause or confounding? (CME). Transfusion 2013;53(1):19–27

Donadee C, Raat NJ, Kanias T, et al. Nitric oxide scavenging by red blood cell microparticles and cell-free hemoglobin as a mechanism for the red cell storage lesion. Circulation 2011;124(4):465–476

Donofrio MT, Moon-Grady AJ, Hornberger LK, et al; American Heart Association Adults With Congenital Heart Disease Joint Committee of the Council on Cardiovascular Disease in the Young and Council on Clinical Cardiology, Council on Cardiovascular Surgery and Anesthesia, and Council on Cardiovascular and Stroke Nursing. Diagnosis and treatment of fetal cardiac disease: a scientific statement from the American Heart Association. Circulation 2014;129(21):2183–2242

Doodeman HJ, van Haelst IM, Egberts TC, et al. The effect of a preoperative erythropoietin protocol as part of a multifaceted blood management program in daily clinical practice (CME). Transfusion 2013;53(9):1930–1939

Douketis JD, Spyropoulos AC, Kaatz S, et al; BRIDGE Investigators. Perioperative bridging anticoagulation in patients with atrial fibrillation. N Engl J Med. Published Online: Jun 22, 2015 (doi: 10 1056/NEJMoa1 501 035)

Dreier J, Vollmer T, Kleesiek K. Novel flow cytometry-based screening for bacterial contamination of donor platelet preparations compared with other rapid screening methods. Clin Chem 2009;55(8):1492–1502

Dunkelgrun M, Hoeks SE, Welten GMJM, et al. Anemia as an independent predictor of perioperative and long-term cardiovascular outcome in patients scheduled for elective vascular surgery. Am J Cardiol 2008;101(8):1196–1200

Dunne JR, Malone D, Tracy JK, Gannon C, Napolitano LM. Perioperative anemia: an independent risk factor for infection, mortality, and resource utilization in surgery. J Surg Res 2002;102(2):237–244

Dunne JR, Malone DL, Tracy JK, Napolitano LM. Allogenic blood transfusion in the first 24 hours after trauma is associated with increased systemic inflammatory response syndrome (SIRS) and death. Surg Infect (Larchmt) 2004;5(4):395–404

Dunne JR, Riddle MS, Danko J, Hayden R, Petersen K. Blood transfusion is associated with infection and increased resource utilization in combat casualties. Am Surg 2006;72(7):619–626

Dyke C, Aronson S, Dietrich W, et al. Universal definition of perioperative bleed-

ing in adult cardiac surgery. J Thorac Cardiovasc Surg 2014;147(5):1458–1463.e1

Eckhardt KU, Lorentz A, Kurtz A. Sauerstoffabhängige Erythropoietinproduktion – Grundlage für die Kompensation von Blutverlusten. In: Schleinzer W, Singbartl G, eds. Fremdblutsparende Maßnahmen in der operativen Medizin. Basel: Karger; 1993:228–239

Edavettal M, Rogers A, Rogers F, Horst M, Leng W. Prothrombin complex concentrate accelerates international normalized ratio reversal and diminishes the extension of intracranial hemorrhage in geriatric trauma patients. Am Surg 2014;80(4):372–376

Edul VS, Enrico C, Laviolle B, Vazquez AR, Ince C, Dubin A. Quantitative assessment of the microcirculation in healthy volunteers and in patients with septic shock. Crit Care Med 2012;40(5):1443–1448

Edward GM, de Haes JCJM, Oort FJ, Lemaire LC, Hollmann MW, Preckel B. Setting priorities for improving the preoperative assessment clinic: the patients' and the professionals' perspective. Br J Anaesth 2008;100(3):322–326

Edward GM, Preckel B, Martijn BS, Oort FJ, de Haes HC, Hollmann MW. The effects of implementing a new schedule at the preoperative assessment clinic. Eur J Anaesthesiol 2010;27(2):209–213

El-Guindy AM. HEAT-PPCI: A clear and welcome win for heparin. Glob Cardiol Sci Pract 2014;1:40–44

El Hachem L, Momeni M, Friedman K, Moshier EL, Chuang LT, Gretz HF 3 rd. Safety, feasibility and learning curve of robotic single-site surgery in gynecology. Int J Med Robot. Published Online: June 11, 2015 (doi: 10 1002/rcs.1675)

El-Sabbagh AM, Toomasian CJ, Toomasian JM, Ulysse G, Major T, Bartlett RH. Effect of air exposure and suction on blood cell activation and hemolysis in an in vitro cardiotomy suction model. ASAIO J 2013;59(5):474–479

Emeklibas N, Kammerer I, Bach J, Sack FU, Hellstern P. Preoperative hemostasis and its association with bleeding and blood component transfusion requirements in cardiopulmonary bypass surgery. Transfusion 2013;53(6):1226–1234

Emmert MY, Salzberg SP, Theusinger OM, et al. How good patient blood management leads to excellent outcomes in Jehovah's witness patients undergoing cardiac surgery. Interact Cardiovasc Thorac Surg 2011;12(2):183–188

English M, Ahmed M, Ngando C, Berkley J, Ross A. Blood transfusion for severe anaemia in children in a Kenyan hospital. Lancet 2002;359(9305):494–495

Ereth MH, Nuttall GA, Orszulak TA, Santrach PJ, Cooney WP IV, Oliver WC Jr. Blood loss from coronary angiography increases transfusion requirements for coronary artery bypass graft surgery. J Cardiothorac Vasc Anesth 2000;14 (2):177–181

Erhard J, Hofmann A. Blutmanagement in der Viszeralchirurgie. Viszeralchirurgie 2005;40:157–164

Erhard J, Schlensak M, Friedrich J. Blood management in surgery—an analysis [article in German]. Zentralbl Chir 2003;128(6):481–486

Estcourt L, Stanworth S, Doree C, et al. Prophylactic platelet transfusion for prevention of bleeding in patients with haematological disorders after chemotherapy and stem cell transplantation. Cochrane Database Syst Rev 2012;(5): CD 004 269

European Medicines Agency (EMA). New recommendations to manage risk of allergic reactions with intravenous iron-containing medicines [press release]. June 28, 2013. http://www.ema. europa.eu/ema/index.jsp?curl=pages/ news_and_events/news/2013/06/ news_detail_001 833.jsp&mid=WC0b01 ac058 004d5c1. Accessed March 12, 2015

Eurostat. Eurostat website. http://ec.europa.eu/eurostat/web/main. Accessed July 31, 2015

Ezekowitz JA, McAlister FA, Armstrong PW. Anemia is common in heart failure and is associated with poor outcomes: insights from a cohort of 12 065 patients with new-onset heart failure. Circulation 2003;107(2):223–225

Fagotti A, Vizzielli G, Fanfani F, et al. Randomized study comparing use of THUNDERBEAT technology vs standard electrosurgery during laparoscopic radical hysterectomy and pelvic lymphadenectomy for gynecologic cancer. J Minim Invasive Gynecol 2014;21 (3):447–453

Fairbanks VF, Klee GG, Wiseman GA, et al. Measurement of blood volume and red cell mass: re-examination of 51Cr and 125I methods. Blood Cells Mol Dis 1996;22(2):169–186

Fan FC, Chen RYZ, Schuessler GB, Chien S. Effects of hematocrit variations on regional hemodynamics and oxygen transport in the dog. Am J Physiol 1980;238(4):H545 –H522

Farmer S, Isbister J, Leahy M. History of transfusion. In: Jabbour N, ed. Transfusion-free Medicine and Surgery. Malden, MA: Wiley-Blackwell; 2013a

Farmer SL, Leahy M. The History of Transfusion and Patient Blood Management: Blackwell; 2014

Farmer SL, Towler SC, Leahy MF, Hofmann A. Drivers for change: Western Australia Patient Blood Management Program (WA PBMP), World Health Assembly (WHA) and Advisory Committee on Blood Safety and Availability (ACBSA). Best Pract Res Clin Anaesthesiol 2013b;27(1):43–58

Farmer SL, Webb D. Your Body, Your Choice. Singapore: Media Masters; 2000

Farrugia A. Falsification or paradigm shift? Toward a revision of the common sense of transfusion. Transfusion 2011;51 (1):216–224

Fenger-Eriksen C, Lindberg-Larsen M, Christensen AQ, Ingerslev J, Sørensen B. Fibrinogen concentrate substitution therapy in patients with massive haemorrhage and low plasma fibrinogen concentrations. Br J Anaesth 2008;101 (6):769–773

Fergusson DA, Hébert P, Hogan DL, et al. Effect of fresh red blood cell transfusions on clinical outcomes in premature, very low-birth-weight infants: the ARIPI randomized trial. JAMA 2012;308(14):1443–1451

Fernandes CJ Jr, Akamine N, De Marco FV, De Souza JA, Lagudis S, Knobel E. Red blood cell transfusion does not increase oxygen consumption in critically ill septic patients. Crit Care 2001;5(6):362–367

Ferraris VA, Brown JR, Despotis GJ, et al; Society of Thoracic Surgeons Blood Conservation Guideline Task Force; Society of Cardiovascular Anesthesiologists Special Task Force on Blood Transfusion; International Consortium for Evidence Based Perfusion. 2011 update to the Society of Thoracic Surgeons and the Society of Cardiovascular Anesthesiologists blood conservation clinical practice guidelines. Ann Thorac Surg 2011a;91(3):944–982

Ferraris VA, Davenport DL, Saha SP, et al. Intraoperative transfusion of small amounts of blood heralds worse postoperative outcome in patients having noncardiac thoracic operations. Ann Thorac Surg 2011b;91:1674–1680

Ferraris VA, Davenport DL, Saha SP, Austin PC, Zwischenberger JB. Surgical outcomes and transfusion of minimal amounts of blood in the operating room. Arch Surg 2012;147(1):49–55

Finlay IG, Edwards TJ, Lambert AW. Damage control laparotomy. Br J Surg 2004;91(1):83–85

Fischer CP, Bochicchio G, Shen J, Patel B, Batiller J, Hart JC. A prospective, randomized, controlled trial of the efficacy and safety of fibrin pad as an adjunct to control soft tissue bleeding during abdominal, retroperitoneal, pelvic, and thoracic surgery. J Am Coll Surg 2013;217(3):385–393

Fischer DP, Zacharowski KD, Meybohm P. Savoring every drop - vampire or mosquito? Crit Care 2014;18(3):306

Fischer SP. Development and effectiveness of an anesthesia preoperative evaluation clinic in a teaching hospital. Anesthesiology 1996;85(1):196–206

Fitzgerald RD, Martin CM, Dietz GE, Doig GS, Potter RF, Sibbald WJ. Transfusing red blood cells stored in citrate phosphate dextrose adenine-1 for 28 days fails to improve tissue oxygenation in rats. Crit Care Med 1997;25(5):726–732

Flamm M, Fritsch G, Seer J, Panisch S, Sönnichsen AC. Non-adherence to guidelines for preoperative testing in a secondary care hospital in Austria: the economic impact of unnecessary and double testing. Eur J Anaesthesiol 2011;28(12):867–873

Flegel WA, Natanson C, Klein HG. Does prolonged storage of red blood cells cause harm? Br J Haematol 2014;165 (1):3–16

Fleisher LA, Beckman JA, Brown KA, et al. 2009 ACCF/AHA focused update on perioperative beta blockade incorporated into the ACC/AHA 2007 guidelines on perioperative cardiovascular evaluation and care for noncardiac surgery: a report of the American college of cardiology foundation/American heart association task force on practice guidelines. Circulation 2009;120(21):e169 –e276

Foley RN, Curtis BM, Parfrey PS. Hemoglobin targets and blood transfusions in hemodialysis patients without symptomatic cardiac disease receiving erythropoietin therapy. Clin J Am Soc Nephrol 2008;3:1669–1675

Fong J, Gurewitsch ED, Kang HJ, Kump L, Mack PF. An analysis of transfusion practice and the role of intraoperative red blood cell salvage during cesarean delivery. Anesth Analg 2007;104 (3):666–672

Food and Drug Administration (FDA). FDA modifies dosing recommendations for erythropoiesis-stimulating agents [press release]. June 24, 2011. http:// www.fda.gov/NewsEvents/Newsroom/ PressAnnouncements/ucm260 670.htm. Accessed March 12, 2015

Forgie MA, Wells PS, Laupacis A, Fergusson D. Preoperative autologous donation decreases allogeneic transfusion but increases exposure to all red blood cell transfusion: results of a meta-analysis. International Study of Perioperative Transfusion (ISPOT) Investigators. Arch Intern Med 1998;158(6):610–616

Forst H, Racenberg J, Schosser R, Messmer K. Right ventricular tissue PO2 in dogs. Effects of hemodilution and acute right coronary artery occlusion. Res Exp Med (Berl) 1987;187(3):159–174

Fowler RA, Berenson M. Blood conservation in the intensive care unit. Crit Care Med 2003;31(12 Suppl) S 715 –S 720

Frank SM, Oleyar MJ, Ness PM, Tobian AA. Reducing unnecessary preoperative blood orders and costs by implementing an updated institution-specific maximum surgical blood order schedule and a remote electronic blood release system. Anesthesiology 2014a;121(3):501–509

Frank SM, Wick EC, Dezern AE, et al. Risk-adjusted clinical outcomes in patients enrolled in a bloodless program. Transfusion 2014b;54(10 Pt 2):2668–2677

Freedman J. The ONTraC Ontario program in blood conservation. Transfus Apher Sci 2014;50(1):32–36

Freedman J. Theme issue on Ontario initiatives in blood conservation and blood management. Transfus Apheresis Sci 2005;33(3):315–316

Freedman J, Luke K, Escobar M, Vernich L, Chiavetta JA. Experience of a network of transfusion coordinators for blood conservation (Ontario Transfusion Coordinators [ONTraC]). Transfusion 2008;48 (2):237–250

Freedman J, Luke K, Monga N, et al. A provincial program of blood conservation: The Ontario Transfusion Coordinators (ONTraC). Transfus Apheresis Sci 2005;33(3):343–349

French CJ, Bellomo R, Finfer SR, Lipman J, Chapman M, Boyce NW. Appropriateness of red blood cell transfusion in Australasian intensive care practice. Med J Aust 2002;177(10):548–551

Frenzel T, Westphal-Varghese B, Westphal M. Role of storage time of red blood cells on microcirculation and tissue oxygenation in critically ill patients. Curr Opin Anaesthesiol 2009;22 (2):275–280

Fries D, Innerhofer P, Reif C, et al. The effect of fibrinogen substitution on reversal of dilutional coagulopathy: an in vitro model. Anesth Analg 2006;102(2):347–351

Friesenecker B, Tsai AG, Dünser MW, et al. Oxygen distribution in microcirculation after arginine vasopressin-induced arteriolar vasoconstriction. Am J Physiol Heart Circ Physiol 2004;287(4): H1792 –H1800

Friesenecker B, Tsai AG, Dünser MW, Martini J, Hasibeder W, Intaglietta M. Lowered microvascular vessel wall oxygen consumption augments tissue pO2 during PgE1-induced vasodilation. Eur J Appl Physiol 2007;99(4):405–414

Friesenecker B, Tsai AG, Martini J, et al. Arginine vasopressin versus norepinephrine: Team work wins the match or there are no simple solutions for complex problems! Commentary posted on June 28, 2006a. http://www.ccforum.com/content/10/3/144/comments#236 554. Accessed July 24, 2015

Friesenecker BE, Tsai AG, Martini J, et al. Arteriolar vasoconstrictive response: comparing the effects of arginine vasopressin and norepinephrine. Crit Care 2006b;10(3):R75

Fritsch G, Flamm M, Hepner DL, Panisch S, Seer J, Soennichsen A. Abnormal preoperative tests, pathologic findings of medical history, and their predictive value for perioperative complications. Acta Anaesthesiol Scand 2012;56 (3):339–350

Funk MB, Guenay S, Lohmann A, et al. Benefit of transfusion-related acute lung injury risk-minimization measures—German haemovigilance data (2006-2010). Vox Sang 2012a;102 (4):317–323

Funk MB, Guenay S, Volz-Zang C, eds. Haemovigilance Report of the Paul-Ehrlich-Institut 2010: Assessment of the Reports of Serious Adverse Transfusion Reactions Pursuant to Section 63 c AMG (Arzneimittelgesetz, German Medicinal Products Act). Langen: Paul-Ehrlich-Institut; 2012b. http://www.pei.de/DE/arzneimittelsicherheit-vigilanz/haemovigilanz/haemovigilanzberichte/haemovigilanzberichte-node.html. Accessed March 12, 2015 </eref>

Gajic O, Dzik WH, Toy P. Fresh frozen plasma and platelet transfusion for non-bleeding patients in the intensive care unit: benefit or harm? Crit Care Med 2006;34(5, Suppl)S 170 –S 173

Gajic O, Rana R, Winters JL, et al. Transfusion-related acute lung injury in the critically ill: prospective nested case-control study. Am J Respir Crit Care Med 2007;176(9):886–891

Ganzoni AM. Intravenous iron-dextran: therapeutic and experimental possibilities [article in German]. Schweiz Med Wochenschr 1970;100(7):301–303

Gauvin F, Champagne MA, Robillard P, Le Cruguel JP, Lapointe H, Hume H. Long-term survival rate of pediatric patients after blood transfusion. Transfusion 2008;48(5):801–808

Gauvin F, Spinella PC, Lacroix J, et al. Association between length of storage of transfused red blood cells and multiple organ dysfunction syndrome in pediatric intensive care patients. Transfusion 2010;50(9):1902–1913

Geisen C, Schmidt M, Klarmann D, Schüttrumpf J, Müller MM, Seifried E. Blood—a special resource [article in German]. Anasthesiol Intensivmed Notfallmed Schmerzther 2012;47(6):398–408

Geldner J, Mertens M, Wappler F, et al. Präoperative Evaluation erwachsener Patienten vor elektiven nicht kardiochirurgischen Eingriffen. Anästh Intensivmed 2010;51:S 788

Généreux P, Cohen DJ, Williams MR, et al. Bleeding complications after surgical aortic valve replacement compared with transcatheter aortic valve replacement: insights from the PARTNER I Trial (Placement of Aortic Transcatheter Valve). J Am Coll Cardiol 2014;63 (11):1100–1109

Gerlach R, Tölle F, Raabe A, Zimmermann M, Siegemund A, Seifert V. Increased risk for postoperative hemorrhage after intracranial surgery in patients with decreased factor XIII activity: implications of a prospective study. Stroke 2002;33 (6):1618–1623

Gibbs L, Kakis A, Weinstein P, Conte JE, Jr. Bone wax as a risk factor for surgical-site infection following neurospinal surgery. Infect Control Hosp Epidemiol 2004;25(4):346–348

Gillebert TC, Brooks N, Fontes-Carvalho R, et al. ESC core curriculum for the general cardiologist (2013). Eur Heart J 2013;34(30):2381–2411

Gladwin MT, Kanias T, Kim-Shapiro DB. Hemolysis and cell-free hemoglobin drive an intrinsic mechanism for human disease. J Clin Invest 2012;122 (4):1205–1208

Glance LG, Dick AW, Mukamel DB, et al. Association between intraoperative blood transfusion and mortality and morbidity in patients undergoing noncardiac surgery. Anesthesiology 2011;114(2):283–292

Gleason E, Grossman S, Campbell C. Minimizing diagnostic blood loss in critically ill patients. Am J Crit Care 1992;1 (1):85–90

Godier A, Ozier Y, Susen S; Groupe d'intérêt en hémostase périopératoire (GIHP). Le ratio transfusionnel PFC/CGR 1/1: un phénomène de mode basé sur des preuves? [1/1 plasma to red blood cell ratio: an evidence-based practice?]. Ann Fr Anesth Reanim 2011;30(5):421–428

Görlinger K, Fries D, Dirkmann D, Weber CF, Hanke AA, Schöchl H. Reduction of Fresh Frozen Plasma Requirements by Perioperative Point-of-Care Coagulation Management with Early Calculated Goal-Directed Therapy. Transfus Med Hemother 2012;39(2):104–113

Gohel MS, Bulbulia RA, Slim FJ, Poskitt KR, Whyman MR. How to approach major surgery where patients refuse blood transfusion (including Jehovah's Witnesses). Ann R Coll Surg Engl 2005;87(1):3–14

Golab HD, Scohy TV, de Jong PL, Takkenberg JJ, Bogers AJ. Intraoperative cell salvage in infants undergoing elective cardiac surgery: a prospective trial. Eur J Cardiothorac Surg 2008;34(2):354–359

Goldman L. Bleeding is rarely good for you. Circulation 2012;126(2):169–171

Gombotz H. Patient Blood Management: A patient-orientated approach to blood replacement with the goal of reducing anemia, blood loss and the need for blood transfusion in elective surgery. Transfus Med Hemother 2012;39(2):67–72

Gombotz H. Patient blood management is key before elective surgery. Lancet 2011;378(9800):1362–1363

Gombotz H, Gries M, Sipurzynski S, Fruhwald S, Rehak P. Preoperative treatment with recombinant human erythropoietin or predeposit of autologous blood in women undergoing primary hip replacement. Acta Anaesthesiol Scand 2000;44(6):737–742

Gombotz H, Hofmann A. Patient Blood Management: three pillar strategy to improve outcome through avoidance of allogeneic blood products [article in German]. Anaesthesist 2013;62(7):519–527

Gombotz H, Hofmann A, Rehak P, Kurz J. Patient blood management (part 1) - patient-specific concept to reduce and avoid anemia, blood loss and transfusion [article in German]. Anasthesiol Intensivmed Notfallmed Schmerzther 2011b;46(6):396–401

Gombotz H, Hofman A, Rehak P, Kurz J. Patient blood management (part 2). Practice: the 3 pillars [article in German]. Anasthesiol Intensivmed Notfallmed Schmerzther 2011a;46(7-8):466–474

Gombotz H, Knotzer H. Preoperative identification of patients with increased risk for perioperative bleeding. Curr Opin Anaesthesiol 2013;26(1):82–90

Gombotz H, Metzler H, Hiotakis K, Dacar D. Open heart surgery in Jehovah's Witnesses [article in German]. Wien Klin Wochenschr 1985;97(12):525–530

Gombotz H, Rehak PH, Hofmann A. Fortsetzung der Studie "Maßnahmen zur Optimierung des Verbrauchs von Blutkomponenten bei ausgewählten operativen Eingriffen in österreichischen Krankenanstalten" 2008–2010. Vienna: Bundesministerium für Gesundheit; 2012

Gombotz H, Rehak PH, Shander A, Hofmann A. Blood use in elective surgery: the Austrian benchmark study. Transfusion 2007;47(8):1468–1480

Gombotz H, Rehak PH, Shander A, Hofmann A. The second Austrian benchmark study for blood use in elective surgery: results and practice change. Transfusion 2014;54(10 Pt 2):2646–2657

Gombotz H, Rigler B, Matzer C, Metzler H, Winkler G, Tscheliessnigg KH. 10 Jahre Herzoperationen bei Zeugen Jehovahs. [10 years' experience with heart surgery in Jehovah's witnesses]. Anaesthesist 1989;38(8):385–390

Gong MN, Thompson BT, Williams P, Pothier L, Boyce PD, Christiani DC. Clinical predictors of and mortality in acute respiratory distress syndrome: potential role of red cell transfusion. Crit Care Med 2005;33(6):1191–1198

Goodnough LT. Current status of perisurgical erythropoietin therapy. In: Maniatis A, Van der Linden P, Hardy JF, eds. Alternatives to Blood Transfusion in Transfusion Medicine. 2nd ed. Oxford: Blackwell Publishing; 2011:348–356

Goodnough LT, Brecher ME, Kanter MH, AuBuchon JP. Transfusion medicine. First of two parts—blood transfusion. N Engl J Med 1999a;340(6):438–447

Goodnough LT, Brecher ME, Kanter MH, AuBuchon JP. Transfusion medicine. Second of two parts—blood conservation. N Engl J Med 1999b;340(7):525–533

Goodnough LT, Levy JH, Murphy MF. Concepts of blood transfusion in adults. Lancet 2013;381(9880):1845–1854

Goodnough LT, Maggio P, Hadhazy E, et al. Restrictive blood transfusion practices are associated with improved patient outcomes. Transfusion 2014a;54(10 Pt 2):2753–2759

Goodnough LT, Maniatis A, Earnshaw P, et al. Detection, evaluation, and management of preoperative anaemia in the elective orthopaedic surgical patient: NATA guidelines. Br J Anaesth 2011;106(1):13–22

Goodnough LT, Shander A. Current status of pharmacologic therapies in patient blood management. Anesth Analg 2013;116(1):15–34

Goodnough LT, Shander A. How I treat warfarin-associated coagulopathy in patients with intracerebral hemorrhage. Blood 2011;117(23):6091–6099

Goodnough LT, Shander A. Patient blood management. Anesthesiology 2012;116(6):1367–1376

Goodnough LT, Shieh L, Hadhazy E, Cheng N, Khari P, Maggio P. Improved blood utilization using real-time clinical decision support. Transfusion 2014b;54(5):1358–1365

Greenberg PL, Tuechler H, Schanz J, et al. Revised international prognostic scoring system for myelodysplastic syndromes. Blood 2012;120(12):2454–2465

Greinacher A, Fendrich K, Brzenska R, Kiefel V, Hoffmann W. Implications of demographics on future blood supply: a population-based cross-sectional study. Transfusion 2011;51(4):702–709

Greinacher A, Fendrich K, Hoffmann W. Demographic changes: The impact for safe blood supply. Transfus Med Hemother 2010;37(3):141–148

Gross I, Shander A, Sweeney J. Patient blood management and outcome, too early or not? Best. Pract. Res. Clin. Anaesthesiol. 2013;27(1):161–172

Grossman PM, Gurm HS, McNamara R, et al; Blue Cross Blue Shield of Michigan Cardiovascular Consortium (BMC 2). Percutaneous coronary intervention complications and guide catheter size: bigger is not better. JACC Cardiovasc Interv 2009;2(7):636–644

Gruen RL, Brohi K, Schreiber M, et al. Haemorrhage control in severely injured patients. Lancet 2012;380(9847):1099–1108

Gunnink SF, Vlug R, Fijnvandraat K, van der Bom JG, Stanworth SJ, Lopriore E. Neonatal thrombocytopenia: etiology, management and outcome. Expert Rev Hematol 2014;7(3):387–395

Guo JR, Jin XJ, Yu J, et al. Acute normovolemic hemodilution effects on perioperative coagulation in elderly patients undergoing hepatic carcinectomy. Asian Pac J Cancer Prev 2013;14(8):4529–4532

Gupta PK, Sundaram A, Mactaggart JN, et al. Preoperative anemia is an independent predictor of postoperative mortality and adverse cardiac events in elderly patients undergoing elective vascular operations. Ann Surg 2013;258(6):1096–1102

Guralnik JM, Eisenstaedt RS, Ferrucci L, Klein HG, Woodman RC. Prevalence of anemia in persons 65 years and older in the United States: evidence for a high rate of unexplained anemia. Blood 2004;104(8):2263–2268

Haas T, Goobie S, Spielmann N, Weiss M, Schmugge M. Improvements in patient blood management for pediatric craniosynostosis surgery using a ROTEM(®) assisted strategy - feasibility and costs. Paediatr Anaesth 2014;24(7):774–780

Haas T, Spielmann N, Mauch J, et al. Comparison of thromboelastometry (ROTEM®) with standard plasmatic coagulation testing in paediatric surgery. Br J Anaesth 2012;108(1):36–41

Habib RH, Zacharias A, Schwann TA, et al. Role of hemodilutional anemia and transfusion during cardiopulmonary bypass in renal injury after coronary revascularization: implications on operative outcome. Crit Care Med 2005;33 (8):1749–1756

Habib RH, Zacharias A, Schwann TA, Riordan CJ, Durham SJ, Shah A. Adverse effects of low hematocrit during cardiopulmonary bypass in the adult: should current practice be changed? J Thorac Cardiovasc Surg 2003;125(6):1438–1450

Habler O. Fluids or blood products? In: Hahn RG, ed. Clinical Fluid Therapy in the Perioperative Setting. Cambridge: Cambridge University Press; 2011:184–192

Habler O, Meier J, Pape A, Kertscho H, Zwissler B. Tolerance to perioperative anemia. Mechanisms, influencing factors and limits [article in German]. Anaesthesist 2006;55(11):1142–1156

Habler OP, Kleen MS, Hutter JW, et al. Effects of hyperoxic ventilation on hemodilution-induced changes in anesthetized dogs. Transfusion 1998;38 (2):135–144

Haiden N, Schwindt J, Cardona F, et al. Effects of a combined therapy of erythropoietin, iron, folate, and vitamin B12 on the transfusion requirements of extremely low birth weight infants. Pediatrics 2006;118(5):2004–2013

Hajjar LA, Vincent JL, Galas FR, et al. Transfusion requirements after cardiac surgery: the TRACS randomized controlled trial. JAMA 2010;304(14):1559–1567

Halabi WJ, Jafari MD, Nguyen VQ, et al. Blood transfusions in colorectal cancer surgery: incidence, outcomes, and predictive factors: an American College of Surgeons National Surgical Quality Improvement Program analysis. Am J Surg 2013;206(6):1024–1033

Hall RI. Anaesthesia for coronary artery surgery—a plea for a goal-directed approach. Can J Anaesth 1993;40 (12):1178–1194

Hamid T, Choudhury TR, Clarke B, Mahadevan VS. Pre-closure of large-sized arterial access sites in adults undergoing transcatheter structural interventions. Cardiol Ther 2015;4(1):59–63

Hamon M, Lemesle G, Tricot O, et al. Incidence, source, determinants, and prognostic impact of major bleeding in outpatients with stable coronary artery disease. J Am Coll Cardiol 2014;64 (14):1430–1436

Hansen E, Bechmann V, Altmeppen J. Intraoperative blood salvage in cancer surgery: safe and effective? Transfus-ApherSci 2002;27(2):153–157

Hansen E, Seyfried T. Cell salvage [article in German]. Anaesthesist 2011;60(4):381–390

Harber CR, Sosnowski KJ, Hegde RM. Highly conservative phlebotomy in adult intensive care—a prospective randomized controlled trial. Anaesth Intensive Care 2006;34(4):434–437

Harder S, Klinkhardt U, Alvarez JM. Avoidance of bleeding during surgery in patients receiving anticoagulant and/or antiplatelet therapy: pharmacokinetic and pharmacodynamic considerations. Clin Pharmacokinet 2004;43(14):963–981

Hardy JD, ed. Complications in Surgery and their Management. 4th ed. Philadelphia, PA: W.B. Saunders; 1981

Hardy JF. Current status of transfusion triggers for red blood cell concentrates. Transfus Apheresis Sci 2004;31(1):55–66

Harnett MJP, Correll DJ, Hurwitz S, Bader AM, Hepner DL. Improving efficiency and patient satisfaction in a tertiary teaching hospital preoperative clinic. Anesthesiology 2010;112(1):66–72

Hartert H. Thrombelastography, a method for physical analysis of blood coagulation [article in German]. Z Gesamte Exp Med 1951;117(2):189–203

Hayden SJ, Albert TJ, Watkins TR, Swenson ER. Anemia in critical illness: insights into etiology, consequences, and management. Am J Respir Crit Care Med 2012;185(10):1049–1057

Haynes AB, Weiser TG, Berry WR, et al; Safe Surgery Saves Lives Study Group. A surgical safety checklist to reduce morbidity and mortality in a global population. N Engl J Med 2009;360 (5):491–499

Hearnshaw SA, Logan RF, Palmer KR, Card TR, Travis SP, Murphy MF. Outcomes following early red blood cell transfusion in acute upper gastrointestinal bleeding. Aliment Pharmacol Ther 2010;32(2):215–224

Hébert PC, Fergusson DA, Stather D, et al; Canadian Critical Care Trials Group. Revisiting transfusion practices in critically ill patients. Crit Care Med 2005;33 (1):7–12

Hébert PC, Van der Linden P, Biro G, Hu LQ. Physiologic aspects of anemia. Crit Care Clin 2004;20(2):187–212

Hébert PC, Wells G, Blajchman MA, et al; Transfusion Requirements in Critical Care Investigators. Canadian Critical Care Trials Group. A multicenter, randomized, controlled clinical trial of transfusion requirements in critical care. Transfusion Requirements in Critical Care Investigators, Canadian Critical Care Trials Group. N Engl J Med 1999a;340(6):409–417

Hébert PC, Wells G, Martin C, et al. Variation in red cell transfusion practice in the intensive care unit: a multicentre cohort study. Crit Care 1999b;3(2):57–63

Helm RE, Rosengart TK, Gomez M, et al. Comprehensive multimodality blood conservation: 100 consecutive CABG operations without transfusion. Ann Thorac Surg 1998;65(1):125–136

Henriksson AE, Svensson JO. Upper gastrointestinal bleeding. With special reference to blood transfusion. Eur J Surg 1991;157(3):193–196

Henry DA, Carless PA, Moxey AJ, et al. Antifibrinolytic use for minimising perioperative allogeneic blood transfusion. Cochrane Database Syst Rev 2011;(1): CD 001 886

Henry DA, Carless PA, Moxey AJ, et al. Pre-operative autologous donation for minimising perioperative allogeneic blood transfusion. Cochrane Database Syst Rev 2002;(2):CD 003 602

Hiippala ST, Myllylä GJ, Vahtera EM. Hemostatic factors and replacement of major blood loss with plasma-poor red cell concentrates. Anesth Analg 1995;81 (2):360–365

Hill GE, Frawley WH, Griffith KE, Forestner JE, Minei JP. Allogeneic blood transfusion increases the risk of postoperative bacterial infection: a meta-analysis. J Trauma 2003;54(5):908–914

Ho C, Sucato DJ, Richards BS. Risk factors for the development of delayed infections following posterior spinal fusion and instrumentation in adolescent idiopathic scoliosis patients. Spine 2007;32 (20):2272–2277

Hoffmann JN, Vollmar B, Laschke MW, Inthorn D, Schildberg FW, Menger MD. Hydroxyethyl starch (130 kD), but not crystalloid volume support, improves microcirculation during normotensive endotoxemia. Anesthesiology 2002;97 (2):460–470

Hofmann A, Farmer S, Shander A. Cost-effectiveness in haemotherapies and transfusion medicine. ISBT Sci Ser 2009;4(2):258–265

Hofmann A, Farmer S, Shander A. Five drivers shifting the paradigm from product-focused transfusion practice to patient blood management. Oncologist 2011;16(Suppl 3):3–11

Hofmann A, Farmer S, Towler SC. Strategies to preempt and reduce the use of blood products: an Australian perspective. Curr Opin Anaesthesiol 2012;25(1):66–73

Hofmann A, Friedman D, Farmer S. Western Australian Patient Blood Management Project 2008–2012: Analysis, Strategy, Implementation and Financial Projections. Perth: Western Australia Department of Health 2007:1–154

Hofmann A, Ozawa S, Farrugia A, Farmer SL, Shander A. Economic considerations on transfusion medicine and patient blood management. Best Pract Res Clin Anaesthesiol 2013;27(1):59–68

Hogervorst E, Rosseel P, van der Bom J, et al. Tolerance of intraoperative hemoglobin decrease during cardiac surgery. Transfusion 2014;54(10 Pt 2):2696–2704

Hohmuth B, Ozawa S, Ashton M, Melseth RL. Patient-centered blood management. J Hosp Med 2014;9 (1):60–65

Hollywood Private Hospital. Western Australia. Ramsey Health Care WA leading the world in blood management [press release]. August 30, 2012. http://www.hollywood.ramsayhealth.com.au/media/rhc-wa-leading-the-world-in-blood-management.aspx. Accessed July 7, 2012

Holst LB, Haase N, Wetterslev J, et al. Lower versus higher hemoglobin threshold for transfusion in septic shock. N Engl J Med 2014;371(15):1381–1391

Holst LB, Petersen MW, Haase N, Perner A, Wetterslev J. Restrictive versus liberal transfusion strategy for red blood cell transfusion: systematic review of randomised trials with meta-analysis and trial sequential analysis. BMJ 2015;350: h1354

Holzer BR, Egger M, Teuscher T, Koch S, Mboya DM, Smith GD. Childhood anemia in Africa: to transfuse or not transfuse? Acta Trop 1993;55(1-2):47–51

Hopewell S, Omar O, Hyde C, Yu LM, Doree C, Murphy MF. A systematic review of the effect of red blood cell transfusion on mortality: evidence from large-scale observational studies published between 2006 and 2010. BMJ Open 2013;3(5):3

Horvath KA, Acker MA, Chang H, et al. Blood transfusion and infection after cardiac surgery. Ann Thorac Surg 2013;95(6):2194–2201

Hourfar MK, Jork C, Schottstedt V, et al; German Red Cross NAT Study Group. Experience of German Red Cross blood donor services with nucleic acid testing: results of screening more than 30 million blood donations for human immunodeficiency virus-1, hepatitis C virus, and hepatitis B virus. Transfusion 2008;48(8):1558–1566

Howard-Quijano K, Schwarzenberger JC, Scovotti JC, et al. Increased red blood cell transfusions are associated with worsening outcomes in pediatric heart transplant patients. Anesth Analg 2013;116(6):1295–1308

Howie SR. Blood sample volumes in child health research: review of safe limits. Bull World Health Organ 2011;89 (1):46–53

Howland WS, Wang KC. A preanesthesia clinic. N Y State J Med 1956;56 (16):2497–2502

Hung M, Ortmann E, Besser M, et al. A prospective observational cohort study to identify the causes of anaemia and association with outcome in cardiac surgical patients. Heart 2015;101(2):107–112

Hutter J, Habler O, Kleen M, et al. Effect of acute normovolemic hemodilution on distribution of blood flow and tissue oxygenation in dog skeletal muscle. J Appl Physiol (1985) 1999;86(3).860–866

Hutton B, Fergusson D, Tinmouth A, McIntyre L, Kmetic A, Hébert PC. Transfusion rates vary significantly amongst Canadian medical centres. Can J Anaesth 2005;52(6):581–590

Ickx BE, Rigolet M, Van Der Linden PJ. Cardiovascular and metabolic response to acute normovolemic anemia. Effects of anesthesia. Anesthesiology 2000;93 (4):1011–1016

Inaba K, Branco BC, Rhee P, et al. Long-term preclinical evaluation of the intracorporeal use of advanced local hemostatics in a damage-control swine model of grade IV liver injury. J Trauma Acute Care Surg 2013;74(2):538–545

Inghilleri G. Prediction of transfusion requirements in surgical patients: a review. TATM 2010;11:10–19

Institute for Patient Blood Management and Bloodless Medicine and Surgery (IPBMBMS) at Englewood Hospital 2012. http://www.englewoodhospital. com/ms_bloodless_home.asp. Accessed March 12, 2015

Irwin DJ, Abrams JY, Schonberger LB, et al. Evaluation of potential infectivity of Alzheimer and Parkinson disease proteins in recipients of cadaver-derived human growth hormone. JAMA Neurol 2013;70(4):462–468

Isbister JP. Clinicians as gatekeepers: what is the best route to optimal blood use? Dev Biol (Basel) 2007;127:9–14

Isbister JP. Risk management in transfusion medicine. Transfus Sci 1994;15(1):3–4

Isbister JP. The paradigm shift in blood transfusion. Med J Aust 1988;148 (6):306–308

Isbister JP, Shander A, Spahn DR, Erhard J, Farmer SL, Hofmann A. Adverse blood transfusion outcomes: establishing causation. Transfus Med Rev 2011;25 (2):89–101

Isil CT, Yazici P, Bakir I. Risk factors and outcome of increased red blood cell transfusion in cardiac surgical patients aged 65 years and older. Thorac Cardiovasc Surg 2015;63(1):39–44

Iyengar A, Scipione CN, Sheth P, et al. Association of complications with blood transfusions in pediatric cardiac surgery patients. Ann Thorac Surg 2013;96(3):910–916

Jackson BR, Busch MP, Stramer SL, AuBuchon JP. The cost-effectiveness of NAT for HIV, HCV, and HBV in whole-blood donations. Transfusion 2003;43 (6):721–729

Jackson WL Jr, Shorr AF. Blood transfusion and nosocomial infection: another brick in the wall. Crit Care Med 2006;34 (9):2488–2489

Jacob M, Chappell D. Reappraising Starling: the physiology of the microcirculation. Curr Opin Crit Care 2013;19(4):282–289

Jagoditsch M, Pozgainer P, Klingler A, et al. Impact of blood transfusions on recurrence and survival after rectal cancer surgery. Dis Colon Rectum 2006;49:1116–1130

Jairath V, Hearnshaw S, Brunskill SJ, et al. Red cell transfusion for the management of upper gastrointestinal haemorrhage. Cochrane Database Syst Rev 2010;9:CD 006 613

Jalal DI, Chonchol M, Targher G. Disorders of hemostasis associated with chronic kidney disease. Semin Thromb Hemost 2010;36(1):34–40

Jans Ø, Jørgensen C, Kehlet H, Johansson PI; Lundbeck Foundation Centre for Fast-track Hip and Knee Replacement Collaborative Group. Role of preoperative anemia for risk of transfusion and postoperative morbidity in fast-track hip and knee arthroplasty. Transfusion 2014;54(3):717–726

Joint Commission (JC). Implementation Guide for Patient Blood Management Performance Measures. Published 2011. http://www.jointcommission.org/assets/1/6/PBM_Implementation_-Guide_2 011 0624.pdf. Accessed March 12, 2015

Johansson PI, Svendsen MS, Salado J, Bochsen L, Kristensen AT. Investigation of the thrombin-generating capacity, evaluated by thrombogram, and clot formation evaluated by thrombelastography of platelets stored in the blood bank for up to 7 days. Vox Sang 2008;94(2):113–118

Johnson P, Fromm D. Effects of bone wax on bacterial clearance. Surgery 1981;89(2):206–209

Jucker M, Walker LC. Pathogenic protein seeding in Alzheimer disease and other neurodegenerative disorders. Ann Neurol 2011;70(4):532–540

Jung W, Ahn CH. A micro blood sampling system for catheterized neonates and pediatrics in intensive care unit. Biomed Microdevices 2013;15(2):241–253

Kaidarova DR, Yugai TA, Sadykova TT. Fibrin sealant hemostatic patch clinical effectiveness evaluation in advanced ovarian cancer patients underwent pelvic lymphadenectomy: institutional experience. Int J Gynecol Cancer 2015;25(Suppl 1):58

Kaleeya Hospital Publication. Blood Conservation Program in Medicine and Surgery – the New Standard of Care. Perth, Western Australia: Fremantle Kaleeya Hospital; 2004

Kammache I, Parrinello G, Marini D, Bonnet D, Agnoletti G. Anaemia is a predictor of early death or cardiac transplantation in children with idiopathic dilated cardiomyopathy. Cardiol Young 2012;22(3):293–300

Kander T, Tanaka KA, Norström E, Persson J, Schött U. The effect and duration of prophylactic platelet transfusions before insertion of a central venous catheter in patients with bone marrow failure evaluated with point-of-care methods and flow cytometry. Anesth Analg 2014;119(4):882–890

Karaca MA, Erbil B, Ozmen MM. Use and effectiveness of prothrombin complex concentrates vs fresh frozen plasma in gastrointestinal hemorrhage due to warfarin usage in the ED. Am J Emerg Med 2014;32(6):660–664

Karam O, Tucci M, Lacroix J, Rimensberger PC; Canadian Critical Care Trials Group and of the Pediatric Acute Lung Injury and Sepsis Investigator Network. International survey on plasma transfusion practices in critically ill children. Transfusion 2014;54(4):1125–1132

Karimi M, Florentino-Pineda I, Weatherred T, et al. Blood conservation operations in pediatric cardiac patients: a paradigm shift of blood use. Ann Thorac Surg 2013;95(3):962–967

Karkouti K, Beattie WS, Wijeysundera DN, et al. Hemodilution during cardiopulmonary bypass is an independent risk factor for acute renal failure in adult cardiac surgery. J Thorac Cardiovasc Surg 2005a;129(2):391–400

Karkouti K, McCluskey SA, Evans L, Mahomed N, Ghannam M, Davey R. Erythropoietin is an effective clinical modality for reducing RBC transfusion in joint surgery. Can J Anaesth 2005b;52(4):362–368

Karkouti K, Wijeysundera DN, Beattie WS; Reducing Bleeding in Cardiac Surgery (RBC) Investigators. Risk associated with preoperative anemia in cardiac surgery: a multicenter cohort study. Circulation 2008a;117(4):478–484

Karkouti K, Wijeysundera DN, Yau TM, et al. Acute kidney injury after cardiac surgery: focus on modifiable risk factors. Circulation 2009;119(4):495–502

Karkouti K, Wijeysundera DN, Yau TM, et al. Advance targeted transfusion in anemic cardiac surgical patients for kidney protection: an unblinded randomized pilot clinical trial. Anesthesiology 2012;116(3):613–621

Karkouti K, Wijeysundera DN, Yau TM, et al. Platelet transfusions are not associated with increased morbidity or mortality in cardiac surgery. Can J Anaesth 2006;53(3):279–287

Karkouti K, Wijeysundera DN, Yau TM, et al. The independent association of massive blood loss with mortality in cardiac surgery. Transfusion 2004;44(10):1453–1462

Karkouti K, Wijeysundera DN, Yau TM, McCluskey SA, Tait G, Beattie WS. The risk-benefit profile of aprotinin versus tranexamic acid in cardiac surgery. Anesthesia & Analgesia 2010;110(1):21–9

Karkouti K, Wijeysundera DN, Yau TM, McCluskey SA, van Rensburg A, Beattie WS. The influence of baseline hemoglobin concentration on tolerance of anemia in cardiac surgery. Transfusion 2008b;48(4):666–672

Karski JM, Mathieu M, Cheng D, Carroll J, Scott GJ. Etiology of preoperative anemia in patients undergoing scheduled cardiac surgery. Can J Anaesth 1999;46(10):979–982

Kassenärztliche Bundesvereinigung (KBV). Rahmenvorgaben nach § 84 Abs. 7 SGB V-Arzneimittel-für das Jahr 2012. Dtsch Arztebl 2011;108:A-2565

Katz RI, Dexter F, Rosenfeld K, et al. Survey study of anesthesiologists' and surgeons' ordering of unnecessary preoperative laboratory tests. Anesth Analg 2011;112(1):207–212

Kemming GI, Meisner FG, Kleen M, et al. Hyperoxic ventilation at the critical haematocrit. Resuscitation 2003;56(3):289–297

Kemming GI, Meisner FG, Meier J, et al. Hyperoxic ventilation at the critical hematocrit: effects on myocardial perfusion and function. Acta Anaesthesiol Scand 2004;48(8):951–959

Kenz HE, Van der Linden P. Transfusion-related acute lung injury. Eur J Anaesthesiol 2014;31(7):345–350

Ker K, Edwards P, Perel P, Shakur H, Roberts I. Effect of tranexamic acid on surgical bleeding: systematic review and cumulative meta-analysis. BMJ 2012a;344:e3054

Ker K, Kiriya J, Perel P, Edwards P, Shakur H, Roberts I. Avoidable mortality from giving tranexamic acid to bleeding trauma patients: an estimation based on WHO mortality data, a systematic literature review and data from the CRASH-2 trial. BMC Emerg Med 2012b;12:3

Kerger H, Saltzman DJ, Menger MD, Messmer K, Intaglietta M. Systemic and subcutaneous microvascular Po2 dissociation during 4-h hemorrhagic shock in conscious hamsters. Am J Physiol 1996;270(3 Pt 2):H827 –H836

Kermode JC, Zheng Q, Milner EP. Marked temperature dependence of the platelet calcium signal induced by human von Willebrand factor. Blood 1999;94(1):199–207

Kertscho H, Lauscher P, Raab L, Zacharowski K, Meier J. Effects of hyperoxic ventilation on 6-h survival at the critical haemoglobin concentration aggravated by experimentally induced tachycardia in anaesthetized pigs. Acta Physiol (Oxf) 2012;204(4):582–591

Kheirabadi BS, Mace JE, Terrazas IB, et al. Safety evaluation of new hemostatic agents, smectite granules, and kaolin-coated gauze in a vascular injury wound model in swine. J Trauma 2010;68(2):269–278

Khorana AA, Francis CW, Blumberg N, Culakova E, Refaai MA, Lyman GH. Blood transfusions, thrombosis, and mortality in hospitalized patients with cancer. Arch Intern Med 2008;168(21):2377–2381

Kikkert WJ, Delewi R, Ouweneel DM, et al. Prognostic value of access site and non-access site bleeding after percutaneous coronary intervention: a cohort study in ST-segment elevation myocardial infarction and comprehensive meta-analysis. JACC Cardiovasc Interv 2014;7 (6):622–630

Kim C, Connell H, McGeorge A, Hu R. Prevalence of preoperative anaemia in patients having first-time cardiac surgery and its impact on clinical outcome. A retrospective observational study. Perfusion 2015a; 30(4):277–283

Kim JH, Park TC, Park GA, et al. A pilot study to investigate the efficacy of fibrin sealant (Tisseel®) in the loop electrosurgical excision procedure. Gynecol Obstet Invest. Published Online: Mar 17, 2015b (doi: 10 1159/0 003 69 391)

Kim K, Park SI, Kim BJ, et al. Efficacy of fibrin sealant in reducing hemorrhage after a loop electrosurgical excision procedure. Gynecol Obstet Invest 2012a;74 (1):1–5

Kim KY, Hwang DW, Park YK, Lee HS. A single surgeon's experience with 54 consecutive cases of multivisceral resection for locally advanced primary colorectal cancer: can the laparoscopic approach be performed safely? Surg Endosc 2012b;26(2):493–500

Kleen M, Habler O, Hutter J, et al. Normovolaemic haemodilution and hyperoxia have no effect on fractal dimension of regional myocardial perfusion in dogs. Acta Physiol Scand 1998;162(4):439–446

Klövekorn WP, Pichlmaier H, Ott E, Bauer H, Sunder-Plassmann L, Messmer K. Acute preoperative hemodilution—possibility for autologous blood transfusion [article in German]. Chirurg 1974;45 (10):452–458

Klövekorn WP, Richter J, Sebening F. Hemodilution in coronary bypass operations. Bibl Haematol 1981;47(47):297–302

Kneyber MC, Hersi MI, Twisk JW, Markhorst DG, Plötz FB. Red blood cell transfusion in critically ill children is independently associated with increased mortality. Intensive Care Med 2007;33 (8):1414–1422

Koch CG. Tolerating anemia: taking aim at the right target before pulling the transfusion trigger. Transfusion 2014; 54:2595–2597

Koch CG, Khandwala F, Li L, Estafanous FG, Loop FD, Blackstone EH. Persistent effect of red cell transfusion on health-related quality of life after cardiac surgery. Ann Thorac Surg 2006a;82(1):13–20

Koch CG, Li L, Duncan AI, et al. Morbidity and mortality risk associated with red blood cell and blood-component transfusion in isolated coronary artery bypass grafting. Crit Care Med 2006b;34 (6):1608–1616

Koch CG, Li L, Duncan AI, et al. Transfusion in coronary artery bypass grafting is associated with reduced long-term survival. Ann Thorac Surg 2006c;81 (5):1650–1657

Koch CG, Li L, Sessler DI, et al. Duration of red-cell storage and complications after cardiac surgery. N Engl J Med 2008;358 (12):1229–1239

Kofidis T, Baraki H, Singh H, et al. The minimized extracorporeal circulation system causes less inflammation and organ damage. Perfusion 2008;23 (3):147–151

Kosiuk J, Koutalas E, Doering M, et al. Comparison of dabigatran and uninterrupted warfarin in patients with atrial fibrillation undergoing cardiac rhythm device implantations. Case-control study. Circ J 2014;78(10):2402–2407

Koster A, Börgermann J, Zittermann A, Lueth JU, Gillis-Januszewski T, Schirmer U. Moderate dosage of tranexamic acid during cardiac surgery with cardiopulmonary bypass and convulsive seizures: incidence and clinical outcome. Br J Anaesth 2013;110(1):34–40

Kotter JP. Leading Change. Boston, MS: Harvard Business School Press; 1996

Kotter JP, Cohen D. The Heart of Change. Boston, MS: Harvard Business School Press; 2002

Kotter JP, Schlesinger LA. Choosing strategies for change. Harv Bus Rev 1979;57 (2):106–114

Kotzé A, Carter LA, Scally AJ. Effect of a patient blood management programme on preoperative anaemia, transfusion rate, and outcome after primary hip or knee arthroplasty: a quality improvement cycle. Br J Anaesth 2012;108 (6):943–952

Kozen BG, Kircher SJ, Henao J, Godinez FS, Johnson AS. An alternative hemostatic dressing: comparison of CELOX, HemCon, and QuikClot. Acad Emerg Med 2008;15(1):74–81

Krafft A, Breymann C. Iron sucrose with and without recombinant erythropoietin for the treatment of severe postpartum anemia: a prospective, randomized, open-label study. J Obstet Gynaecol Res 2011;37(2):119–124

Kreimeier U, Messmer K. Hemodilution in clinical surgery: state of the art 1996. World J Surg 1996;20(9):1208–1217

Kreimeier U, Messmer K. Perioperative hemodilution. Transfus Apheresis Sci 2002;27(1):59–72

Kretschmer V, Gombotz H, Rump G. Transfusionsmedizin – Klinische Hämotherapie. Stuttgart: Thieme; 2008

Kröncke T, David M. Uterine artery embolization (UAE) for fibroid treatment – results of the 5th radiological gynecological expert meeting. Geburtshilfe Frauenheilkd 2015;75(5):439–441

Kronecker H. Kritisches und Experimentelles über lebensrettende Infusionen von Kochsalzlösungen bei Hunden. Correspondenzblatt für Schweizer Ärzte 1886;16:447–455

Kuehlein T, Sghedoni D, Visentin G, et al. Quartäre Prävention, eine Aufgabe für Hausärzte. PrimaryCare 2010;10:350–354

Kulier A, Gombotz H. Perioperative anemia [article in German]. Anaesthesist 2001;50(2):73–86

Kulier A, Levin J, Moser R, et al; Investigators of the Multicenter Study of Perioperative Ischemia Research Group; Ischemia Research and Education Foundation. Impact of preoperative anemia on outcome in patients undergoing coronary artery bypass graft surgery. Circulation 2007;116(5):471–479

Kungys G, Rose DD, Fleming NW. Stroke volume variation during acute normovolemic hemodilution. Anesth Analg 2009;109(6):1823–1830

Lackritz EM, Campbell CC, Ruebush TK II, et al. Effect of blood transfusion on survival among children in a Kenyan hospital. Lancet 1992;340(8818):524–528

Lacroix J, Hébert PC, Fergusson DA, et al. Age of transfused blood in critically ill adults. N Engl J Med 2015;372 (15):1410–1418

Lacroix J, Hébert PC, Hutchison JS, et al; TRIPICU Investigators; Canadian Critical Care Trials Group; Pediatric Acute Lung Injury and Sepsis Investigators Network. Transfusion strategies for patients in pediatric intensive care units. N Engl J Med 2007;356(16):1609–1619

Laios A, Baharuddin N, Iliou K, Gubara E, O'Sullivan G. Uterine artery embolization for treatment of symptomatic fibroids; a single institution experience. Hippokratia 2014;18(3):258–261

LaPar DJ, Crosby IK, Ailawadi G, et al; Investigators for the Virginia Cardiac Surgery Quality Initiative. Blood product conservation is associated with improved outcomes and reduced costs after cardiac surgery. J Thorac Cardiovasc Surg 2013;145(3):796–804

Lau K, Shah H, Kelleher A, Moat N. Coronary artery surgery: cardiotomy suction or cell salvage? J Cardiothorac Surg 2007;2:46

Lau YC, Lip GY. Which drug should we use for stroke prevention in atrial fibrillation? Curr Opin Cardiol 2014;29 (4):293–300

Lauscher P, Kertscho H, Meissner A, Zacharowski K, Habler O, Meier J. Hyperoxic ventilation improves survival in pigs during endotoxaemia at the critical hemoglobin concentration. Resuscitation 2011;82(4):473–480

Lauscher P, Mirakaj V, Rosenberger P, Meier J. Practical guidelines for blood transfusions in Germany [article in German]. Anasthesiol Intensivmed Notfallmed Schmerzther 2012;47(6):410–417

Laux G, Koerner T, Rosemann T, Beyer M, Gilbert K, Szecsenyi J. The CONTENT project: a problem-oriented, episode-based electronic patient record in primary care. Inform Prim Care 2005;13 (4):249–255

Lauzier F, Cook D, Griffith L, Upton J, Crowther M. Fresh frozen plasma transfusion in critically ill patients. Crit Care Med 2007;35(7):1655–1659

Lawrence VA, Silverstein JH, Cornell JE, Pederson T, Noveck H, Carson JL. Higher Hb level is associated with better early functional recovery after hip fracture repair. Transfusion 2003;43(12):1717–1722

Leahy MF, Mukhtar SA. From blood transfusion to patient blood management: a new paradigm for patient care and cost assessment of blood transfusion practice. Intern Med J 2012;42(3):332–338

Leahy MF, Roberts H, Mukhtar SA, et al; Western Australian Patient Blood Management Program. A pragmatic approach to embedding patient blood management in a tertiary hospital. Transfusion 2014;54(4):1133–1145

Leal-Noval SR, Jara-López I, García-Garmendia JL, et al. Influence of erythrocyte concentrate storage time on postsurgical morbidity in cardiac surgery patients. Anesthesiology 2003;98 (4):815–822

Lechner K, Jäger U. How I treat autoimmune hemolytic anemias in adults. Blood 2010;116(11):1831–1838

Lee JC, Peitzman AB. Damage-control laparotomy. Curr Opin Crit Care 2006;12 (4):346–350

Lemaire R. Strategies for blood management in orthopaedic and trauma surgery. J Bone Joint Surg Br 2008;90 (9):1128–1136

Levi M, Eerenberg E, Kamphuisen PW. Bleeding risk and reversal strategies for old and new anticoagulants and antiplatelet agents. J Thromb Haemost 2011;9(9):1705–1712

Levine GN, Bates ER, Blankenship JC, et al. ACCF/AHA/SCAI guideline for percutaneous coronary intervention: Executive summary: a report of the American College of Cardiology Foundation/American Heart Association Task Force on Practice Guidelines and the Society for Cardiovascular Angiography and Interventions. Circulation 2011;124 (23):2574–2609

Levy JH, Szlam F, Tanaka KA, Sniecienski RM. Fibrinogen and hemostasis: a primary hemostatic target for the management of acquired bleeding. Anesth Analg 2012;114(2):261–274

Levy PS, Quigley RL, Gould SA. Acute dilutional anemia and critical left anterior descending coronary artery stenosis impairs end organ oxygen delivery. J Trauma 1996;41(3):416–423

Lewis KM, Spazierer D, Slezak P, Baumgartner B, Regenbogen J, Gulle H. Swelling, sealing, and hemostatic ability of a novel biomaterial: A polyethylene glycol-coated collagen pad. J Biomater Appl 2014;29(5):780–788

Lhermusier T, Baker NC, Waksman R. Overview of the 2014 Food and Drug Administration Cardiovascular and Renal Drugs Advisory Committee meeting regarding cangrelor. Am J Cardiol 2015;115(8):1154–1161

Lidder PG, Sanders G, Whitehead E, et al. Pre-operative oral iron supplementation reduces blood transfusion in colorectal surgery - a prospective, randomised, controlled trial. Ann R Coll Surg Engl 2007;89(4):418–421

Lier H, Böttiger BW, Hinkelbein J, Krep H, Bernhard M. Coagulation management in multiple trauma: a systematic review. Intensive Care Med 2011;37 (4):572–582

Likosky DS, Al-Attar PM, Malenka DJ, et al. Geographic variability in potentially discretionary red blood cell transfusions after coronary artery bypass graft surgery. J Thor Cardiovasc Surg 2014;148(6):3084–3089

Lin DM, Lin ES, Tran M-H. Efficacy and Safety of Erythropoietin and Intravenous Iron in Perioperative Blood Management: A Systematic Review. Transfusion Medicine Reviews 2013;27 (4):221–234

Lin PC, Hsu CH, Huang CC, Chen WS, Wang JW. The blood-saving effect of tranexamic acid in minimally invasive total knee replacement: is an additional pre-operative injection effective? J Bone Joint Surg Br 2012;94(7):932–936

Lin Y, Stanford S, Birchall J et al. Recombinant factor VIIa for the prevention and treatment of bleeding in patients without haemophilia. Cochrane Database Syst Rev2011; 16(2): CD 005 0011

Lin Y, Yang YM, Zhu J, Tan HQ, Liang Y, Li JD. Anaemia and prognosis in acute coronary syndromes: a systematic review and meta-analysis. J Int Med Res 2012;40(1):43–55

Lindbom L, Arfors KE. Mechanisms and site of control for variation in the number of perfused capillaries in skeletal muscle. Int J Microcirc Clin Exp 1985;4(1):19–30

Linder BJ, Thompson RH, Leibovich BC, et al. The impact of perioperative blood transfusion on survival after nephrectomy for non-metastatic renal cell carcinoma (RCC). BJU Int 2013;114(3):368–374

Lion N, Crettaz D, Rubin O, Tissot JD. Stored red blood cells: a changing universe waiting for its map(s). J Proteomics 2010;73(3):374–385

Lippi G, Plebani M. Identification errors in the blood transfusion laboratory: a still relevant issue for patient safety. Transfus Apheresis Sci 2011;44(2):231–233

Litton E, Baker S, Erber W, et al; Australian and New Zealand Intensive Care Society Clinical Trials Group. The IRONMAN trial: a protocol for a multicentre randomised placebo-controlled trial of intravenous iron in intensive care unit patients with anaemia. Crit Care Resusc 2014;16(4):285–290

Litton E, Xiao J, Ho KM. Safety and efficacy of intravenous iron therapy in reducing requirement for allogeneic blood transfusion: systematic review and meta-analysis of randomised clinical trials. BMJ 2013;347:f4822

Liu L, Wang Z, Jiang S, et al. Perioperative allogenenic blood transfusion is associated with worse clinical outcomes for hepatocellular carcinoma: a meta-analysis. PLoS ONE 2013;8(5):e64 261

Liumbruno GM, Grazzini G, Rafanelli D. Post-operative blood salvage in patient blood management: is it really cost-effective and safe? Blood Transfus 2013;11(2):175–177

Lu J, Liao LM, Geng YX, et al. A double-blind, randomized, controlled study to explore the efficacy of rFVIIa on intraoperative blood loss and mortality in patients with severe acute pancreatitis. Thromb Res 2014;133(4):574–578

Luan H, Ye F, Wu L, Zhou Y, Jiang J. Perioperative blood transfusion adversely affects prognosis after resection of lung cancer: a systematic review and a meta-analysis. BMC Surg 2014;14:34

Luddington RJ. Thrombelastography/thromboelastometry. Clin Lab Haematol 2005;27(2):81–90

Ludwig H, Fritz E. Anemia of cancer patients: patient selection and patient stratification for epoetin treatment. Semin Oncol 1998;25(3 Suppl 7):35–38

Ludwig H, Van Belle S, Barrett-Lee P, et al. The European Cancer Anaemia Survey (ECAS): a large, multinational, prospective survey defining the prevalence, incidence, and treatment of anaemia in cancer patients. Eur J Cancer 2004;40 (15):2293–2306

Lunde J, Stensballe J, Wikkelsø A, Johansen M, Afshari A. Fibrinogen concentrate for bleeding—a systematic review. Acta Anaesthesiol Scand 2014;58(9):1061–1074

Lundholm C, Forsgren C, Johansson ALV, Chattingius S, Altman D. Hysterectomy on benign indications in Sweden 1987–2003: A nationwide trend analysis. Acta Obstetricia et Gynecologica Scandinavica 2009;88(1):52–58

Mackenzie CF, Moon-Massat PF, Shander A, Javidroozi M, Greenburg AG. When blood is not an option: factors affecting survival after the use of a hemoglobin-based oxygen carrier in 54 patients with life-threatening anemia. Anesth Analg 2010;110(3):685–693

Maddox FW, Dickinson TA, Rilla D, et al. Institutional variability of intraoperative red blood cell utilization in coronary artery bypass graft surgery. Am J Med Qual 2009;24:403–411

Madi-Jebara SN, Sleilaty GS, Achouh PE, et al. Postoperative intravenous iron used alone or in combination with low-dose erythropoietin is not effective for correction of anemia after cardiac surgery. J Cardiothorac Vasc Anesth 2004;18 (1):59–63

Madjdpour C, Spahn DR. Allogeneic red blood cell transfusions: efficacy, risks, alternatives and indications. Br J Anaesth 2005;95(1):33–42

Madsen LP, Rasmussen MK, Bjerregaard LL, Nøhr SB, Ebbesen F. Impact of blood sampling in very preterm infants. Scand J Clin Lab Invest 2000;60 (2):125–132

Magee G, Zbrozek A. Fluid overload is associated with increases in length of stay and hospital costs: pooled analysis of data from more than 600 US hospitals. Clinicoecon Outcomes Res 2013;5:289–296

Mainous AG 3rd, Tanner RJ, Hulihan MM, Amaya M, Coates TD. The impact of chelation therapy on survival in transfusional iron overload: a meta-analysis of myelodysplastic syndrome. Br J Haematol 2014;167(5):720–723

Maisano F, Kjaergard HK, Bauernschmitt R, et al. TachoSil surgical patch versus conventional haemostatic fleece material for control of bleeding in cardiovascular surgery: a randomised controlled trial. Eur J Cardiothorac Surg 2009;36:708–714

Malone DL, Dunne J, Tracy JK, Putnam AT, Scalea TM, Napolitano LM. Blood transfusion, independent of shock severity, is associated with worse outcome in trauma. J Trauma 2003;54(5):898–907

Malone DL, Hess JR, Fingerhut A. Massive transfusion practices around the globe and a suggestion for a common massive transfusion protocol. J Trauma 2006; 60 (6, Suppl):S 91 –S 96

Mangano DT; Multicenter Study of Perioperative Ischemia Research Group. Aspirin and mortality from coronary bypass surgery. N Engl J Med 2002;347 (17):1309–1317

Manns BJ, Tonelli M. The new FDA labeling for ESA—implications for patients and providers. Clin J Am Soc Nephrol 2012;7(2):348–353

Marik PE, Cavallazzi R, Vasu T, Hirani A. Dynamic changes in arterial waveform derived variables and fluid responsiveness in mechanically ventilated patients: a systematic review of the literature. Crit Care Med 2009;37(9):2642–2647

Marik PE, Corwin HL. Efficacy of red blood cell transfusion in the critically ill: a systematic review of the literature. Crit Care Med 2008;36(9):2667–2674

Marik PE, Sibbald WJ. Effect of stored-blood transfusion on oxygen delivery in patients with sepsis. JAMA 1993;269 (23):3024–3029

Markar SR, Kutty R, Edmonds L, Sadat U, Nair S. A meta-analysis of minimally invasive versus traditional open vein harvest technique for coronary artery bypass graft surgery. Interact Cardiovasc Thorac Surg 2010;10(2):266–270

Martini J, Cabrales P, Acharya SA, Intaglietta M, Tsai AG. Survival time in severe hemorrhagic shock after perioperative hemodilution is longer with PEG-conjugated human serum albumin than with HES 130/0.4: a microvascular perspective. Crit Care 2008;12(2):R54

Martini J, Cabrales P, Tsai AG, Intaglietta M. Mechanotransduction and the homeostatic significance of maintaining blood viscosity in hypotension, hypertension and haemorrhage. J Intern Med 2006;259(4):364–372

Martyn V, Farmer SL, Wren MN, et al. The theory and practice of bloodless surgery. Transfus Apher Sci 2002;27 (1):29–43

Mauri L, Kereiakes DJ, Yeh RW, et al; DAPT Study Investigators. Twelve or 30 months of dual antiplatelet therapy after drug-eluting stents. N Engl J Med. 2014;371(23):2155–2166

May TA, Clancy M, Critchfield J, et al. Reducing unnecessary inpatient laboratory testing in a teaching hospital. Am J Clin Pathol 2006;126(2):200–206

Mazzoni MC, Borgstrom P, Arfors KE, Intaglietta M. The efficacy of iso- and hyperosmotic fluids as volume expanders in fixed-volume and uncontrolled hemorrhage. Ann Emerg Med 1990;19 (4):350–358

McCartney S, Guinn N, Roberson R, Broomer B, White W, Hill S. Jehovah's Witnesses and cardiac surgery: a single institution's experience. Transfusion 2014;54(10 Pt 2):2745–2752

McDonagh JR, Seth M, LaLonde TA, et al. Radial PCI and the obesity paradox: Insights from blue cross blue shield of michigan cardiovascular consortium (BMC 2). Catheter Cardiovasc Interv. Published Online: May 22, 2015 (doi: 10 1002/ccd.26 015)

McGrath T, Koch CG, Xu M, et al. Platelet transfusion in cardiac surgery does not confer increased risk for adverse morbid outcomes. Ann Thorac Surg 2008;86(2):543–553

McIntire LV, Frangos JA, Rhee BG, Eskin SG, Hall ER. The effect of fluid mechanical stress on cellular arachidonic acid metabolism. Ann N Y Acad Sci 1987;516:513–524

McIntyre L, Hébert PC, Wells G, et al; Canadian Critical Care Trials Group. Is a restrictive transfusion strategy safe for resuscitated and critically ill trauma patients? J Trauma 2004;57(3):563–568

McLean E, Cogswell M, Egli I, Wojdyla D, de Benoist B. Worldwide prevalence of anaemia, WHO Vitamin and Mineral Nutrition Information System, 1993-2005. Public Health Nutr 2009;12 (4):444–454

McQuilten ZK, Andrianopoulos N, Wood EM, et al. Transfusion practice varies widely in cardiac surgery: Results from a national registry. J Thorac Cardiovasc Surg 2014;147(5):1684–1690.e1

Mehran R, Pocock SJ, Nikolsky E, et al. A risk score to predict bleeding in patients with acute coronary syndromes. J Am Coll Cardiol 2010;55(23):2556–2566

Meier J, Gombotz H. Pillar III—optimisation of anaemia tolerance. Best Pract Res Clin Anaesthesiol 2013;27(1):111–119

Meier J, Kemming GI, Kisch-Wedel H, Wölkhammer S, Habler OP. Hyperoxic ventilation reduces 6-hour mortality at the critical hemoglobin concentration. Anesthesiology 2004;100(1):70–76

Meier J, Meininger D, Zacharowski K. Patient blood management: from blood-sparing techniques to the rationale use of blood products. Curr Opin Anaesthesiol 2012;25(1):48–49

Meier J, Messmer K, Habler O. Hyperoxic hemodilution. In: Hardy JF, Van der Linden P, Maniatis A, eds. Alternatives to Blood Transfusion in Transfusion Medicine. 2nd ed. Oxford: Blackwell Publishing; 2011:450–457

Meier J, Pape A, Loniewska D, et al. Norepinephrine increases tolerance to acute anemia. Crit Care Med 2007;35 (6):1484–1492

Meißner A, Schlenke P. Massive bleeding and massive transfusion. Transfus Med Hemother 2012;39(2):73–84

Mercuriali F, Inghilleri G. Proposal of an algorithm to help the choice of the best transfusion strategy. Curr Med Res Opin 1996;13(8):465–478

Meremikwu M, Smith HJ. Blood transfusion for treating malarial anaemia. Cochrane Database Syst Rev 2000;(2): CD 001 475

Messmer C, Yalcin O, Palmer AF, Cabrales P. Small-volume resuscitation from hemorrhagic shock with polymerized human serum albumin. Am J Emerg Med 2012;30(8):1336–1346

Messmer K. Blood rheology factors and capillary blood flow. In: Gutierrez G, Vincent JL, eds. Tissue Oxygen Utilization. Berlin: Springer; 1991:103–113

Messmer K, Sunder-Plassmann L, Jesch F, Görnandt L, Sinagowitz E, Kessler M. Oxygen supply to the tissues during limited normovolemic hemodilution. Res Exp Med (Berl) 1973;159(3):152–166

Messmer K, Sunder-Plassmann L, Klövekorn WP, et al. Circulatory significance of hemodilution: rheological changes and limitations. Adv Microrcirc 1972;4:1–77

Meybohm P, Zacharowski K, Weber CF. Point-of-care coagulation management in intensive care medicine. Crit Care 2013;17(2):218–227

Miao X, Liu J, Zhao M, et al. Evidence-based use of FFP: the influence of a priming strategy without FFP during CPB on postoperative coagulation and recovery in pediatric patients. Perfusion 2015;30 (2):140–147

Miao X, Liu J, Zhao M, et al. The influence of cardiopulmonary bypass priming without FFP on postoperative coagulation and recovery in pediatric patients with cyanotic congenital heart disease. Eur J Pediatr 2014;173(11):1437–1443

Miceli A, Romeo F, Glauber M, de Siena PM, Caputo M, Angelini GD. Preoperative anemia increases mortality and postoperative morbidity after cardiac surgery. J Cardiothorac Surg 2014;9:137

Mikat M, Peters J, Zindler M, Arndt JO. Whole body oxygen consumption in awake, sleeping, and anesthetized

dogs. Anesthesiology 1984;60(3):220–227

Mikkola R, Gunn J, Heikkinen J, et al. Use of blood products and risk of stroke after coronary artery bypass surgery. Blood Transfus 2012;10(4):490–501

Milsom J, Trencheva K, Monette S, et al. Evaluation of the safety, efficacy, and versatility of a new surgical energy device (THUNDERBEAT) in comparison with Harmonic ACE, LigaSure V, and EnSeal devices in a porcine model. J Laparoendosc Adv Surg Tech A 2012;22(4):378–386

Mircescu G, Gârneata L, Capusa C, Ursea N. Intravenous iron supplementation for the treatment of anaemia in pre-dialyzed chronic renal failure patients. Nephrol Dial Transplant 2006;21 (1):120–124

Mirhashemi S, Breit GA, Chavez Chavez RH, Intaglietta M. Effects of hemodilution on skin microcirculation. Am J Physiol 1988;254(3 Pt 2):H411–H416

Mitra B, Cameron PA, Gruen RL. Aggressive fresh frozen plasma (FFP) with massive blood transfusion in the absence of acute traumatic coagulopathy. Injury 2012;43(1):33–37

Mitra B, Mori A, Cameron PA, Fitzgerald M, Paul E, Street A. Fresh frozen plasma (FFP) use during massive blood transfusion in trauma resuscitation. Injury 2010;41(1):35–39

Moore FA, Moore EE, Sauaia A. Blood transfusion. An independent risk factor for postinjury multiple organ failure. Arch Surg 1997;132(6):620–625

Morais S, Ortega-Andreu M, Rodriguez-Merchan EC, et al. Blood transfusion after primary total knee arthroplasty can be significantly minimised through a multimodal blood-loss prevention approach. Int Orthop 2014;38(2):347–354

Morales R, Duran-Aniotz C, Castilla J, Estrada LD, Soto C. De novo induction of amyloid-β deposition in vivo. Mol Psychiatry 2012;17(12):1347–1353

Morita Y, Chin-Yee I, Yu P, Sibbald WJ, Martin CM. Critical oxygen delivery in conscious septic rats under stagnant or anemic hypoxia. Am J Respir Crit Care Med 2003;167(6):868–872

Morton J, Anastassopoulos KP, Patel ST, et al. Frequency and outcomes of blood products transfusion across procedures and clinical conditions warranting inpatient care: an analysis of the 2004 healthcare cost and utilization project nationwide inpatient sample database. Am J Med Qual 2010;25(4):289–296

Moscucci M, Rogers EK, Montoye C, et al. Association of a continuous quality im-

provement initiative with practice and outcome variations of contemporary percutaneous coronary interventions. Circulation 2006;113(6):814–822

Moskowitz DM, McCullough JN, Shander A, et al. The impact of blood conservation on outcomes in cardiac surgery: is it safe and effective? Ann Thorac Surg 2010;90(2):451–458

Moskowitz KA, Manly D, Mackman N. Effect of topical hemostatic agents on clotting times in a whole blood model of dilutional coagulopathy. J Thromb Haemost 2009;7(Supp 2):1161

Mozzarelli A, Ronda L, Faggiano S, Bettati S, Bruno S. Haemoglobin-based oxygen carriers: research and reality towards an alternative to blood transfusions. Blood Transfus 2010;8(Suppl 3):s59–s68

Müller MC, Arbous MS, Spoelstra-de Man AM, et al. Transfusion of fresh-frozen plasma in critically ill patients with a coagulopathy before invasive procedures: a randomized clinical trial. Transfusion 2015;55(1):26–35

Mukhopadhaya N, Manyonda IT. The hysterectomy story in the United Kingdom. J Midlife Health 2013;4(1):40–41

Mukhopadhyay A, Yip HS, Prabhuswamy D, et al. The use of a blood conservation device to reduce red blood cell transfusion requirements: a before and after study. Crit Care 2010;14(1):R7

Mukhtar SA, Leahy MF, Koay K, et al. Effectiveness of a patient blood management data system in monitoring blood use in Western Australia. Anaesth Intensive Care 2013;41(2):207–215

Mulaj M, Faraoni D, Willems A, Sanchez Torres C, Van der Linden P. Predictive factors for red blood cell transfusion in children undergoing noncomplex cardiac surgery. Ann Thorac Surg 2014;98 (2):662–667

Muñoz M, Garcia-Erce JA, Bisbe E. Iron deficiency: causes, diagnosis and management. In: Maniatis A, Van der Linden P, Hardy JF, eds. Alternatives to Blood Transfusion in Transfusion Medicine. 2nd ed. Oxford: Blackwell Publishing; 2011:333–347

Muñoz M, García-Erce JA, Cuenca J, Bisbe E, Naveira E; AWGE (Spanish Anaemia Working Group). On the role of iron therapy for reducing allogeneic blood transfusion in orthopaedic surgery. Blood Transfus 2012;10(1):8–22

Muñoz M, García-Erce JA, Villar I, Thomas D. Blood conservation strategies in major orthopaedic surgery: efficacy, safety and European regulations. Vox Sang 2009;96(1):1–13

Muñoz M, Gómez-Ramírez S, Campos A. Iron supplementation for perioperative anaemia in patient blood management. EMJ Hema 2014a;1:123–132

Muñoz M, Gómez-Ramírez S, Cuenca J, et al. Very-short-term perioperative intravenous iron administration and postoperative outcome in major orthopedic surgery: a pooled analysis of observational data from 2547 patients. Transfusion 2014b;54(2):289–299

Murphy GJ, Patel NN, Sterne JAC. Red blood cell transfusion trigger in cardiac surgery. In: Juffermans N, Walsh T, eds. Transfusion in the Intensive Care Unit. Cham: Springer International Publishing; 2015a:35–44

Murphy GJ, Pike K, Rogers CA, et al. Liberal or restrictive transfusion after cardiac surgery. N Engl J Med 2015b;372 (11):997–1008

Murphy GJ, Reeves BC, Rogers CA, Rizvi SI, Culliford L, Angelini GD. Increased mortality, postoperative morbidity, and cost after red blood cell transfusion in patients having cardiac surgery. Circulation 2007;116(22):2544–2552

Murphy MF, Wallington TB, Kelsey P, et al; British Committee for Standards in Haematology, Blood Transfusion Task Force. Guidelines for the clinical use of red cell transfusions. Br J Haematol 2001;113 (1):24–31

Murphy S, Gardner FH. Effect of storage temperature on maintenance of platelet viability—deleterious effect of refrigerated storage. N Engl J Med 1969;280 (20):1094–1098

Musallam KM, Tamim HM, Richards T, et al. Preoperative anaemia and postoperative outcomes in non-cardiac surgery: a retrospective cohort study. Lancet 2011;378(9800):1396–1407

Myers E, O'Grady P, Dolan AM. The influence of preclinical anaemia on outcome following total hip replacement. Arch Orthop Trauma Surg 2004;124 (10):699–701

Myers JW, Gilmore BA, Powers KA, Kim PJ, Attinger CE. The utility of the surgical safety checklist for wound patients. Int Wound J. Published Online: Jan 14, 2015 (doi: 10 1111/iwj.12 391)

Mylankal KJ, Wyatt MG. Control of major haemorrhage and damage control surgery. Surgery 2013;31(11):574–581

Nadler SB, Hidalgo JH, Bloch T. Prediction of blood volume in normal human adults. Surgery 1962;51(2):224–232

Nandi A, Wallace S, Moore J. Use of FloSeal to stop persistent intraoperative bleeding during caesarean section. J Obstet Gynaecol 2012;32(1):34–35

Napolitano LM, Kurek S, Luchette FA, et al; EAST Practice Management Workgroup;

American College of Critical Care Medicine (ACCM) Taskforce of the Society of Critical Care Medicine (SCCM). Clinical practice guideline: red blood cell transfusion in adult trauma and critical care. J Trauma 2009;67(6):1439–1442

Natanson C, Kern SJ, Lurie P, Banks SM, Wolfe SM. Cell-free hemoglobin-based blood substitutes and risk of myocardial infarction and death: a meta-analysis. JAMA 2008;299(19):2304–2312

National Blood Authority of Australia (NBA). Annual Report 2008–2009. 2009. http://www.nba.gov.au/publications/annualreport.htm. Accessed March 12, 2015

National Blood Authority of Australia (NBA). Annual Reports. http://www.blood.gov.au/about-nba#annual-report. Accessed July 24, 2015

National Blood Authority of Australia (NBA). Patient Blood Management Guidelines. Module 1: Critical Bleeding/Massive Transfusion. Published 2011. http://www.blood.gov.au/pbm-module-1. Accessed April 9, 2015

National Blood Authority of Australia (NBA). Patient Blood Management Guidelines. Module 2: Perioperative. Published 2012. http://www.blood.gov.au/pbm-module-2. Accessed March 12, 2015

National Blood Authority of Australia (NBA). Patient Blood Management Guidelines. Module 5: Obstetrics and Maternity. Published 2015. http://www.blood.gov.au/pbm-module-5. Accessed July 12, 2015

National Blood Authority of Australia (NBA). Patient Blood Management Steering Committee. Committee Terms of Reference. September 2014. www.blood.gov.au/system/files/documents/pbmsc-governance-arrangements-sept-2014.pdf. Accessed July 7, 2015

National Comprehensive Cancer Network (NCCN). NCCN Guidelines®. Updated 2015. http://www.nccn.org/professionals/physician_gls/f_guidelines.asp. Accessed July 7, 2015

National CJD Research & Surveillance Unit (NCJDRSU), University of Edinburgh. Variand CJD Cases Worldwide. Updated February 2015. www.cjd.ed.ac.uk/documents/worldfigs.pdf. Accessed March 17, 2015

Ndrepepa G, Berger PB, Mehilli J, et al. Periprocedural bleeding and 1-year outcome after percutaneous coronary interventions: appropriateness of including bleeding as a component of a quadruple end point. J Am Coll Cardiol 2008;51(7):690–697

Nelson DR, Buxton TB, Luu QN, Rissing JP. The promotional effect of bone wax on

experimental Staphylococcus aureus osteomyelitis. J Thorac Cardiovasc Surg 1990;99(6):977–980

Nemergut EC, Littlewood KE, de Souza DG. Preoperative hematocrit levels and outcomes after noncardiac surgery. JAMA 2007;298(13):1512–1513, author reply 1513–1514

Nepple KG, Sandhu GS, Rogers CG, et al. Description of a multicenter safety checklist for intraoperative hemorrhage control while clamped during robotic partial nephrectomy. Patient Saf Surg 2012;6:8

Nguyen BV, Bota DP, Mélot C, Vincent JL. Time course of hemoglobin concentrations in nonbleeding intensive care unit patients. Crit Care Med 2003;31 (2):406–410

Nicolau JC, Moreira HG, Baracioli LM, et al. The bleeding risk score as a mortality predictor in patients with acute coronary syndrome. Arq Bras Cardiol 2013;101(6):511–518

Niranjan G, Asimakopoulos G, Karagounis A, Cockerill G, Thompson M, Chandrasekaran V. Effects of cell saver autologous blood transfusion on blood loss and homologous blood transfusion requirements in patients undergoing cardiac surgery on- versus off-cardiopulmonary bypass: a randomised trial. Eur J Cardiothorac Surg 2006;30(2):271–277

Nissenson AR, Goodnough LT, Dubois RW. Anemia: not just an innocent bystander? Arch Intern Med 2003;163 (12):1400–1404

Norfolk D, ed. Handbook of Transfusion Medicine. 5th ed. Norwich: TSO; 2013. http://www.transfusionguidelines.org.uk/transfusion-handbook. Accessed June 6, 2014

Nübling CM, Heiden M, Chudy M, et al. Experience of mandatory nucleic acid test (NAT) screening across all blood organizations in Germany: NAT yield versus breakthrough transmissions. Transfusion 2009;49(9):1850–1858

Nuttall GA, Henderson N, Quinn M, et al. Excessive bleeding and transfusion in a prior cardiac surgery is associated with excessive bleeding and transfusion in the next surgery. Anesth Analg 2006;102(4):1012–1017

O'Gara PT, Kushner FG, Ascheim DD, et al; CF/AHA Task Force. 2013 ACCF/AHA guideline for the management of ST-elevation myocardial infarction: executive summary: a report of the American College of Cardiology Foundation/American Heart Association Task Force on Practice Guidelines. Circulation 2013;127(4):529–555

Obladen M, Sachsenweger M, Stahnke M. Blood sampling in very low birth weight infants receiving different levels of intensive care. Eur J Pediatr 1988;147 (4):399–404

Österreichische Gesellschaft für Anästhesie (ÖGARI). Reanimation und Intensivmedizin. Fragebogen vor Operationen in Anästhesie. 2012a. http://www.oegari.at/web_files/dateiarchiv/205/Anamnesebogen%20ÖGARI%20vers%201.1.pdf. Accessed October 18, 2010

Österreichische Gesellschaft für Anästhesie (ÖGARI). Reanimation und Intensivmedizin. Österreichische Quellleitlinie zur präoperativen Patientenevaluierung. Published 2012b. http://www.oegari.at/web_files/dateiarchiv/205/Quellleitlinie%20Praeop.PatientInnenevaluierung%20Januar%202 012.pdf. Accessed March 12, 2015

Ogilvie MP, Pereira BMT, McKenney MG, et al. First report on safety and efficacy of hetastarch solution for initial fluid resuscitation at a level 1 trauma center. J Am Coll Surg 2010;210(5):870–880, 880–882

Oliver E, Carrio ML, Rodríguez-Castro D, et al. Relationships among haemoglobin level, packed red cell transfusion and clinical outcomes in patients after cardiac surgery. Intensive Care Med 2009;35(9):1548–1555

Oliver JC, Griffin RL, Hannon T, Marques MB. The success of our patient blood management program depended on an institution-wide change in transfusion practices. Transfusion 2014;54(10 Pt 2):2617–2624

Oriani G, Pavesi M, Oriani A, Bollina I. Acute normovolemic hemodilution. Transfus Apheresis Sci 2011;45 (3):269–274

Osborn JJ, Cohn K, Hait M, et al. Hemolysis during perfusion. Sources and means of reduction. J Thorac Cardiovasc Surg 1962;43:459–464

Osselaer JC, Doyen C, Defoin L, et al. Universal adoption of pathogen inactivation of platelet components: impact on platelet and red blood cell component use. Transfusion 2009;49 (7):1412–1422

Otsuki DA, Fantoni DT, Margarido CB, et al. Hydroxyethyl starch is superior to lactated Ringer as a replacement fluid in a pig model of acute normovolaemic haemodilution. Br J Anaesth 2007;98 (1):29–37

Ott DA, Cooley DA. Cardiovascular surgery in Jehovah's Witnesses. Report of 542 operations without blood transfusion. JAMA 1977;238(12):1256–1258

Otto JM, O'Doherty AF, Hennis PJ, et al. Association between preoperative haemoglobin concentration and cardiopulmonary exercise variables: a multicentre study. Perioper Med (Lond) 2013;2 (1):18

Ottosen C, Lingman G, Ottosen L. Three methods for hysterectomy: a randomised, prospective study of short term outcome. BJOG 2000;107(11):1380–1385

Page C, Retter A, Wyncoll D. Blood conservation devices in critical care: a narrative review. Ann Intensive Care 2013;3:14

Palmer SC, Saglimbene V, Mavridis D, et al. Erythropoiesis-stimulating agents for anaemia in adults with chronic kidney disease: a network meta-analysis. Cochrane Database Syst Rev 2014;(12): CD 010 590

Palmer T, Wahr JA, O'Reilly M, Greenfield ML. Reducing unnecessary cross-matching: a patient-specific blood ordering system is more accurate in predicting who will receive a blood transfusion than the maximum blood ordering system. Anesth Analg 2003;96(2):369–375

Palmerini T, Généreux P, Mehran R, et al. Association among leukocyte count, mortality, and bleeding in patients with non-ST-segment elevation acute coronary syndromes (from the Acute Catheterization and Urgent Intervention Triage StrategY [ACUITY] trial). Am J Cardiol 2013;111(9):1237–1245

Palmieri TL, Caruso DM, Foster KN, et al; American Burn Association Burn Multicenter Trials Group. Effect of blood transfusion on outcome after major burn injury: a multicenter study. Crit Care Med 2006;34(6):1602–1607

Palmieri TL, Greenhalgh DG, Sen S. Prospective comparison of packed red blood cell-to-fresh frozen plasma transfusion ratio of 4: 1 versus 1: 1 during acute massive burn excision. J Trauma Acute Care Surg 2013;74(1):76–83

Pandey S, Vyas GN. Adverse effects of plasma transfusion. Transfusion 2012;52 (Suppl 1):65S– 79S

Paone G, Likosky DS, Brewer R, et al. Transfusion of 1 and 2 units of red blood cells is associated with increased morbidity and mortality. Ann Thorac Surg 2014;97:87–94

Pape A, Kertscho H, Stein P, et al. Neuromuscular blockade with rocuronium bromide increases the tolerance of acute normovolemic anemia in anesthetized pigs. Eur Surg Res 2012a;48 (1):16–25

Pape A, Kutschker S, Kertscho H, et al. The choice of the intravenous fluid influences the tolerance of acute normovolemic anemia in anesthetized domestic pigs. Crit Care 2012b;16(2):R69

Pape A, Steche M, Laout M, et al. The limit of anemia tolerance during hyperoxic ventilation with pure oxygen in anesthetized domestic pigs. Eur Surg Res 2013;51(3-4):156–169

Park DW, Chun BC, Kwon SS, et al. Red blood cell transfusions are associated with lower mortality in patients with severe sepsis and septic shock: a propensity-matched analysis. Crit Care Med 2012;40(12):3140–3145

Parsons EC, Kross EK, Ali NA, et al. Red blood cell transfusion is associated with decreased in-hospital muscle strength among critically ill patients requiring mechanical ventilation. J Crit Care 2013;28(6):1079–1085

Pasquier P, Gayat E, Rackelboom T, et al. An observational study of the fresh frozen plasma: red blood cell ratio in postpartum hemorrhage. Anesth Analg 2013;116(1):155–161

Patel KV. Epidemiology of anemia in older adults. Semin Hematol 2008;45(4):210–217

Patel MS, Carson JL. Anemia in the preoperative patient. Med Clin North Am 2009;93(5):1095–1104

Pattakos G, Koch CG, Brizzio ME, et al. Outcome of patients who refuse transfusion after cardiac surgery: a natural experiment with severe blood conservation. Arch Intern Med 2012;172(15):1154–1160

Paul-Ehrlich-Institut (PEI). Report on notifications pursuant to Section 21 TFG (German Transfusion Act) for 2013 - tables. Updated July 30, 2015. http://www.pei.de/EN/information/blood-supply/reports/report-blood-supply-2012-2014-21tfg-content.html? nn=3 251 266. Accessed July 31, 2015

Paul-Ehrlich-Institut (PEI). TRALI: Keine Einführung von Risiko-minimierender Maßnahmen bei der Herstellung von Thrombozytenkonzentraten. November 2011. http://www.pei.de/cln_227/nn_154 580/DE/arzneimittelsicherheit-vigilanz/archiv-sicherheitsinformationen/2011/ablage2011/2011-11-16-haemovigilanz-trali-keine-massnahmen-tk.html?__nnn=true. Accessed October 17, 2012

Pawlik W, Shepherd AP, Jacobson ED. Effect of vasoactive agents on intestinal oxygen consumption and blood flow in dogs. J Clin Invest 1975;56(2):484–490

Pawlik WW, Shepherd AP, Mailman D, Shanbour LL, Jacobson ED. Effects of dopamine and epinephrine on intestinal blood flow and oxygen uptake. Adv Exp Med Biol 1976;75:511–516

Payne KA, Desrosiers MP, Caro JJ, et al. Clinical and economic burden of infused iron chelation therapy in the United States. Transfusion 2007;47 (10):1820–1829

Pedersen AB, Mehnert F, Overgaard S, Johnsen SP. Allogeneic blood transfusion and prognosis following total hip replacement: a population-based follow up study. BMC Musculoskelet Disord 2009;10:167

Pekelharing J, Furck A, Banya W, Macrae D, Davidson SJ. Comparison between thromboelastography and conventional coagulation tests after cardiopulmonary bypass surgery in the paediatric intensive care unit. Int J Lab Hematol 2014;36:465–471

Perazzo P, Viganò M, De Girolamo L, et al. Blood management and transfusion strategies in 600 patients undergoing total joint arthroplasty: an analysis of pre-operative autologous blood donation. Blood Transfus 2013;11(3):370–376

Perel P, Prieto-Merino D, Shakur H, Roberts I. Development and validation of a prognostic model to predict death in patients with traumatic bleeding, and evaluation of the effect of tranexamic acid on mortality according to baseline risk: a secondary analysis of a randomised controlled trial. Health Technol Assess 2013;17(24):1–45

Perez-de-Sá V, Roscher R, Cunha-Goncalves D, Larsson A, Werner O. Mild hypothermia has minimal effects on the tolerance to severe progressive normovolemic anemia in Swine. Anesthesiology 2002;97(5):1189–1197

Petricevic M, Biocina B, Milicic D, et al. Activated coagulation time vs. intrinsically activated modified rotational thromboelastometry in assessment of hemostatic disturbances and blood loss after protamine administration in elective cardiac surgery: analysis from the clinical trial (NCT 0 128 1397). J Cardiothorac Surg 2014;9:129

Pfanner G, Koscielny J, Pernerstorfer T, et al. Präoperative Blutungsanamnese. Anästhesist 2007;56:604

Pieracci FM, Barie PS. Iron and the risk of infection. Surg Infect (Larchmt) 2005;6 (Suppl 1):S 41 –S 46

Pieracci FM, Henderson P, Rodney JR, et al. Randomized, double-blind, placebo-controlled, trial of effects of enteral iron supplementation on anemia and risk of infection during surgical critical illness. Surg Infect (Larchmt) 2009;10 (1):9–19

Pisters R, Lane DA, Nieuwlaat R, de Vos CB, Crijns HJ, Lip GY. A novel user-friendly score (HAS-BLED) to assess 1-year risk of major bleeding in patients with atrial fibrillation: the Euro Heart Survey. Chest 2010;138(5):1093–1100

Poeran J, Rasul R, Suzuki S, et al. Tranexamic acid use and postoperative outcomes in patients undergoing total hip or knee arthroplasty in the United States: retrospective analysis of effectiveness and safety. BMJ 2014;349: g4829

Polderman KH. Mechanisms of action, physiological effects, and complications of hypothermia. Crit Care Med 2009;37 (7 Suppl)S 186 –S 202

Poldermans D, Bax JJ, Boersma E, et al; Task Force for Preoperative Cardiac Risk Assessment and Perioperative Cardiac Management in Non-cardiac Surgery; European Society of Cardiology (ESC). Guidelines for pre-operative cardiac risk assessment and perioperative cardiac management in non-cardiac surgery. Eur Heart J 2009;30 (22):2769–2812

Pollack CV Jr, Reilly PA, Eikelboom J, et al. Idarucizumab for dabigatran reversal. N Engl J Med. Published Online: Jun 22, 2015 (doi: 10 1056/NEJMoa1 502 000)

Price TH. Standards for Blood Banks and Transfusion Services. 26th ed. Bethesda, MD: AABB; 2009

Prick BW, Duvekot JJ, van der Moer PE, et al. Cost-effectiveness of red blood cell transfusion vs. non-intervention in women with acute anaemia after postpartum haemorrhage. Vox Sang 2014;107(4):381–388

Pries AR, Fritzsche A, Ley K, Gaehtgens P. Redistribution of red blood cell flow in microcirculatory networks by hemodilution. Circ Res 1992;70(6):1113–1121

Puetz J. Fresh frozen plasma: the most commonly prescribed hemostatic agent. J Thromb Haemost 2013;11 (10):1794–1799

Puetz J, Witmer C, Huang YS, Raffini L. Widespread use of fresh frozen plasma in US children's hospitals despite limited evidence demonstrating a beneficial effect. J Pediatr 2012;160(2):210–215. e1

Pybus S, MacCormac A, Houghton A, Martlew V, Thachil J. Inappropriateness of fresh frozen plasma for abnormal coagulation tests. J R Coll Physicians Edinb 2012;42(4):294–300

Qaseem A, Humphrey LL, Fitterman N, Starkey M, Shekelle P. Clinical Guidelines Committee of the American College of Physicians. Treatment of anemia in patients with heart disease: a clinical practice guideline from the American College of Physicians. Ann Intern Med 2013;159(11):770–9

Queensland Government (Queensland Health). Blood and blood product management. Updated August 2014. https://www.health.qld.gov.au/clinical-practice/guidelines-procedures/patient-safety/blood-management/blood-product/default.asp. Accessed July 24, 2015

Räsänen J. Supply-dependent oxygen consumption and mixed venous oxyhemoglobin saturation during isovolemic hemodilution in pigs. Chest 1992;101 (4):1121–1124

Raheman F. Unnecessary interventions. If less is more, how much is zero? BMJ 2009;339:b3500

Raison T. I Need to Know about Patient Blood Management. Transfusion Fact Sheet Volume 4, Number 3. Published 2012. http://resources.transfusion.com. au/cdm/ref/collection/p16 691coll1/id/ 259. Accessed July 7, 2015

Rana R, Fernández-Pérez ER, Khan SA, et al. Transfusion-related acute lung injury and pulmonary edema in critically ill patients: a retrospective study. Transfusion 2006;46(9):1478–1483

Ranucci M, Aronson S, Dietrich W, et al. Patient blood management during cardiac surgery: do we have enough evidence for clinical practice? J Thorac Cardiovasc Surg 2011a;142:249.e1–32

Ranucci M, Baryshnikova E, Castelvecchio S, Pelissero G; Surgical and Clinical Outcome Research (SCORE) Group. Major bleeding, transfusions, and anemia: the deadly triad of cardiac surgery. Ann Thorac Surg 2013;96(2):478–485

Ranucci M, Di Dedda U, Castelvecchio S, Menicanti L, Frigiola A, Pelissero G; Surgical and Clinical Outcome Research (SCORE) Group. Impact of preoperative anemia on outcome in adult cardiac surgery: a propensity-matched analysis. Ann Thorac Surg 2012;94(4):1134–1141

Ranucci M, La Rovere MT, Castelvecchio S, et al. Postoperative anemia and exercise tolerance after cardiac operations in patients without transfusion: what hemoglobin level is acceptable? Ann Thorac Surg 2011b;92(1):25–31

Rao SV, Jollis JG, Harrington RA, et al. Relationship of blood transfusion and clinical outcomes in patients with acute coronary syndromes. JAMA 2004;292(13):1555–1562

Rao SV, O'Grady K, Pieper KS, et al. Impact of bleeding severity on clinical outcomes among patients with acute coronary syndromes. Am J Cardiol 2005;96 (9):1200–1206

Rao SV, Sherwood MW. Isn't it about time we learned how to use blood transfusion in patients with ischemic heart disease? J Am Coll Cardiol 2014;63 (13):1297–1299

Rawn J. The silent risks of blood transfusion. Curr Opin Anaesthesiol 2008;21 (5):664–668

Redlin M, Habazettl H, Schoenfeld H, et al. Red blood cell storage duration is associated with various clinical outcomes in pediatric cardiac surgery. Transfus Med Hemother 2014;41:146–151

Reeves BC, Murphy GJ. Increased mortality, morbidity, and cost associated with red blood cell transfusion after cardiac surgery. Curr Opin Cardiol 2008;23 (6):607–612

Refaai MA, Blumberg N. The transfusion dilemma—weighing the known and newly proposed risks of blood transfusions against the uncertain benefits. Best Pract Res Clin Anaesthesiol 2013a;27(1):17–35

Refaai MA, Blumberg N. Transfusion immunomodulation from a clinical perspective: an update. Expert Rev Hematol 2013b;6(6):653–663

Regueira T, Djafarzadeh S, Brandt S, et al. Oxygen transport and mitochondrial function in porcine septic shock, cardiogenic shock, and hypoxaemia. Acta Anaesthesiol Scand 2012;56(7):846–859

Reitsma S, Slaaf DW, Vink H, van Zandvoort MA, oude Egbrink MG. The endothelial glycocalyx: composition, functions, and visualization. Pflugers Arch 2007;454(3):345–359

Rennke S, Fang MC. Hazards of hospitalization: more than just "never events". Arch Intern Med 2011;171(18):1653–1654

Restellini S, Kherad O, Jairath V, Martel M, Barkun AN. Red blood cell transfusion is associated with increased rebleeding in patients with nonvariceal upper gastrointestinal bleeding. Aliment Pharmacol Ther 2013;37(3):316–322

Reynolds JD, Ahearn GS, Angelo M, Zhang J, Cobb F, Stamler JS. S-nitrosohemoglobin deficiency: a mechanism for loss of physiological activity in banked blood. Proc Natl Acad Sci U S A 2007;104(43): 17 058–17 062

Richardson TQ, Guyton AC. Effects of polycythemia and anemia on cardiac output and other circulatory factors. Am J Physiol 1959;197:1167–1170

Riedl R, Engels EA, Warren JL, Berghold A, Ricker W, Pfeiffer RM. Blood transfusions and the subsequent risk of cancers in the United States elderly. Transfusion 2013;53(10):2198–2206

Rinder CS. Platelet physiology: cellular and protein interactions. In: Spiess BD, Spence RK, Shander A, eds. Perioperative Transfusion Medicine, 2nd ed. Baltimore, MD: Lippincott Williams & Wilkins; 2006:93–102

Rinder HM, Murphy M, Mitchell JG, Stocks J, Ault KA, Hillman RS. Progressive platelet activation with storage: evidence for shortened survival of activated platelets after transfusion. Transfusion 1991;31(5):409–414

Riskin DJ, Tsai TC, Riskin L, et al. Massive transfusion protocols: the role of aggressive resuscitation versus product ratio in mortality reduction. J Am Coll Surg 2009;209(2):198–205

Rizzo JD, Brouwers M, Hurley P, et al; American Society of Clinical Oncology; American Society of Hematology. American Society of Clinical Oncology/American Society of Hematology clinical practice guideline update on the use of epoetin and darbepoetin in adult patients with cancer. J Clin Oncol 2010;28(33):4996–5010

Rizzo JD, Somerfield MR, Hagerty KL, et al; American Society of Clinical Oncology; American Society of Hematology. Use of epoetin and darbepoetin in patients with cancer: 2007 American Society of Clinical Oncology/American Society of Hematology clinical practice guideline update. J Clin Oncol 2008;26(1):132–149

Roback JD. Vascular effects of the red blood cell storage lesion. Hematology Am Soc Hematol Educ Program 2011;2011 (1):475–479

Rock GA, Shumak KH, Buskard NA, et al; Canadian Apheresis Study Group. Comparison of plasma exchange with plasma infusion in the treatment of thrombotic thrombocytopenic purpura. N Engl J Med 1991;325(6):393–397

Rock WA Jr, Meeks GR. Managing anemia and blood loss in elective gynecologic surgery patients. J Reprod Med 2001;46(5 Suppl)507–514

Rodman T, Close HP, Purcell MK. The oxyhemoglobin dissociation curve in anemia. Ann Intern Med 1960;52:295–309

Rogers MA, Blumberg N, Saint S, Langa KM, Nallamothu BK. Hospital variation in transfusion and infection after cardiac surgery: a cohort study. BMC Med 2009;7:37

Rogers MA, Blumberg N, Saint SK, Kim C, Nallamothu BK, Langa KM. Allogeneic blood transfusions explain increased mortality in women after coronary artery bypass graft surgery. Am Heart J 2006;152(6):1028–1034

Rohde JM, Dimcheff DE, Blumberg N, et al. Health care-associated infection after red blood cell transfusion: a systematic review and meta-analysis. JAMA 2014;311(13):1317–1326

Rohrer MJ, Natale AM. Effect of hypothermia on the coagulation cascade. Crit Care Med 1992;20(10):1402–1405

Rollins KE, Trim NL, Luddington RJ, et al. Coagulopathy associated with massive cell salvage transfusion following aortic surgery. Perfusion 2012;27(1):30–33

Romagnoli E, Biondi-Zoccai G, Sciahbasi A, et al. Radial versus femoral randomized investigation in ST-segment elevation acute coronary syndrome: the RIFLE-STEACS (Radial Versus Femoral Randomized Investigation in ST-Elevation Acute Coronary Syndrome) study. J Am Coll Cardiol 2012;60(24):2481–2489

Rosencher N, Bellamy L, Chabbouh T, et al. Blood conservation approaches in orthopedic surgery [article in French]. Transfus Clin Biol 2008;15:294–302

Rosencher N, Kerkkamp HE, Macheras G, et al; OSTHEO Investigation. Orthopedic Surgery Transfusion Hemoglobin European Overview (OSTHEO) study: blood management in elective knee and hip arthroplasty in Europe. Transfusion 2003;43(4):459–469

Rosengart TK, Helm RE, DeBois WJ, Garcia N, Krieger KH, Isom OW. Open heart operations without transfusion using a multimodality blood conservation strategy in 50 Jehovah's Witness patients: implications for a "bloodless" surgical technique. J Am Coll Surg 1997;184(6):618–629

Rossaint R, Bouillon B, Cerny V, et al; Task Force for Advanced Bleeding Care in Trauma. Management of bleeding following major trauma: an updated European guideline. Crit Care 2010;14(2): R52

Roth WK, Buhr S, Drosten C, Seifried E. NAT and viral safety in blood transfusion. Vox Sang 2000;78(Suppl 2):257–259

Roth WK, Busch MP, Schuller A, et al. International survey on NAT testing of blood donations: expanding implementation and yield from 1999 to 2009. Vox Sang 2012;102(1):82–90

Roth WK, Weber M, Seifried E. Feasibility and efficacy of routine PCR screening of blood donations for hepatitis C virus, hepatitis B virus, and HIV-1 in a blood-bank setting. Lancet 1999;353(9150): 359–363

Rothwell SW, Maglasang P, Krishnamurti C. Survival of fresh human platelets in a rabbit model as traced by flow cytometry. Transfusion 1998;38(6):550–556

Roubille F, Morena M, Leray-Moragues H, Canaud B, Cristol JP, Klouche K. Pharmacologic therapies for chronic and acute decompensated heart failure: specific insights on cardiorenal syndromes. Blood Purif 2014;37(Suppl 2):20–33

Roubinian NH, Escobar GJ, Liu V, et al; NHLBI Recipient Epidemiology and Donor Evaluation Study (REDS-III).

Trends in red blood cell transfusion and 30-day mortality among hospitalized patients. Transfusion 2014b;54(10 Pt 2):2678–2686

Roubinian NH, Murphy EL, Swain BE, Gardner MN, Liu V, Escobar GJ; NHLBI Recipient Epidemiology and Donor Evaluation Study-III (REDS-III); Northern California Kaiser Permanente DOR Systems Research Initiative. Predicting red blood cell transfusion in hospitalized patients: role of hemoglobin level, comorbidities, and illness severity. BMC Health Serv Res 2014a;14:213

SA Health. BloodSafe website. 2012, Updated July 2015. http://www.sahealth.sa.gov.au/wps/wcm/connect/public+content/sa+health+internet/clinical+resources/clinical+programs/blood+products+and+programs/bloodsafe. Accessed July 24, 2015

Sabatine MS, Morrow DA, Giugliano RP, et al. Association of hemoglobin levels with clinical outcomes in acute coronary syndromes. Circulation 2005;111 (16):2042–2049

Sadani DT, Urbaniak SJ, Bruce M, Tighe JE. Repeat ABO-incompatible platelet transfusions leading to haemolytic transfusion reaction. Transfus Med 2006;16(5):375–379

Sadeghi M, Atefyekta R, Azimaraghi O, et al. A randomized, double blind trial of prophylactic fibrinogen to reduce bleeding in cardiac surgery. Braz J Anestesiol 2014;64(4):253–257

Sahler J, Spinelli S, Phipps R, Blumberg N. CD 40 ligand (CD 154) involvement in platelet transfusion reactions. Transfus Clin Biol 2012;19(3):98–103

Sakr Y, Lobo S, Knuepfer S, et al. Anemia and blood transfusion in a surgical intensive care unit. Crit Care 2010;14(3): R92

Salazar Vázquez BY, Wettstein R, Cabrales P, et al. Microvascular experimental evidence on the relative significance of restoring oxygen carrying capacity vs. blood viscosity in shock resuscitation. Biochim Biophys Acta 2008;1784: 1421–1427

Salim A, Hadjizacharia P, DuBose J, et al. Role of anemia in traumatic brain injury. J Am Coll Surg 2008;207(3):398–406

Salisbury AC, Reid KJ, Alexander KP, et al. Diagnostic blood loss from phlebotomy and hospital-acquired anemia during acute myocardial infarction. Arch Intern Med 2011;171(18):1646–1653

Salpeter SR, Buckley JS, Chatterjee S. Impact of more restrictive blood transfusion strategies on clinical outcomes: a meta-analysis and systematic review. Am J Med 2014;127:124–131.e3

Samsel RW, Schumacker PT. Determination of the critical O2 delivery from experimental data: sensitivity to error. J Appl Physiol (1985) 1988;64(5):2074–2082

Sanchez-Giron F, Alvarez-Mora F. Reduction of blood loss from laboratory testing in hospitalized adult patients using small-volume (pediatric) tubes. Arch Pathol Lab Med 2008;132(12):1916–1919

Sanguis Study Group (SSG). Use of blood products for elective surgery in 43 European hospitals. Transfus Med 1994;4 (4):251–268

Santos AA, Silva JP, Silva Lda F, Sousa AG, Piotto RF, Baumgratz JF. Therapeutic options to minimize allogeneic blood transfusions and their adverse effects in cardiac surgery: a systematic review. Rev Bras Cir Cardiovasc 2014;29 (4):606–621

Sargin D, Friedrichs H, El-Kordi A, Ehrenreich H. Erythropoietin as neuroprotective and neuroregenerative treatment strategy: comprehensive overview of 12 years of preclinical and clinical research. Best Pract Res Clin Anaesthesiol 2010;24(4):573–594

Sarode R, Refaai MA, Matevosyan K, Burner JD, Hampton S, Rutherford C. Prospective monitoring of plasma and platelet transfusions in a large teaching hospital results in significant cost reduction. Transfusion 2010;50(2):487–492

Savonitto S, D'Urbano M, Caracciolo M, et al. Urgent surgery in patients with a recently implanted coronary drug-eluting stent: a phase II study of 'bridging' antiplatelet therapy with tirofiban during temporary withdrawal of clopidogrel. Br J Anaesth 2010;104(3):285–291

Schmid-Schönbein H, Gallasch G, von Gosen J, Volger E, Klose HJ. Red cell aggregation in blood flow. II. Effect on apparent viscosity of blood. Klin Wochenschr 1976;54(4):159–167

Schmidt H, Kongsgaard U, Kofstad J, Geiran O, Refsum HE. Autotransfusion after open heart surgery: the oxygen delivery capacity of shed mediastinal blood is maintained. Acta Anaesthesiol Scand 1995;39(6):754–758

Schmidt M, Korn K, Nübling CM, et al. First transmission of human immunodeficiency virus Type 1 by a cellular blood product after mandatory nucleic acid screening in Germany. Transfusion 2009;49(9):1836–1844

Schmidt M, Nübling CM, Scheiblauer H, et al. Anti-HBc screening of blood donors: a comparison of nine anti-HBc tests. Vox Sang 2006;91(3):237–243

Schrezenmeier H, Seifried E. Buffy-coat-derived pooled platelet concentrates and apheresis platelet concentrates: which product type should be preferred? Vox Sang 2010;99(1):1–15

Schrezenmeier H, Walther-Wenke G, Müller TH, et al. Bacterial contamination of platelet concentrates: results of a prospective multicenter study comparing pooled whole blood-derived platelets and apheresis platelets. Transfusion 2007;47(4):644–652

Scott BH, Seifert FC, Grimson R. Blood transfusion is associated with increased resource utilisation, morbidity and mortality in cardiac surgery. Ann Card Anaesth 2008;11(1):15–19

Scottish Arthroplasty Project (SAP). Annual Report 2009. Scottish Arthroplasty Steering Committee. Published 2009. http://www.arthro.scot.nhs.uk/Reports/Scottish_Arthroplasty_Project_Report_2009. Accessed March 12, 2015

Segal JB, Dzik WH; Transfusion Medicine/Hemostasis Clinical Trials Network. Paucity of studies to support that abnormal coagulation test results predict bleeding in the setting of invasive procedures: an evidence-based review. Transfusion 2005;45(9):1413–1425

Seghatchian J, Krailadsiri P. Platelet storage lesion and apoptosis: are they related? Transfus Apheresis Sci 2001;24(1):103–105

Seifried E, Klueter H, Weidmann C, et al. How much blood is needed? Vox Sang 2011;100(1):10–21

Sekhon MS, McLean N, Henderson WR, Chittock DR, Griesdale DE. Association of hemoglobin concentration and mortality in critically ill patients with severe traumatic brain injury. Crit Care 2012;16(4):R128

Seltsam A, Müller TH. UVC irradiation for pathogen reduction of platelet concentrates and plasma. Transfus Med Hemother 2011;38(1):43–54

Sena MJ, Douglas G, Gerlach T, Grayson JK, Pichakron KO, Zierold D. A pilot study of the use of kaolin-impregnated gauze (Combat Gauze) for packing high-grade hepatic injuries in a hypothermic coagulopathic swine model. J Surg Res 2013;183(2):704–709

Shah M, Martin A, Myers B, MacSweeney S, Richards T. Recognising anaemia and malnutrition in vascular patients with critical limb ischaemia. Ann R Coll Surg Engl 2010;92(6):495–498

Shah NH, LePendu P, Bauer-Mehren A, et al. Proton pump inhibitor usage and the risk of myocardial infarction in the general population. PLoS One 2015;10 (6):e0124653

Shakur H, Roberts I, Bautista R, et al; CRASH-2 trial collaborators. Effects of tranexamic acid on death, vascular occlusive events, and blood transfusion in trauma patients with significant haemorrhage (CRASH-2): a randomised, placebo-controlled trial. Lancet 2010; 376(9734):23–32

Shander A. The cost of blood: multidisciplinary consensus conference for a standard methodology. Transfus Med Rev 2005;19(1):66–78

Shander A, Fink A, Javidroozi M, et al; International Consensus Conference on Transfusion Outcomes Group. Appropriateness of allogeneic red blood cell transfusion: the International Consensus Conference on Transfusion Outcomes. Transfus Med Rev 2011a;25 (3):232–246.e53

Shander A, Gernsheimer T. Are we begging a question or begging an answer? Anesth Analg 2014;119(4):755–757

Shander AS, Goodnough LT. Blood transfusion as a quality indicator in cardiac surgery. JAMA 2010;304(14):1610–1611

Shander A, Goodnough LT, Javidroozi M, et al. Iron deficiency anemia—bridging the knowledge and practice gap. Transfus Med Rev 2014b;28(3):156–166

Shander A, Hofmann A, Gombotz H, Theusinger OM, Spahn DR. Estimating the cost of blood: past, present, and future directions. Best Pract Res Clin Anaesthesiol 2007;21(2):271–289

Shander A, Hofmann A, Isbister J, Van Aken H. Patient blood management—the new frontier. Best Pract Res Clin Anaesthesiol 2013;27(1):5–10

Shander A, Hofmann A, Ozawa S, Theusinger OM, Gombotz H, Spahn DR. Activity-based costs of blood transfusions in surgical patients at four hospitals. Transfusion 2010;50(4):753–765

Shander A, Javidroozi M, Ashton ME. Drug-induced anemia and other red cell disorders: a guide in the age of polypharmacy. Curr Clin Pharmacol 2011c;6 (4):295–303

Shander A, Javidroozi M, Naqvi S, et al. An update on mortality and morbidity in patients with very low postoperative hemoglobin levels who decline blood transfusion (CME). Transfusion 2014c;54(10 Pt 2):2688–2695

Shander A, Javidroozi M, Ozawa S, Hare GM. What is really dangerous: anaemia or transfusion? Br J Anaesth 2011b;107 (Suppl 1):i41–i59

Shander A, Javidroozi M, Perelman S, Puzio T, Lobel G. From bloodless surgery to patient blood management. Mt Sinai J Med 2012a;79(1):56–65

Shander A, Michelson EA, Sarani B, Flaherty ML, Shulman IA. Use of plasma in the management of central nervous system bleeding: evidence-based consensus recommendations. Adv Ther 2014a;31 (1):66–90

Shander A, Moskowitz DM, Javidroozi M. Blood conservation in practice: an overview. Br J Hosp Med (Lond) 2009;70 (1):16–21

Shander A, Perelman S. The long and winding road of acute normovolemic hemodilution. Transfusion 2006;46(7):1075–1079

Shander A, Sazama K. Clinical consequences of iron overload from chronic red blood cell transfusions, its diagnosis, and its management by chelation therapy. Transfusion 2010;50(5):1144–1155

Shander A, Van Aken H, Colomina MJ, et al. Patient blood management in Europe. Br J Anaesth 2012b;109(1):55–68

Sharma P, Barajas FJ, Krishnamoorthy P, Campo LM, Blumenthal E, Spinnell M. Transfusion-free management of gastrointestinal bleeding: the experience of a bloodless institute. J Clin Gastroenterol 2015;49(3):206–211

Shaw RE, Johnson CK, Ferrari G, et al. Blood transfusion in cardiac surgery does increase the risk of 5-year mortality: results from a contemporary series of 1714 propensity-matched patients. Transfusion 2014;54(4):1106–1113

Shaz BH, Hillyer CD, Waters JH. Patient blood management: key for accountable care organizations. JAMA Surg 2013;148(6):491–492

Shehata N, Burns LA, Nathan H, et al. A randomized controlled pilot study of adherence to transfusion strategies in cardiac surgery. Transfusion 2012;52 (1):91–99

Shepard KV, Bukowski RM. The treatment of thrombotic thrombocytopenic purpura with exchange transfusions, plasma infusions, and plasma exchange. Semin Hematol 1987;24(3):178–193

Shiba H, Misawa T, Fujiwara Y, et al. Negative impact of fresh-frozen plasma transfusion on prognosis of pancreatic ductal adenocarcinoma after pancreatic resection. Anticancer Res 2013;33 (9):4041–4047

Shorr AF, Duh MS, Kelly KM, Kollef MH; CRIT Study Group. Red blood cell transfusion and ventilator-associated pneumonia: A potential link? Crit Care Med 2004;32(3):666–674

Shorr AF, Jackson WL, Kelly KM, Fu M, Kollef MH. Transfusion practice and blood stream infections in critically ill patients. Chest 2005;127(5):1722–1728

Shrestha LB, Heisler EJ. The Changing Demographic Profile of the United States. Congressional Research Service Report for Congress. March 31, 2011. http://www.fas.org/sgp/crs/misc/RL32701.pdf; Accessed May 14, 2014

Shrivastava M. The platelet storage lesion. Transfus Apheresis Sci 2009;41(2):105–113

Siegal D, Yudin J, Kaatz S, Douketis JD, Lim W, Spyropoulos AC. Periprocedural heparin bridging in patients receiving vitamin K antagonists: systematic review and meta-analysis of bleeding and thromboembolic rates. Circulation 2012;126(13):1630–1639

Silverboard H, Aisiku I, Martin GS, Adams M, Rozycki G, Moss M. The role of acute blood transfusion in the development of acute respiratory distress syndrome in patients with severe trauma. J Trauma 2005;59(3):717–723

Simms ER, Hennings DL, Hauch A, et al. Impact of infusion rates of fresh frozen plasma and platelets during the first 180 minutes of resuscitation. J Am Coll Surg 2014;219(2):181–188

Simpson E, Lin Y, Stanworth S, Birchall J, Doree C, Hyde C. Recombinant factor VIIa for the prevention and treatment of bleeding in patients without haemophilia. Cochrane Database Syst Rev 2012;3(3):CD005011

Singbartl G. Preoperative autologous blood donation - part I. Only two clinical parameters determine efficacy of the autologous predeposit. Minerva Anestesiol 2007;73(3):143–151

Singbartl G, Schreiber J, Singbartl K. Preoperative autologous blood donation versus intraoperative blood salvage: intraindividual analyses and modeling of efficacy in 1103 patients. Transfusion 2009;49(11):2374–2383

Sinha R, Sanjay M, Rupa B, Kumari S. Robotic surgery in gynecology. J Minim Access Surg 2015;11(1):50–59

Sireis W, Rüster B, Daiss C, et al. Extension of platelet shelf life from 4 to 5 days by implementation of a new screening strategy in Germany. Vox Sang 2011; 101(3):191–199

Smith BD, La Celle PL. Blood viscosity and thrombosis: clinical considerations. Prog Hemost Thromb 1982;6:179–201

Snyder-Ramos SA, Möhnle P, Weng YS, et al; Investigators of the Multicenter Study of Perioperative Ischemia; MCSPI Research Group. The ongoing variability in blood transfusion practices in cardiac surgery. Transfusion 2008;48(7):1284–1299

Sølbeck S, Ostrowski SR, Johansson PI. A review of the clinical utility of INR to monitor and guide administration of prothrombin complex concentrate to orally anticoagulated patients. Thromb J 2012;10(1):5

Sonzogni V, Crupi G, Poma R, et al. Erythropoietin therapy and preoperative autologous blood donation in children undergoing open heart surgery. Br J Anaesth 2001;87(3):429–434

So-Osman C, Cicilia J, Brand A, Schipperus M, Berning B, Scherjon S. Triggers and appropriateness of red blood cell transfusions in the postpartum patient—a retrospective audit. Vox Sang 2010;98 (1):65–69

So-Osman C, Nelissen RG, Koopman-van Gemert AW, et al. Patient blood management in elective total hip- and knee-replacement surgery (Part 1): a randomized controlled trial on erythropoietin and blood salvage as transfusion alternatives using a restrictive transfusion policy in erythropoietin-eligible patients. Anesthesiology 2014;120 (4):839–851

Sood R, Sood A, Ghosh AK. Non-evidence-based variables affecting physicians' test-ordering tendencies: a systematic review. Neth J Med 2007;65(5):167–177

Soper NJ, Swanström LL, Eubanks WS, eds. Mastery of Endoscopic and Laparoscopic Surgery. 3rd ed. Philadelphia, PA: Lippincott Williams & Wilkins; 2009

Soto C. In vivo spreading of tau pathology. Neuron 2012;73(4):621–623

Soutoul JH, Pierre F. Refusal of blood because of being Jehovah's witnesses or for fear of AIDS. Deontologic and legal aspects [article in French]. J Gynecol Obstet Biol Reprod (Paris) 1988;17 (8):965–980

Sowade O, Warnke H, Scigalla P, et al. Avoidance of allogeneic blood transfusions by treatment with epoetin beta (recombinant human erythropoietin) in patients undergoing open-heart surgery. Blood 1997;89(2):411–418

Spahn DR. Anemia and patient blood management in hip and knee surgery: a systematic review of the literature. Anesthesiology 2010;113(2):482–495

Spahn DR, Bouillon B, Cerny V, et al. Management of bleeding and coagulopathy following major trauma: an updated European guideline. Crit Care 2013a;17 (2):R76

Spahn DR, Cerny V, Coats TJ, et al. Management of bleeding following major trauma: a European guideline. Critical care (London) 2007;11(1):R17

Spahn DR, Ganter MT. Towards early individual goal-directed coagulation management in trauma patients. Br J Anaesth 2010;105(2):103–105

Spahn DR, Goodnough LT. Alternatives to blood transfusion. Lancet 2013;381 (9880):1855–1865

Spahn DR, Korte W. Novel oral anticoagulants: new challenges for anesthesiologists in bleeding patients. Anesthesiology 2012;116(1):9–11

Spahn DR, Leone BJ, Reves JG, Pasch T. Cardiovascular and coronary physiology of acute isovolemic hemodilution: a review of nonoxygen-carrying and oxygen-carrying solutions. Anesth Analg 1994;78(5):1000–1021

Spahn DR, Moch H, Hofmann A, Isbister JP. Patient blood management: the pragmatic solution for the problems with blood transfusions. Anesthesiology 2008;109(6):951–953

Spahn DR, Shander A, Hofmann A. The chiasm: transfusion practice versus patient blood management. Best Pract Res Clin Anaesthesiol 2013b;27(1):37–42

Spahn DR, Theusinger OM, Hofmann A. Patient blood management is a win-win: a wake-up call. Br J Anaesth 2012;108 (6):889–892

Spahn DR, van Brempt R, Theilmeier G, et al; European Perflubron Emulsion Study Group. Perflubron emulsion delays blood transfusions in orthopedic surgery. Anesthesiology 1999;91 (5):1195–1208

Sparling EA, Nelson CL, Lavender R, Smith J. The use of erythropoietin in the management of Jehovah's Witnesses who have revision total hip arthroplasty. J Bone Joint Surg Am 1996;78 (10):1548–1552

Spertus J. "TITRe"ing the approach to transfusions after cardiac surgery. N Engl J Med 2015;372:1069-70

Spiess BD. Red cell transfusions and guidelines: a work in progress. Hematol Oncol Clin North Am 2007;21(1):185–200

Spiess BD. Risks of transfusion: outcome focus. Transfusion 2004b; 44(12, Suppl):4S- 14S

Spiess BD, ed. The Relationship between Coagulation, Inflammation and Endothelium—A Pyramid Towards Outcome. Baltimore: Lippincott Williams & Wilkins; 2000

Spiess BD. Transfusion of blood products affects outcome in cardiac surgery. Semin Cardiothorac Vasc Anesth 2004a;8(4):267–281

Spiess BD, Royston D, Levy JH, et al. Platelet transfusions during coronary artery bypass graft surgery are associated with serious adverse outcomes. Transfusion 2004;44(8):1143–1148

Spitzer RF, Caccia N, Kives S, Allen LM. Hysteroscopic unification of a complete obstructing uterine septum: case report and review of the literature. Fertil Steril 2008;90(5):2016.e17–2016.e20

Sriram K, Tsai AG, Cabrales P, et al. PEG-albumin supraplasma expansion is due to increased vessel wall shear stress induced by blood viscosity shear thinning. Am J Physiol Heart Circ Physiol 2012;302(12):H2489 –H2497

Stainsby D, Russell J, Cohen H, Lilleyman J. Reducing adverse events in blood transfusion. Br J Haematol 2005;131(1):8–12

Stamou SC, White T, Barnett S, Boyce SW, Corso PJ, Lefrak EA. Comparisons of cardiac surgery outcomes in Jehovah's versus Non-Jehovah's Witnesses. Am J Cardiol 2006;98(9):1223–1225

Stang A, Merrill RM, Kuss O. Hysterectomy in Germany: a DRG-based nationwide analysis, 2005-2006. Dtsch Arztebl Int 2011;108(30):508–514

Stansbury LG, Dutton RP, Stein DM, Bochicchio GV, Scalea TM, Hess JR. Controversy in trauma resuscitation: do ratios of plasma to red blood cells matter? Transfus Med Rev 2009;23(4):255–265

Stanworth SJ. Thrombocytopenia, bleeding and use of platelet transfusions in sick neonates. Hematology Am Soc Hematol Educ Program 2012;2012(1):512–516

Stanworth SJ, Estcourt LJ, Llewelyn CA, Murphy MF, Wood EM; TOPPS Study Investigators. Impact of prophylactic platelet transfusions on bleeding events in patients with hematologic malignancies: a subgroup analysis of a randomized trial. Transfusion 2014;54 (10):2385–2393

Stanworth SJ, Walsh TS, Prescott RJ, Lee RJ, Watson DM, Wyncoll D; Intensive Care Study of Coagulopathy (ISOC) investigators. A national study of plasma use in critical care: clinical indications, dose and effect on prothrombin time. Crit Care 2011;15(2):R108

Stein JI, Gombotz H, Rigler B, Metzler H, Suppan C, Beitzke A. Open heart surgery in children of Jehovah's Witnesses: extreme hemodilution on cardiopulmonary bypass. Pediatr Cardiol 1991;12 (3):170–174

Steingrímsson S, Gustafsson R, Gudbjartsson T, Mokhtari A, Ingemansson R, Sjögren J. Sternocutaneous fistulas after cardiac surgery: incidence and late outcome during a ten-year follow-up. Ann Thorac Surg 2009;88(6):1910–1915

Steinmetz HT, Tsamaloukas A, Schmitz S, et al. A new concept for the differential diagnosis and therapy of anaemia in cancer patients. Support Care Cancer 2010;19(2):261–269

Stephen N. Review of the Australian Blood Banking and Plasma Product Sector. A report to the Commonwealth Minister for Health and Aged Care. Canberra: Department of Health and Aged Care; 2001

Stone GW, Clayton TC, Mehran R, et al. Impact of major bleeding and blood transfusions after cardiac surgery: analysis from the Acute Catheterization and Urgent Intervention Triage strategY (ACUITY) trial. Am Heart J 2012;163 (3):522–529

Stover EP, Siegel LC, Parks R, et al; Institutions of the Multicenter Study of Perioperative Ischemia Research Group. Variability in transfusion practice for coronary artery bypass surgery persists despite national consensus guidelines: a 24-institution study. Anesthesiology 1998;88(2):327–333

Subherwal S, Bach RG, Chen AY, et al. Baseline risk of major bleeding in non-ST-segment-elevation myocardial infarction: the CRUSADE (Can Rapid risk stratification of Unstable angina patients Suppress ADverse outcomes with Early implementation of the ACC/AHA Guidelines) Bleeding Score. Circulation 2009;119(14):1873–1882

Sudmann B, Bang G, Sudmann E. Histologically verified bone wax (beeswax) granuloma after median sternotomy in 17 of 18 autopsy cases. Pathology 2006;38(2):138–141

Sugai Y, Sugai K, Fuse A. Current status of bacterial contamination of autologous blood for transfusion. Transfus Apheresis Sci 2001;24(3):255–259

Surgenor DM, Wallace EL, Churchill WH, Hao SH, Chapman RH, Poss R. Red cell transfusions in total knee and total hip replacement surgery. Transfusion 1991;31(6):531–537

Svitek V, Lonsky V, Anjum F. Pathophysiological aspects of cardiotomy suction usage. Perfusion 2010;25(3):147–152

Tafur AJ, McBane R II, Wysokinski WE, et al. Predictors of major bleeding in periprocedural anticoagulation management. J Thromb Haemost 2012;10 (2):261–267

Takagi H, Sekino S, Kato T, Matsuno Y, Umemoto T. Intraoperative autotransfusion in abdominal aortic aneurysm surgery: meta-analysis of randomized controlled trials. Arch Surg 2007;142 (11):1098–1101

Tavares M, DiQuattro P, Nolette N, Conti G, Sweeney J. Reduction in plasma transfusion after enforcement of transfusion guidelines. Transfusion 2011;51 (4):754–761

Taylor RW, O'Brien J, Trottier SJ, et al. Red blood cell transfusions and nosocomial infections in critically ill patients. Crit Care Med 2006;34(9):2302–2309

Tettamanti M, Lucca U, Gandini F, et al. Prevalence, incidence and types of mild anemia in the elderly: the "Health and Anemia" population-based study. Haematologica 2010;95(11):1849–1856

Thavendiranathan P, Bagai A, Ebidia A, Detsky AS, Choudhry NK. Do blood tests cause anemia in hospitalized patients? The effect of diagnostic phlebotomy on hemoglobin and hematocrit levels. J Gen Intern Med 2005;20(6):520–524

Theusinger OM, Kind SL, Seifert B, Borgeat L, Gerber C, Spahn DR. Patient blood management in orthopaedic surgery: a four-year follow-up of transfusion requirements and blood loss from 2008 to 2011 at the Balgrist University Hospital in Zurich, Switzerland. Blood Transfus 2014b;12(2):195–203

Theusinger OM, Spahn DR, Ganter MT. Transfusion in trauma: why and how should we change our current practice? Curr Opin Anaesthesiol 2009;22 (2):305–312

Theusinger OM, Stein P, Spahn DR. Applying 'Patient Blood Management' in the trauma center. Curr Opin Anaesthesiol 2014a;27(2):225–232

Thomas D, Thompson J, Ridler B, eds. A Manual for Blood Conservation. Harley: TFM Publishing; 2005

Thomas L. Labor und Diagnose. Frankfurt: TH-Books Verlagsgesellschaft mbH; 2008

Thomas L, Thomas C. Anemia in iron deficiency and disorders of iron metabolism [article in German]. Dtsch Med Wochenschr 2002;127(30):1591–1594

Thomson A, Farmer S, Hofmann A, et al. Patient Blood Management – a new paradigm for transfusion medicine? ISBT Sci Ser 2009;4(2):423–435

Thürmann P, Holt-Noreiks S, Nink K, et al. Arzneimittelversorgung älterer Patienten. In: Günster C, Klose J, Schmacke N, eds. Versorgungsreport 2012. Stuttgart: Schattauer; 2012

Tinmouth A, Fergusson D, Yee IC, Hébert PC; ABLE Investigators; Canadian Critical Care Trials Group. Clinical consequences of red cell storage in the critically ill. Transfusion 2006;46 (11):2014–2027

To AC, Armstrong G, Zeng I, Webster MW. Noncardiac surgery and bleeding after percutaneous coronary intervention. Circ Cardiovasc Interv 2009;2(3):213–221

Top AP, Ince C, de Meij N, van Dijk M, Tibboel D. Persistent low microcircula-

tory vessel density in nonsurvivors of sepsis in pediatric intensive care. Crit Care Med 2011;39(1):8–13

Torres Filho IP, Spiess BD, Pittman RN, Barbee RW, Ward KR. Experimental analysis of critical oxygen delivery. Am J Physiol Heart Circ Physiol 2005;288 (3):H1071–H1079

Toulon P, Ozier Y, Ankri A, Fléron MH, Leroux G, Samama CM. Point-of-care versus central laboratory coagulation testing during haemorrhagic surgery. A multicenter study. Thromb Haemost 2009;101(2):394–401

Towler S. Patient Blood Management. Engaging Clinicians and Patients Western Australian Style. Presented at: United Kingdom British Blood Transfusion Society Scientific Meeting; September 24, 2014; Harrogate, United Kingdom. https://www.bbts.org.uk/whatwedo/annualconference/pres/. Accessed March 12, 2015

Trentino KM, Farmer SL, Swain SG, et al. Increased hospital costs associated with red blood cell transfusion. Transfusion 2015;55(5):1082–1089

Trzeciak S, Dellinger RP, Parrillo JE, et al. Microcirculatory Alterations in Resuscitation and Shock Investigators. Early microcirculatory perfusion derangements in patients with severe sepsis and septic shock: relationship to hemodynamics, oxygen transport, and survival. Ann Emerg Med 2007;49:88–98; 98.e1-2

Tsai AG, Friesenecker B, Cabrales P, Hangai-Hoger N, Intaglietta M. The vascular wall as a regulator of tissue oxygenation. Curr Opin Nephrol Hypertens 2006;15(1):67–71

Tsai AG, Friesenecker B, Intaglietta M. Capillary flow impairment and functional capillary density. Int J Microcirc Clin Exp 1995;15(5):238–243

Tsai AG, Friesenecker B, McCarthy M, Sakai H, Intaglietta M. Plasma viscosity regulates capillary perfusion during extreme hemodilution in hamster skinfold model. Am J Physiol 1998;275(6 Pt 2): H2170–H2180

Tsai AG, Hofmann A, Cabrales P, Intaglietta M. Perfusion vs. oxygen delivery in transfusion with "fresh" and "old" red blood cells: the experimental evidence. Transfus Apheresis Sci 2010;43(1):69–78

Tsai AG, Intaglietta M. Evidence of flow-motion induced changes in local tissue oxygenation. Int J Microcirc Clin Exp 1993;12(1):75–88

Tsui AK, Dattani ND, Marsden PA, et al. Reassessing the risk of hemodilutional anemia: Some new pieces to an old puzzle. Can J Anaesth 2010;57(8):779–791

Turgeon AF, Fergusson DA, Doucette S, et al. Red blood cell transfusion practices amongst Canadian anesthesiologists: a survey. Can J Anaesth 2006;53(4):344–352

Tynan K. Patient blood management program: reducing anaemia, transfusions and length of stay for knee patients. Posted January 23, 2013. https://www.healthroundtable.org/GetNews/tabid/1457/itemid/172/amid/5205/default.aspx. Accessed January 25, 2015

United States Department of Health & Human Services (USDHHS). Advisory Committee on Blood Safety and Availability – Recommendations: June 2011. Published 2011. http://www.hhs.gov/ash/bloodsafety/advisorycommittee/recommendations/resolutions.html. Accessed March 12, 2015

Valentine SL, Bateman ST. Identifying factors to minimize phlebotomy-induced blood loss in the pediatric intensive care unit. Pediatr Crit Care Med 2012;13(1):22–27

Vamvakas EC. Establishing causation in transfusion medicine and related tribulations. Transfus Med Rev 2011;25(2):81–88

Vamvakas EC. Reasons for moving toward a patient-centric paradigm of clinical transfusion medicine practice. Transfusion 2013;53(4):888–901

Vamvakas EC, Carven JH. Allogeneic blood transfusion and postoperative duration of mechanical ventilation: effects of red cell supernatant, platelet supernatant, plasma components and total transfused fluid. Vox Sang 2002;82(3):141–149

van de Watering L. Red cell storage and prognosis. Vox Sang 2011b;100(1):36–45

van de Watering L; Biomedical Excellence for Safer Transfusion (BEST) Collaborative. Pitfalls in the current published observational literature on the effects of red blood cell storage. Transfusion 2011a;51(8):1847–1854

van der Heijden M, Verheij J, van Nieuw Amerongen GP, Groeneveld AB. Crystalloid or colloid fluid loading and pulmonary permeability, edema, and injury in septic and nonseptic critically ill patients with hypovolemia. Crit Care Med 2009;37(4):1275–1281

Van der Linden P. The physiology of acute isovolaemic anaemia. Acta Anaesthesiol Belg 2002;53(2):97–103

Van der Linden P, De Hert S, Mathieu N, et al. Tolerance to acute isovolemic hemodilution. Effect of anesthetic depth. Anesthesiology 2003;99(1):97–104

Van der Linden P, Gilbart E, Paques P, Simon C, Vincent JL. Influence of hematocrit on tissue O2 extraction capabilities during acute hemorrhage. Am J Physiol 1993;264(6 Pt 2):H1942–H1947

Van der Linden P, Schmartz D, De Groote F, et al. Critical haemoglobin concentration in anaesthetized dogs: comparison of two plasma substitutes. Br J Anaesth 1998;81(4):556–562

Van der Linden P, Schmartz D, Gilbart E, Engelman E, Vincent JL. Effects of propofol, etomidate, and pentobarbital on critical oxygen delivery. Crit Care Med 2000;28(7):2492–2499

van der Meer PF, Tomson B, Brand A. In vivo tracking of transfused platelets for recovery and survival studies: an appraisal of labeling methods. Transfus Apheresis Sci 2010;42(1):53–61

van der Poel CL, Janssen MP, Behr-Gross ME. The Collection, Testing and Use of Blood and Blood Components in Europe – 2008 Report. Strasbourg: Council of Europe; 2011

van Gelder FE, de Graaff JC, van Wolfswinkel L, van Klei WA. Preoperative testing in noncardiac surgery patients: a survey amongst European anaesthesiologists. Eur J Anaesthesiol 2012;29(10):465–470

Van PY, Hamilton GJ, Kremenevskiy IV, et al. Lyophilized plasma reconstituted with ascorbic acid suppresses inflammation and oxidative DNA damage. J Trauma 2011;71(1):20–25

Van Mieghem NM, Nuis RJ, Tzikas A, et al. Prevalence and prognostic implications of baseline anaemia in patients undergoing transcatheter aortic valve implantation. EuroIntervention 2011;7(2):184–191

van Straten AH, Bekker MW, Soliman Hamad MA, et al. Transfusion of red blood cells: the impact on short-term and long-term survival after coronary artery bypass grafting, a ten-year follow-up. Interact Cardiovasc Thorac Surg 2010;10(1):37–42

van Woerkens ECSM, Trouwborst A, van Lanschot JJB. Profound hemodilution: what is the critical level of hemodilution at which oxygen delivery-dependent oxygen consumption starts in an anesthetized human? Anesth Analg 1992;75(5):818–821

Vassallo RR Jr. Preparation, preservation and storage of platelet concentrates. In: Simon TL, ed. Rossi's Principles of Transfusion Medicine. Hoboken, NJ: Wiley-Blackwell; 2009:187–198

Vassallo RR, Fung M, Rebulla P, et al; International Collaboration for Guideline De-

velopment, Implementation and Evaluation for Transfusion Therapies. Utility of cross-matched platelet transfusions in patients with hypoproliferative thrombocytopenia: a systematic review. Transfusion 2014;54(4):1180–1191

Veelo DP, Vlaar AP, Dongelmans DA, et al. Correction of subclinical coagulation disorders before percutaneous dilatational tracheotomy. Blood Transfus 2012;10(2):213–220

Vegting IL, van Beneden M, Kramer MH, Thijs A, Kostense PJ, Nanayakkara PW. How to save costs by reducing unnecessary testing: lean thinking in clinical practice. Eur J Intern Med 2012;23(1):70–75

Velibey Y, Erbay A, Ozkurt E, Usta E, Akin F. Acute myocardial infarction associated with blood transfusion: case report and literature review. Transfus Apheresis Sci 2014;50(2):260–262

Ventura HO, Mehra MR. Bloodletting as a cure for dropsy: heart failure down the ages. J Card Fail 2005;11(4):247–252 Erratum in: J Card Fail. 2005 Jun;11(5):404

Verheij J, van Lingen A, Beishuizen A, et al. Cardiac response is greater for colloid than saline fluid loading after cardiac or vascular surgery. Intensive Care Med 2006;32(7):1030–1038

Verheugt FW, Steinhubl SR, Hamon M, et al. Incidence, prognostic impact, and influence of antithrombotic therapy on access and nonaccess site bleeding in percutaneous coronary intervention. JACC Cardiovasc Interv 2011;4(2):191–197

Vermeulen Windsant IC, de Wit NC, Sertorio JT, et al. Blood transfusions increase circulating plasma free hemoglobin levels and plasma nitric oxide consumption: a prospective observational pilot study. Crit Care 2012;16(3):R95

Vestergaard RF, Jensen H, Vind-Kezunovic S, Jakobsen T, Søballe K, Hasenkam JM. Bone healing after median sternotomy: a comparison of two hemostatic devices. J Cardiothorac Surg 2010;5:117

Vestergaard RF, Nielsen PH, Terp KA, Søballe K, Andersen G, Hasenkam JM. Effect of hemostatic material on sternal healing after cardiac surgery. Ann Thorac Surg 2014;97(1):153–160

Vida VL, De Franceschi M, Barzon E, Padalino MA, Scattolin F, Stellin G. The use fibrinogen/thrombin-coated equine collagen patch in children requiring re-operations for congenital heart disease. A single center clinical experience. J Cardiovasc Surg (Torino) 2014;55(3):401–406

253

Vignali A, Braga M, Gianotti L, et al. A single unit of transfused allogeneic blood increases postoperative infections. Vox Sang 1996;71(3):170–175

Villanueva C, Colomo A, Bosch A. Transfusion for acute upper gastrointestinal bleeding. N Engl J Med 2013b;368 (14):1362–1363

Villanueva C, Colomo A, Bosch A, et al. Transfusion strategies for acute upper gastrointestinal bleeding. N Engl J Med 2013a;368(1):11–21

Villela NR, Salazar Vázquez BY, Intaglietta M. Microcirculatory effects of intravenous fluids in critical illness: plasma expansion beyond crystalloids and colloids. Curr Opin Anaesthesiol 2009;22 (2):163–167

Villela NR, Tsai AG, Cabrales P, Intaglietta M. Improved resuscitation from hemorrhagic shock with Ringer's lactate with increased viscosity in the hamster window chamber model. J Trauma 2011;71 (2):418–424

Vincent JL, Baron JF, Reinhart K, et al; ABC (Anemia and Blood Transfusion in Critical Care) Investigators. Anemia and blood transfusion in critically ill patients. JAMA 2002;288(12):1499–1507

Vincent JL, Piagnerelli M. Transfusion in the intensive care unit. Crit Care Med 2006;34(5 Suppl):S 96 –S 101

Vincent JL, Rossaint R, Riou B, et al. Recommendations on the use of recombinant activated factor VII as an adjunctive treatment for massive bleeding-a European perspective. Crit Care 2006;10(4):R120

Vivacqua A, Koch CG, Yousuf AM, et al. Morbidity of bleeding after cardiac surgery: is it blood transfusion, reoperation for bleeding, or both? Ann Thorac Surg 2011;91(6):1780–1790

Vlahakes GJ. The value of phase 4 clinical testing. N Engl J Med 2006;354(4):413–415

Vogiatzi G, Briasoulis A, Tousoulis D, Papageorgiou N, Stefanadis C. Is there a role for erythropoietin in cardiovascular disease? Expert Opin Biol Ther 2010;10 (2):251–264

Vogt AW, Henson LC. Unindicated preoperative testing: ASA physical status and financial implications. J Clin Anesth 1997;9(6):437–441

Vonk AB, Meesters MI, Garnier RP, et al. Intraoperative cell salvage is associated with reduced postoperative blood loss and transfusion requirements in cardiac surgery: a cohort study. Transfusion 2013;53(11):2782–2789

Vuille-Lessard E, Boudreault D, Girard F, Ruel M, Chagnon M, Hardy JF. Postoperative anemia does not impede functional outcome and quality of life early after hip and knee arthroplasties. Transfusion 2012;52(2):261–270

Vuylsteke A, Pagel C, Gerrard C, et al. The Papworth Bleeding Risk Score: a stratification scheme for identifying cardiac surgery patients at risk of excessive early postoperative bleeding. Eur J Cardiothorac Surg 2011;39(6):924–930

Wade CE, Eastridge BJ, Jones JA, et al. Use of recombinant factor VIIa in US military casualties for a five-year period. J Trauma 2010;69(2):353–359

Wald ML. Blood industry shrinks as transfusions decline. New York Times. Published August 22, 2014. http://www.nytimes.com/2014/08/23/business/blood-industry-hurt-by-surplus.html Accessed March 12, 2015

Wallis JP. Preventing ABO incompatible blood transfusion. Br J Haematol 2006;132(4):531, author reply 532

Wallis JP, Wells AW, Chapman CE. Changing indications for red cell transfusion from 2000 to 2004 in the North of England. Transfus Med 2006;16(6):411–417

Walsh M, Garg AX, Devereaux PJ, Argalious M, Honar H, Sessler DI. The association between perioperative hemoglobin and acute kidney injury in patients having noncardiac surgery. Anesth Analg 2013;117(4):924–931

Walsh TS, Garrioch M, Maciver C, et al; Audit of Transfusion in Intensive Care in Scotland Study Group. Red cell requirements for intensive care units adhering to evidence-based transfusion guidelines. Transfusion 2004;44 (10):1405–1411

Walsh TS, Maciver CR; Scottish Critical Care Trials Group and Scottish National Blood Transfusion Service Clinical Effectiveness Group. A clinical scenario-based survey of transfusion decisions for intensive care patients with delayed weaning from mechanical ventilation. Transfusion 2009;49(12):2661–2667

Wang G, Bainbridge D, Martin J, Cheng D. The efficacy of an intraoperative cell saver during cardiac surgery: a meta-analysis of randomized trials. Anesth Analg 2009;109(2):320–330

Wang T, Luo L, Huang H, et al. Perioperative blood transfusion is associated with worse clinical outcomes in resected lung cancer. Ann Thorac Surg 2014;97 (5):1827–1837

Wang TY, Xiao L, Alexander KP, et al. Antiplatelet therapy use after discharge among acute myocardial infarction patients with in-hospital bleeding. Circulation 2008;118(21):2139–2145

Warmuth M, Mad P, Wild C. Systematic review of the efficacy and safety of fibrinogen concentrate substitution in adults. Acta Anaesthesiol Scand 2012;56(5):539–548

Watrowski R. Hemostatic gelatine-thrombin matrix (Floseal®) facilitates hemostasis and organ preservation in laparoscopic treatment of tubal pregnancy. Arch Gynecol Obstet 2014;290(3):411–415

Watson GA, Sperry JL, Rosengart MR, et al; Inflammation and Host Response to Injury Investigators. Fresh frozen plasma is independently associated with a higher risk of multiple organ failure and acute respiratory distress syndrome. J Trauma 2009;67(2):221–230

Watts DD, Trask A, Soeken K, Perdue P, Dols S, Kaufmann C. Hypothermic coagulopathy in trauma: effect of varying levels of hypothermia on enzyme speed, platelet function, and fibrinolytic activity. J Trauma 1998;44(5):846–854

Weber CF, Görlinger K, Meininger D, et al. Point-of-care testing: a prospective, randomized clinical trial of efficacy in coagulopathic cardiac surgery patients. Anesthesiology 2012;117(3):531–547

Weber CF, Zacharowski K, Meybohm P, et al. Hemotherapy algorithms for coagulopathic cardiac surgery patients. Clin Lab 2014;60(6):1059–1063

Weber CF, Zacharowski K. Perioperative point of care coagulation testing. Dtsch Arztebl Int 2012;109(20):369–375

Weber EW, Slappendel R, Hémon Y, et al. Effects of epoetin alfa on blood transfusions and postoperative recovery in orthopaedic surgery: the European Epoetin Alfa Surgery Trial (EEST). Eur J Anaesthesiol 2005;22(4):249–257

Weber WP, Zwahlen M, Reck S, et al. The association of preoperative anemia and perioperative allogeneic blood transfusion with the risk of surgical site infection. Transfusion 2009;49(9):1964–1970

Weinberg ED. Iron availability and infection. Biochim Biophys Acta 2009;1790 (7):600–605

Weinberg JA, McGwin G Jr, Marques MB, et al. Transfusions in the less severely injured: does age of transfused blood affect outcomes? J Trauma 2008;65 (4):794–798

Weinberg I, Kaufman J, Jaff MR. Inferior vena cava filters. JACC Cardiovasc Interv 2013;6(6):539–547

Weiskopf RB, Feiner J, Hopf HW, et al. Oxygen reverses deficits of cognitive function and memory and increased heart rate induced by acute severe isovolemic anemia. Anesthesiology 2002;96(4):871–877

Weiskopf RB, Silverman TA. Balancing potential risks and benefits of hemoglobin-based oxygen carriers. Transfusion 2013;53(10):2327–2333

Weiskopf RB, Viele MK, Feiner J, et al. Human cardiovascular and metabolic response to acute, severe isovolemic anemia. JAMA 1998;279(3):217–221

Wells AW, Mounter PJ, Chapman CE, Stainsby D, Wallis JP. Where does blood go? Prospective observational study of red cell transfusion in north England. BMJ 2002;325(7368):803

Welsby IJ, Jiao K, Ortel TL, et al. The kaolin-activated Thrombelastograph predicts bleeding after cardiac surgery. J Cardiothorac Vasc Anesth 2006;20(4):531–535

Welsh KJ, Padilla A, Dasgupta A, Nguyen AN, Wahed A. Thromboelastography is a suboptimal test for determination of the underlying cause of bleeding associated with cardiopulmonary bypass and may not predict a hypercoagulable state. Am J Clin Pathol 2014;142(4):492–497

Weltert L, D'Alessandro S, Nardella S, et al. Preoperative very short-term, high-dose erythropoietin administration diminishes blood transfusion rate in off-pump coronary artery bypass: a randomized blind controlled study. J Thorac Cardiovasc Surg 2010;139 (3):621–627

Westbrook A, Pettilä V, Nichol A, et al; Blood Observational Study Investigators of ANZICS-Clinical Trials Group. Transfusion practice and guidelines in Australian and New Zealand intensive care units. Intensive Care Med 2010;36 (7):1138–1146

Westenbrink BD, Kleijn L, de Boer RA, et al; IMAGINE Investigators. Sustained postoperative anaemia is associated with an impaired outcome after coronary artery bypass graft surgery: insights from the IMAGINE trial. Heart 2011;97(19):1590–1596

Whitaker BI, Hinkins S. The 2011 National Blood Collection and Utilization Survey Report. Washington, DC: United States Department of Health and Human Services; 2011. http://www.hhs.gov/ash/bloodsafety/2011-nbcus.pdf. Accessed March 12, 2015

White PF. Comparative evaluation of intravenous agents for rapid sequence induction—thiopental, ketamine, and midazolam. Anesthesiology 1982;57 (4):279–284

Whiteman MK, Hillis SD, Jamieson DJ, et al. Inpatient hysterectomy surveillance in the United States, 2000-2004. Am J Obstet Gynecol 2008;198(1):34. e1–34.e7

Wick M, Pinggera W, Lehmann P. Clinical Aspects and Laboratory-Iron Metabolism, Anemias. Vienna: Springer; 2011

Widman J, Isacson J. Lateral position reduces blood loss in hip replacement surgery: a prospective randomized study of 74 patients. Int Orthop 2001;25(4):226–227

Wikkelsø A, Lunde J, Johansen M, et al. Fibrinogen concentrate in bleeding patients. Cochrane Database Syst Rev 2013;(8):CD 008 864

Willems A, Van Lerberghe C, Gonsette K, et al. The indication for perioperative red blood cell transfusions is a predictive risk factor for severe postoperative morbidity and mortality in children undergoing cardiac surgery. Eur J Cardiothorac Surg 2014;45(6):1050–1057

Williams ML, He X, Rankin JS, Slaughter MS, Gammie JS. Preoperative hematocrit is a powerful predictor of adverse outcomes in coronary artery bypass graft surgery: a report from the Society of Thoracic Surgeons Adult Cardiac Surgery Database. Ann Thorac Surg 2013;96(5):1628–1634

Wolf RF, Peng J, Friese P, Gilmore LS, Burstein SA, Dale GL. Erythropoietin administration increases production and reactivity of platelets in dogs. Thromb Haemost 1997;78(6):1505–1509

Wong CJ, Vandervoort MK, Vandervoort SL, et al. A cluster randomized controlled trial of a blood conservation algorithm in patients undergoing total hip joint arthroplasty. Transfusion 2007;47 (5):832–841

Wood C, Maher P, Hill D. Bleeding associated with vaginal hysterectomy. Aust N Z J Obstet Gynaecol 1997;37(4):457–461

Wood JC. Guidelines for quantifying iron overload. Hematology Am Soc Hematol Educ Program 2014;2014(1):210–215

Woodward JL, Roper E. Political activity of American citizens. Am Polit Sci Rev 1950;XLIV:872–885

World Health Organization (WHO). Global Database on Blood Safety 2011. Geneva: WHO; 2012

World Health Organization (WHO). Global Database on Blood Safey 2011. Summary Report 2011. Published 2011a. http://www.who.int/bloodsafety/global_database/GDBS_Summary_Report_2011.pdf. Accessed June 11, 2015

World Health Organization (WHO). Global Database on Blood Safety Report 2004–2005. Geneva: WHO; 2008

World Health Organization (WHO). Global Forum for Blood Safety: Patient Blood Management. Priorities for Action. Published 2011b. http://www.who.int/bloodsafety/collaboration/who_gfbs_2011_03_priorities_for_action.pdf. Accessed March 12, 2015

World Health Organization (WHO). Nutritional Anaemias. Report of a WHO scientific group. WHO Technical Report Series No. 405. Geneva: WHO; 1968

World Health Organization (WHO). Recommendation of the Executive Board to the Sixty-third World Health Assembly for the Adoption of Resolution on Availability, Safety and Quality of Blood Products. Published 2010a. http://apps.who.int/gb/ebwha/pdf_files/EB126/B126_R14-en.pdf. Accessed March 12, 2015

World Health Organization (WHO), Sixty-Third World Health Assembly. Resolution WHA 63.12: Availability, Safety and Quality of Blood Products. Published 2010b. http://apps.who.int/gb/ebwha/pdf_files/WHA63/A63_R12-en.pdf. Accessed March 12, 2015

World Health Organization (WHO) Executive Board. Availability, Safety and Quality of Blood Products. 126th Session. Provisional agenda item 4.16. Published 2009. http://apps.who.int/gb/ebwha/pdf_files/EB126/B126_19Add1-en.pdf. Accessed March 12, 2015

World Health Organization (WHO) Regional Office for Europe. Demographic Change, Life Expectancy and Mortality Trends in Europe: Fact Sheet. Published 2012. http://www.euro.who.int/__data/assets/pdf_file/0003/185 214/Demographic-change,-life-expectancy-Fact-Sheet.pdf; Accessed March 12, 2015

Wu WC, Rathore SS, Wang Y, Radford MJ, Krumholz HM. Blood transfusion in elderly patients with acute myocardial infarction. N Engl J Med 2001;345 (17):1230–1236

Wysham WZ, Roque DR, Soper JT. Use of topical hemostatic agents in gynecologic surgery. Obstet Gynecol Surv 2014;69 (9):557–563

Xenos ES, Vargas HD, Davenport DL. Association of blood transfusion and venous thromboembolism after colorectal cancer resection. Thromb Res 2012;129 (5):568–572

Yalcin O, Ortiz D, Tsai AG, Johnson PC, Cabrales P. Microhemodynamic aberrations created by transfusion of stored blood. Transfusion 2014;54(4):1015–1027

255

Yao HS, Wang Q, Wang WJ, Hu ZQ. Intra-operative allogeneic red blood cell transfusion in ampullary cancer outcome after curative pancreatoduode-nectomy: a clinical study and meta-analysis. World J Surg 2008;32 (9):2038–2046

Yazicioğlu L, Eryilmaz S, Sirlak M, et al. Recombinant human erythropoietin administration in cardiac surgery. J Thorac Cardiovasc Surg 2001;122(4):741–745

Yoo YC, Shim JK, Kim JC, Jo YY, Lee JH, Kwak YL. Effect of single recombinant human erythropoietin injection on transfusion requirements in preoperatively anemic patients undergoing valvular heart surgery. Anesthesiology 2011;115(5):929–937

Yu J, Mehran R, Grinfeld L, et al. Sex-based differences in bleeding and long term adverse events after percutaneous coronary intervention for acute myocardial infarction: Three year results from the HORIZONS-AMI trial. Catheter Cardiovasc Interv 2015;85(3):359–368

Zeller MP, Al-Habsi KS, Heddle NM. Prophylactic platelet transfusions: should they be a treatment of the past? Curr Opin Hematol 2014;21(6):521–527

Zhou XD, Tao LJ, Li J, Wu LD. Do we really need tranexamic acid in total hip arthroplasty? A meta-analysis of nineteen randomized controlled trials. ArchOrthopTrauma Surg 2013;133(7):1017–27

Zilberberg MD, Carter C, Lefebvre P, et al. Red blood cell transfusions and the risk of acute respiratory distress syndrome among the critically ill: a cohort study. Crit Care 2007;11(3):R63

Zollinger A, Hager P, Singer T, Friedl HP, Pasch T, Spahn DR. Extreme hemodilution due to massive blood loss in tumor surgery. Anesthesiology 1997;87 (4):985–987

Zufferey PJ, Miquet M, Quenet S, et al; tranexamic acid in hip-fracture surgery (THIF) study. Tranexamic acid in hip fracture surgery: a randomized controlled trial. Br J Anaesth 2010;104(1):23–30

Index

Page numbers in *italics* refer to illustrations; those in **bold** refer to tables

A